HISTORY OF EMOTIONS

Editors
Susan J. Matt
Peter N. Stearns

A list of books in this series appears at the end of this book.

Emotional Bodies

The Historical Performativity of Emotions

Edited by
Dolores Martín-Moruno
and Beatriz Pichel

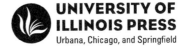

© 2019 by the Board of Trustees
of the University of Illinois
All rights reserved
1 2 3 4 5 C P 5 4 3 2 1
♾ This book is printed on acid-free paper.

Publication has been supported in part by the
Fonds Général de l'Université de Genève

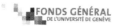

Library of Congress Cataloging-in-Publication Data
Names: Martín-Moruno, Dolores, editor. | Pichel,
   Beatriz, editor.
Title: Emotional bodies : the historical performativity
   of emotions / edited by Dolores Martín-Moruno
   and Beatriz Pichel.
Description: Urbana : University of Illinois Press,
   [2019] | Series: History of emotions | Includes
   bibliographical references and index. |
Identifiers: LCCN 2019023474 (print) | LCCN
   2019023475 (ebook) | ISBN 9780252042898
   (hardcover) | ISBN 9780252084713 (paperback) |
   ISBN 9780252051753 (ebook)
Subjects: LCSH: Emotions—Social aspects—History.
Classification: LCC BF531 .E49825 2019 (print) | LCC
   BF531 (ebook) | DDC 152.4—dc23
LC record available at https://lccn.loc.gov/2019023474
LC ebook record available at https://lccn.loc.gov
   /2019023475

Contents

Acknowledgments   vii

Introduction   1

PART I. DISEASED BODIES UNDER CONSTRUCTION

1. Hysteria or Tetanus? Ambivalent Embodiments and the Authenticity of Pain   *Rob Boddice*   19

2. The Criminal of Passion: Its Construction in Italian Legal and Medical Discourses, 1860s–1920s   *Gian Marco Vidor*   36

3. Locating Cancer: Body Image and Emotions from a Psychosomatic Perspective (1950–1959)   *Pilar León-Sanz*   53

PART II. PERFORMING EMOTIONAL BODIES

4. The Language of Children's Pain (1870–1900)   *Leticia Fernández-Fontecha*   77

5. Photographing the Emotional Body: The Question of Expressions in the Theater and the Psychological Sciences   *Beatriz Pichel*   97

6. Yolanda: Youth, Heroin, and AIDS through the Lens of Photographic Practices   *María Rosón*   120

PART III. MAKING SOCIAL BODIES

7. Making a Collective Emotional Body: Francis of Assisi Celebrating Christmas in Greccio (1223)   *Piroska Nagy*   151

8. Fearful Female Bodies: The *Pétroleuses* of the Paris Commune   *Dolores Martín-Moruno*   175

PART IV. HUMANITARIAN BODIES IN ACTION

9. Performing Compassion in Wartime: Humanitarian Narratives in the Spanish Civil Wars of the 1870s   *Jon Arrizabalaga*   199

10. Humanitarian Emotions through History: Imaging Suffering and Performing Aid   *Emma Hutchison*   219

11. Compassion Fatigue: The Changing Nature of Humanitarian Emotions   *Bertrand Taithe*   242

Afterword   263

Selected Bibliography   267

Contributors   275

Index   279

Acknowledgments

WE WOULD LIKE TO THANK our colleagues who have accompanied us throughout this emotional journey, which started with the organization of an international conference in 2014 at the Louis Jeantet Auditorium in Geneva: Jon Arrizabalaga, Rob Boddice, Damien Boquet, Andrea Carlino, François Delaporte, Otniel Dror, Guillermo de Eugenio, Leticia Fernández Fontecha, Emma Hutchison, Pilar León Sanz, Patrizia Lombardo, Sophie Milquet, Rafael Mandressi, Piroska Nagy, Stephanie Olsen, Marc Ratcliff, Antonio Rodríguez, Miriam Ronca, María Rosón, Bertrand Taithe, Gian Marco Vidor, Sophie Wahnich and Paul White. This workshop and the present book have been possible thanks to the financial support of the Swiss National Science Foundation, the Rectorate of the University of Geneva, the Institute for Ethics, History, and the Humanities, the Fonds Generals de l'Université de Genève, and the Wellcome Trust.

We feel very grateful for having received strong, affective support from some colleagues working on Women and Gender Studies: Aline Acevedo, Francesca Arena, Camille Bajeux, Julien Debonneville, Yali Chen, Delphine Gardey, Jo Labanyi, Marylène Lieber, Marie Leyder, Rosa María Medina-Domenech, Teresa Ortíz, Lorena Parini, Carolina Topini, and Marylène Vuille. We met other historians of emotions before 2014, who have been crucial for the completion of this book, such as Fay Bound Alberti, Thomas Dixon, and Colin Jones. The support of colleagues at the Photographic History Research Centre, De Montfort University (Kelley Wilder, Elizabeth Edwards, Gil Pasternak, and Jenifer Chao) has been and continues to be invaluable.

The completion of this book would have not been possible without feminist friends working behind the scenes: Fanny Hernández Brotons, María Gómez

Garrido, Esther Lorenzo, Eva Botella Ordinas and Violeta Ruíz Cuenca. We are very proud of them for having shown us the importance of mutual care while growing up in the academia. We should make a special mention to Leticia Fernández Fontecha, who has inspired the journey represented by this book by suggesting us to read Maggie Nelson's *The Argonauts*.

We would like to dedicate *Emotional Bodies* to those who have taught us that history is not just a cold discipline dealing with the past. If we love history, this is because it is something more than theoretical exercise. Thanks to all who have conveyed us their passion for this political practice, whose aim is to destabilize our present society. We firmly believe that historical research constitutes a weapon useful in the fight for the future of those generations who will inhabit this world by promoting an emotion that we need more than ever before: HOPE.

Introduction

WHAT DO EMOTIONS DO? Do they materialize in our bodies? And if so, how are we, as individuals and collectivities, made and unmade by the work of emotions? This edited collection aims to answer these questions through eleven case studies dating from the Middle Ages to the twentieth-first century. Topics include nineteenth-century criminology, photographic cameras and exhibitions, humanitarian relief work and advocacy strategies, religious and revolutionary experiences, as well as medical understandings of pain. This wide variety of contributions allows us to provide a colorful picture of what we call in this volume "emotional bodies." We propose "emotional bodies" as an analytical tool to understand how the performativity of emotional practices is at the origin of particular configurations of bodies, both individual and collective. In this introduction we discuss this concept by linking the work on emotional practices as developed by anthropologists, cultural historians, and sociologists such as Monique Scheer, Jo Labanyi, and Sarah Ahmed with the feminist materialism of Judith Butler and Karen Barad. But first, a short detour to Roland Barthes's discourse on love will allow us to explain the bodily effects of the performativity of emotions.

What Love Does

In 1977 Roland Barthes published a compilation of fragments, which included literary and philosophical quotations, conversations with friends, and even his own personal experiences about feeling love. He organized those reflections according to what he considered the central figures that make up the discourse of "someone speaking within himself, amorously, confronting the other (the loved object) who does not speak."[1] Like a kind of mirror, Barthes's *A Lover's Discourse* captures the bodily gestures of the person who reports feeling love: "the *I*."[2] Among the typical gestures through which we recognize "the lover at work," he distinguishes the singularity of the utterance *"Je-t'-aime*/I-love-you," as it enables us to carry that feeling from the self to the other by means of speaking these three words.

> *I-love-you* is without nuance. It suppresses explanations, adjustments, degrees, scruples. In a way—exorbitant paradox of language—to say *I-love-you* is to proceed as if there were no theater of speech, and this word is always *true* (has no referent other than its utterance: it is a performative).[3]

What did Barthes really mean when he referred to "I-love-you" as a performative? By employing this term, Barthes was inscribing his fragments in a long-standing tradition of philosophers such as John L. Austin, who had already explored the enigmatic effects of some words that do not simply describe reality but also have the power of transforming it.[4] "I love you" belongs to this type of performative utterance that only acquires meaning "in its immediate saying," when the speaker gives words the power of doing things.[5] Performative utterances are, therefore, not true or false, but happy or infelicitous, depending on the success of the action. This is why a love pronouncement is unforeseeable, because it always depends on the reaction of the person we want to reciprocate us.

For sure, we can consider "I love you" just as a marketed formula ready to be consumed on Valentine's Day.[6] This phrase is a cliché that hides, under the anonymity of the two personal pronouns, gender, class and ethnic stereotypes about what is considered a true romance in our early-twenty-first-century globalized world.[7] We must not forget that "I love you" might sound like a frontal attack on women's sexual liberation.[8] As Kate Millet criticized, "love has been the opium of women, as religion for masses. While we loved, men ruled."[9] Indeed, one can wonder why still today our hegemonic female side *hys-te-ri-ca-lly* insists on claiming our love, when our male side reminds us that "I love you" just means: I want only to have sex with you.

Even though Barthes imagines "So do I" as the most expected answer to our love's announcement, it never has an automatic response.[10] We may anticipate various replies to our demand, but the tragedy of these three words is that they have "no perfect answer."[11] Besides the many reactions that can be triggered by an "I love you," what it is certain is that its illocutionary force makes us vulnerable in a radical way. We expose ourselves to judgment, to shame, and even to the possibility of scaring the other, who might then run away. "There is a chance," writes Judith Butler, "that our speech act will be refused, and when and if it is, we are ourselves refused, and we feel that refusal in a bodily way."[12] We say, indeed, that our heart is broken. In so saying, we are pointing out the organ in which love feelings have inhabited since Ancient Greece in order to describe, physically and metaphorically, how our whole body has been rejected by the stillness following our words.[13]

When we say "I love you," what is really at stake is a kind of alchemical transmutation between words and the body, which results in the coming into being of a new person: an *I* who declares herself or himself in love—or, in other words, a body which comes into existence thanks to love's performative effects.[14] "I love you" is such a physical force that we can compare its articulation with the motion of the lips when having an orgasm. Indeed, the movement described by this utterance shows to what extent love is related to the muscular contractions of a body full of feeling.[15] Thus, "I love you" allows the "I" to travel toward the "you" through the inflexion of the verb "to love," from "here" to "there," where the lover is waiting to finally meet the beloved one.

"*Je-t-'aime*/I love you" is, therefore, a declaration, which—rephrasing Jacques Derrida's words—"has caused more than one to say that [. . .] one begins truly to love after or at the earliest from the moment when love is declared and not before."[16] "I love you" is like an optical illusion. It resembles in many aspects Judith Butler's definition of gender: because it is "an expectation that ends up producing the very phenomenon that it is anticipating."[17] It is not for nothing that love always emerges as a relational force that makes us feel like a natural woman or man, depending on whom we are mirroring our desire.[18]

Even if "I love you" leads us to feel our vulnerability in a feral way, we are condemned to its foolish perpetual repetition in order to better cope with the emptiness into which our bodily existence is delivered from the moment we are born.[19] The film *The Eternal Sunshine of the Spotless Mind* beautifully pictures the necessity of erasing the memories from our brains in order to play, once again, the role of somebody who falls in love as an innocent child.[20] This is why Barthes wrote that "*Je-t'-aime*/I-love-you" perfectly exemplifies a performative: because it is the saying of a certain doing whose irresponsible reiteration provides to each lover "inflections which will be forever new."[21]

Love turns us into emotional bodies, but its performative force is not particular to this feeling. As the chapters in this book will demonstrate, emotions are always a doing that transforms the subject in myriad ways. The next section will delve into the intimate relationship between emotions, performativity, and bodies in order to introduce the theoretical grounding of the concept "emotional bodies."

Doing Emotions; or, How Emotions Do Us

For us, editors of this volume, "I love you" is a paradigmatic example of doing emotions or how emotions do us, while shaping our bodies in the most intricate ways: both private and public, personal and political. Back in 2013 we decided to organize a workshop on this very topic, as a result of the discussions that we maintained between Geneva, Paris, London, Leicester, and Madrid. Back then, we suggested the category "emotional body" as an analytical tool to investigate new methodological avenues to account for the performative effects of emotions and their material effects. Like Butler's notion of gender, we viewed emotions as a form of action that did us by repetition, rather than "as an expression of a determinate underlying psychological or psychosocial phenomenon."[22]

Looking into what emotions do, rather than what they are, led us to break with the initial affiliation of emotion history with what Lucien Febvre referred to in 1941 as the "history of sensibilities."[23] In spite of its many virtues, the French Annales School presupposed that our past affective life may be approached as collective systems of beliefs, perceptions, and representations (*mentalités*). Instead of thinking about how emotions have been regarded in the past, we set to examine the daily effects of feeling, doing, and communicating emotions. By shifting the focus away from intellectual history, our aim was to capture emotional experience "from below," as it had been lived by people.[24] This book takes up those discussions, which we started several years ago, in order to explore the potential advantages and challenges of considering emotions as a practical engagement with the world. From then on, our work has been very much indebted to methodological contributions, such as Peter and Carol Stearns's "emotionology," Barbara Rosenwein's "emotional communities," and William Reddy's "emotional regimes," which have enabled us to better contemplate the role emotions have played as an integral part of the past social life.[25] All of these scholars have emphasized, from very different positions, the importance of the "language of emotion" as being "not simply passive, descriptive, but constitutive" in their expressive form.[26] In particular, Reddy has proposed the term "emotives" to refer to those emotional statements, which, like performative utterances, are able to change its referent.[27]

This book particularly follows the "practice turn" that emotion research has undergone since the 1980s in order to elude dichotomies such as mind and body, experience and expression, or nature and culture.[28] We are referring to the work of anthropologists such as Michelle Rosaldo, who introduced the term "embodied thoughts" in order to think about feelings "not as substances" but rather as "social practices organized by stories that we both enact and tell."[29] Sarah Ahmed's *The Cultural Politics of Emotions* shook the foundations of sociology by approaching emotions as practices that shape the surface of collective bodies.[30] Fay Bound Alberti's edited volume, *Emotions, Bodies and Disease*, has also been deeply influential among historians of medicine, providing key elements to study emotions as practices from the point of view of the patient.[31] We do not forget our Hispanophile colleagues, Luisa Elena Delgado, Pura Fernández, and Jo Labanyi, who have established the grounds for including the performativity of emotions into the historical agenda after the publication of *Engaging Emotions in Spanish Culture and Society*.[32] Precisely, Labanyi's article "Doing Emotions: Affect, Culture and Materiality" has been a very inspirational source to seize the possibilities of performativity. Unlike Labanyi, we have preferred to avoid the use of the term "affect" in this book to avoid the application of any biological or psychological contemporary framework when studying the past.[33]

Last but not least, this book owes a great deal to Monique Scheer's pioneering article "Are Emotions a Kind of Practice?" In it, Scheer defines emotional practices as "things that people do in order to have emotions or doing emotions in a performative sense."[34] Little matters if we are dealing with speech acts such as "I love you" or with other kinds of practices such as taking photographs, diagnosing patients' suffering, or helping war victims. As Scheer puts it, "practice is action, as [...] it refers to a nexus between sayings and doings."[35] For us, as for Scheer, the performative nature of emotions is necessarily linked to the body. Appropriating Bourdieu's notion of *habitus*, the "embodied history, internalized as a second nature," Scheer explains that practices are aimed at mobilizing emotions "where there are none, to focus diffuse arousals and give them an intelligible shape, or to change or remove emotions already there."[36] At the same time, showing that emotions are always "materially produced," "physically practiced or fabricated [...] within particular social conditions," demonstrates that they always happen in a body, which is also culturally produced.[37] According to Scheer's definition, "I love you" can be regarded as a way of naming emotions that is supposed to affect another person's feelings by touching him or her through one's declaration. The performative effects of this declaration will shape the identity of those *bodies that matter* in the love's story.[38] The very moment when emotions as practices give a new meaning to a body is the starting point of this book.

We argue that the benefit of approaching emotions as practices is that it allows a deeper and richer reflection on emotions and bodies. *Emotional Bodies* started as a project aimed to examine bodily emotional practices but has ended up offering new ways to think about bodies, performativity, and emotions in ways we did not anticipate. Thinking about the performative effects of emotions has led us to a necessary interrogation of the notion of the body and particularly whether we can consider our bodies as separate substances from the outer world. Historians of emotions working on experiences and expressions have often made use of the framework established by the history of the body in the 1990s.[39] Leading historians such as Roy Porter understood the body as something that is culturally and historically conditioned, a porous entity that cannot be reduced to its biology.[40] While we agree with this approach to human bodies, we also would like to challenge the assumption that all bodies are human. In this book, we propose to consider the performativity of emotions in both human and nonhuman bodies from a materialist and feminist point of view.

Feminist scholars such as Judith Butler, Donna Haraway, and Karen Barad have been calling into question what we know about the body and its materiality since the 1990s. Most famously, Haraway has blurred the boundaries between humans and nonhumans in her work on cyborgs and companion species.[41] In her writing, the human body is not only an organism that has been historically and culturally shaped by practices and systems of beliefs. What Haraway and others are questioning is the very nature of the body, or what exactly we can call "bodies." As Barad explains, bodies are not just "objects with inherent boundaries and properties; they are material and discursive phenomena." This means that "all bodies—not merely human bodies—come to matter through the world iterative intra-activity; its performativity."[42] Applying Niels Bohr's quantum model to the study of matter, bodies become configurations of matter that do not exist externally to their observation and their illusory fixation into a linguistic substance after the intervention of discursive practices.[43] Hers is a "performative metaphysics" inspired by Butler's conception of gender, in which "the formation of the subject" is also linked "to the production of the matter of bodies."[44] Performativity has led her to go far beyond a representational model in order to assert an "agential realism," concluding that there do not exist any ontological differences between subjects and objects in the world: they are just phenomena that were already interconnected before being separated by the human eye and language.[45]

As Katie Barclay has recently argued, historians of emotions can benefit greatly from this approach that radically rethinks the materiality of emotions. In particular, Barclay defends the application of new materialism in relation to the sources that historians choose by asking themselves about their production.[46] For us, it allows one to deploy the material performativity of emotions to its final consequences to desacralize "the atoms that make up the biological body."[47] If performativity is at the origin of matter, then the performativity of emotions creates *Emotional Bodies*: particular configurations of matter in which the doing of emotions is a driving force.

The bodies with which this book deals are, therefore, not simply what we understand as "the physical structure, including the bones, flesh, and organs, of a person or an animal."[48] Bodies are here defined by the result of the performative work of emotions. This is why the chapters in this book constantly change the scale of observation, zooming in and out from a micro to a macro perspective, in order to imagine an "alternative imagining of matter" as corporeal.[49] Under these parameters, emotional bodies emerge throughout the different sections of this book not only as actors like Susan Bickford, the woman suffering from hysteria whom Rob Boddice studies in chapter 1, but also as fictional collectives, such as the women incendiaries of the Paris Commune that Dolores Martín-Moruno revisits in chapter 8—and even as transnational agencies like those Bertrand Taithe analyses in chapter 11. It is the looseness of the body that enables us to think about the outer world not solely as a space inhabited by objects that only exist "in order to be mastered."[50] Objects also reclaim their own agency in the material production of bodies—for instance, in chapter 5, where Beatriz Pichel explores the effects of photographic cameras and artificial lighting on the patients photographed at La Salpêtrière.[51] Thus, the shifting meaning of the bodies that matter here is the consequence of our materialist posthumanist approach: a perspective which facilitates thinking about the performativity of emotions beyond the representational theory and the linguistic turn. This epistemological posthumanist position responds to a political and ethical choice in our present world and not to an intended justification of our views by appealing to any kind of scientific truth.[52]

Moreover, this materialist approach to the performativity of emotions involves necessarily rethinking the subject of emotions and, therefore, what "subjectivity" means.[53] As Caroline Braunmühl has argued, "rather than speaking of *doing emotions*, ... we should think of emotions as *(un-)doing us*."[54] We cannot presuppose an already constituted subject that does things such as emotions but rather should consider that the subject is the product of the doing of emotions. In this sense, it is not only the matter of the subject (the body) that is configured through the performativity of emotions but also the identity of the subject itself. Returning to our beloved example, the performative "I love you" is not simply configuring the lover's subjectivity in its utterance but is also exposing it to what one cannot control: the potential harm of receiving a negative response. Bodies, in this sense are literally *undone* after the refusal of their love's pronouncement. As Braunmühl suggests, "emotions" are, in this sense, "a fundamentally decentering force, depriving us of (self-)control as much as of self-identity."[55]

Throughout this book we explore identities linked with the construction of both individual and collective bodies. As Barbara Rosenwein has demonstrated, emotions construct communities, but we cannot take for granted any previous identity.[56] While the emphasis of most of the chapters is on what brings communities together, we also recognize the role of emotions in resisting identities and shaping subaltern subjects.[57] This prominence of the doing of emotions over the identity of the subjects also means that agency is a key characteristic of *emotional bodies*, which are understood in this collection of essays as either human or nonhuman actors. After all, "empirically speaking, we are made of star stuff. Why aren't we talking more about that? Materials never leave this world. They just keep recycling, recombining."[58]

Material Entanglements in This Volume

Emotional Bodies brings together specialists from a wide range of disciplines: the history of medicine, political studies, international relations, photographic history, religious history, gender studies, humanitarian studies, legal history, the history of childhood, and art history. A multidisciplinary perspective is necessary to articulate the category "emotional bodies" as a notion flexible enough to be applied alongside different fields, theories, and enactments of emotions across a long life span, from the Middle Ages to the present. The wide range of topics these chapters explore demonstrate that the performative effects of emotions are to be found everywhere: from early religious communities to current photographic practices, from social upheavals to psychological research.

As a result of this approach, the chapters engage with crucial debates in the history of emotions. First, the book provides a long-term vision of emotions without assuming a linear history. Continuities and discontinuities in the history of emotions are at the heart of chapters, which are able to account for how change can happen, as Piroska Nagy argues in chapter 7. The preeminence of the nineteenth and the twentieth centuries also contributes to the understanding of the history of emotions as a "history of the present," which aims at destabilizing our well-established contemporary evidence about what emotions are supposed to be.[59] Second, the broad scope of the book expands the range of sources habitually used in the history of emotions to include nontextual sources such as photographs and cameras.[60] The myriad case studies make creative use of sources to examine different kinds of practices in a variety of cultural contexts involving scientific theories like those Pilar León Sanz examines in chapter 2, relief practices such as those Jon Arrizabalaga analyzes in chapter 9, and the humanitarian images Emma Hutchison deals with in chapter 10.

Going from the micro to the macro level, this book is organized around individual, social, and transnational bodies. Chapters 1 through 6 discuss how individual emotions have been conceived, experienced, embodied, and performed. In contrast, chapters 7 through 11 examine collectives grouped together physically, such as the humanitarian transnational bodies. Distinguishing between individual and collective bodies offers a vantage point for the study of performativity, as it allows detailed accounts of the specific effects of doing emotions in different historical settings. However, we cannot take these two categories as completely opposite. Some questions, such as how emotional performances reflect and shape social change, are explored across the different sections of the book. The distinction between individual and collective bodies is, thereby, one of perspective rather than nature when dealing with the historical performativity of emotions.

In the end, writing a book collectively is like taking a long journey. Since 2013, this project on the historical performativity of emotions has led us into new and exciting directions we had never imagined before. In many aspects, *Emotional Bodies* resembles to the utterance of "I love you," as it has given us the possibility of becoming otherwise, thanks to the work we have accomplished in emotion history. The understanding of emotions this book has inspired is the result of our discussions on how to become politically engaged when writing history today. This is why we regard this book not merely as an intellectual exercise but more specifically as a practical one that has been nourished by our own personal experiences as female scholars. Rephrasing Simone de Beauvoir's words: no one is born, but rather becomes a woman in academia.[61] Our commitment to gender studies and particularly to feminism is intellectual but also, in a way, emotional. We firmly believe that "the personal is political."[62] We reject the idea of authors as disembodied brains writing from nowhere. Our knowledge is situated and comes from a partial perspective.[63] For us, vindicating and owning our emotions is a way to resist to stereotypes and survive in a male-dominated world, even if this epistemological decision places us in an irremediably vulnerable position.[64]

Although we have decided to maintain the original title of our workshop, we are completely aware that this book finally appears as something radically different from what we expected in 2013. Like Roland Barthes's "*Je-t'-aime*/I-love-you," *Emotional Bodies* appears as a type of work conducted by the *Argonauts*: those sailors who should change all the parts of their boat over time but insisted in calling in it "Argo."[65] This is why we would like to introduce this book as the result of a shared reflections about love and friendship: because each of us is destined to renew her/his own ship during the "voyage without changing its name" and "to give to one and the same phrase inflections which will be forever new."⁶⁶

Notes

1. Roland Barthes, *A Lover's Discourse: Fragments*, trans. Richard Howard (New York: Hill and Wang, 1978), 3.
2. Ibid., 122.
3. Ibid., 143.
4. On the philosophical discussion of performative utterances, see J. L. Austin, *How to Do Things with Words: The William James Lectures delivered at Harvard University in 1955* (Oxford: Clarendon, 1962); John R. Searle, "How Performatives Work," *Linguistics and Philosophy* 12 no. 5 (1989): 535–58. Other perspectives to consider the meaning of performative and performance are Jean-François Lyotard, *La condition postmoderne: Rapport sur le savoir* (Paris: Minuit, 1978); and Jacques Derrida, *L'université sans condition* (Paris: Galilée, 2011). On the meaning of performativity in gender studies, see Judith Butler, *Gender Trouble: Feminism and the Subversion of Identity* (London: Routledge, 1990); Shoshana Felman, *The Scandal of the Speaking Body: Don Juan with J. L. Austin; or, Seduction in Two Languages* (Stanford, Calif.: Stanford University Press, 2002); and Eve Kosofsky Sedgwick, *Touching Feeling: Affect Pedagogy, Performativity* (Durham, N.C.: Duke University Press, 2003).
5. Barthes, *Lover's Discourse*, 149.
6. Eva Illouz, *Consuming the Romantic Utopia: Love and the Cultural Contradictions of Capitalism* (Berkeley: University of California Press, 1977). See also Eva Illouz, *Why Love Hurts: A Sociological Explanation* (Cambridge: Polity, 2011).
7. Judith Butler, "Response: Performative Reflections on Love and Commitment," *Women's Studies Quarterly* 39, nos. 1–2 (2011): 237.
8. Anna G. Jónasdóttir and Ann Ferguson, eds., *Love: A Question for Feminism in the Twenty-First Century* (London: Routledge, 2014).
9. Kate Millet's assertion is discussed in Julia Huehn, "'Je t'aime . . . moi non plus': Deconstructing Love in *Open Confession to a Man from a Woman*," *Women's Writing* 13, no. 2 (2006): 225–45.
10. Barthes, *Lover's Discourse*, 150.
11. Ibid.
12. Butler, "Response," 237.
13. On the heart as the anatomical site of love feelings, see Fay Bound Alberti, *Matters of the Heart: History, Medicine and Emotion* (Oxford: Oxford University Press, 2010). See also Fay Bound Alberti, *This Mortal Coil: The Human Body in History and Culture* (Oxford: Oxford University Press, 2016), 92–111.
14. On "I love you" as a performative that establishes the condition of a new per-

son, see Lisa Fletcher, *Historical Romance Fiction: Heterosexuality and Performativity* (London: Routledge, 2008), 25–36.

15. Jacques Lacan, *Conférence à Genève sur le symptôme* (Paris: Bloc notes de la psychoanalyse, 1985).

16. An English translation of Jacques Derrida's citation can be found in Julian Wolfreys, ed., *The J. Hillis Miller Reader* (Stanford, Calif.: Stanford University Press, 2005).

17. Butler, *Gender Trouble*, xv.

18. Ibid., 212. She refers to Aretha Franklin's song "(You Make Me Feel Like) A Natural Woman" (USA: Atlantic, 1967) to introduce her definition of gender as free floating rather than a fixed substance.

19. Friedrich Nietzsche, *Also Sprach Zarathustra* (Berlin: Walter de Gruyter, 1883–1885), 27.

20. Michel Gondry, *The Eternal Sunshine of the Spotless Mind* (Universal Studios, 2004). About the relationship between forgiveness and promise, see Friedrich Nietzsche, *Zur Genealogie der Moral: Eine Streitschrift* (Leipzig: Neumann, 1887).

21. Maggie Nelson, *The Argonauts* (Minneapolis, Minn.: Graywolf, 2015), 5. On the iterability of performative utterances, see Judith Butler, *Excitable Speech: A Politics of the Performative* (New York: Routledge, 1997).

22. Catherine Lutz, "Feminist Theories and the Science of Emotion," in *Science and Emotions after 1945: A Transatlantic Perspective*, ed. Frank Biess and Daniel M. Gross (Chicago: Chicago University Press, 2014), 357.

23. Lucien Febvre, "Sensibility and History: How to Reconstitute the Emotional Life of the Past?" in *A New Kind of History: From the Writings of Febvre*, ed. Peter Burke, trans. K. Folca (London: Routledge and Keagan Paul, 1973), 12–26.

24. For understanding the history of emotions as a history of experience, see Rob Boddice, "The History of Emotions: Past, Present and Future," in *Revista de Estudios Sociales* 62 (2017): 10–15; *The History of Emotions* (Manchester: Manchester University Press, 2018); and *A History of Feelings* (London: Reaktion, 2019), 188–91. On the expression "history from below," see Edward Palmer Thompson, *The Making of the English Working-Class* (London: Gollancz, 1963). About Thompson's historiographical approach in the present, see Katrina Navicas, "A Return to Materialism? Putting Social History Back into Place," in *New Directions in Social and Cultural History*, ed. Sasha Handley, Rohan McWilliam, and Lucy Noakes (London: Bloomsbury, 2018), 93.

25. Peter Stearns and Carol Stearns, "Emotionology: Clarifying the History of Emotions and Emotional Standards," *American Historical Review* 90, no. 4, (1985): 813–36; Barbara H. Rosenwein, *Emotional Communities in the Middle Ages* (Ithaca, N.Y.: Cornell University Press, 2007); and William M. Reddy, *The Navigation of Feeling: A Framework for the History of Emotions* (Cambridge: Cambridge University Press, 2001).

26. Katie Barclay, "New Materialism and the New History of Emotions," *Emotions: History, Culture, Society* 1, no. 1 (2017): 166. For a review of the significance of these

works in shaping the history of emotions as a field, see Boddice, *History of Emotions*, 1–7.

27. Reddy, *Navigation of Feeling*, 63–111.

28. Boddice, *History of Emotions*, 120–24.

29. Michelle Z. Rosaldo, "Toward an Anthropology of Self and Feeling," in *Culture Theory: Essay on Mind, Self, and Emotion*, ed. Richard A. Shweder and Robert A. LeVine (Cambridge: Cambridge University Press, 1995), 143.

30. Sara Ahmed, *The Cultural Politics of Emotion* (New York: Routledge, 2004).

31. Fay Bound Alberti, ed., *Medicine, Emotion and Disease, 1700–1950* (Basingstoke: Palgrave Macmillan, 2005).

32. Luisa Elena Delgado, Pura Fernández, and Jo Labanyi, eds., *Engaging the Emotions in Spanish Culture and History* (Nashville, Tenn.: Vanderbilt University Press, 2016).

33. Jo Labanyi, "Doing Things: Emotions, Affect and Materiality," *Journal of Spanish Cultural Studies* 11, nos. 3–4 (2010): 223–33. For a critical view on affect theory, see Ruth Leys, "The Turn to Affect: A Critique," *Critical Inquiry* 37, no. 3 (2011): 434–72.

34. Monique Scheer, "Are Emotions a Kind of Practice (and Is That What Makes Them Have a History?): A Bourdieuian Approach to Understanding Emotion," *History and Theory* 51, no. 2 (2012): 209. See also Jan Plamper, *The History of Emotions: An Introduction* (Oxford: Oxford University Press, 2015), 313–14.

35. Scheer, "Are Emotions," 200.

36. Pierre Bourdieu, *The Logic of Practice*, trans. Richard Nice (Stanford, Calif.: Stanford University Press, 1990), 56. Scheer, "Are Emotions," 194.

37. Pascal Eitler and Monique Scheer, "Emotionengeschichte als Körpergeschichte: Eine heuristische Perspektive auf religiöse Konversionen im 19. und 20. Jahrhundert," *Geschichte und Gesellschaft* 35, no. 2 (2009): 291. See also Plamper, *History of Emotions*, 136.

38. Judith Butler, *Bodies That Matter: On the Discursive Limits of "Sex"* (New York: Routledge, 1993).

39. Roger Cooter, "The Turn of the Body: History and the Politics of the Corporeal," *Arbor* 743 (2010): 393–405.

40. Roy Porter, *Bodies Politic: Disease, Death and Doctors in Britain, 1650–1900* (London: Reaktion, 2001). For further reading, see Mark S. R. Jenner and Bertrand O. Taithe, "The Historiographical Body," in *Companion to Medicine in the Twentieth Century*, ed. Roger Cooter and John Pickstone (Routledge: New York, 2003), 187–216.

41. Donna Haraway, *Primate Visions: Gender, Race, and Nature in the World of Modern Science* (New York: Routledge, 1989), and Donna Haraway, *The Companion Species Manifesto: Dogs, People, and Significant Otherness* (Chicago: Chicago University Press, 2003). To go further, see Delphine Gardey, "Donna Haraway: Poétique et politique du vivant," *Cahiers du genre*, no. 55 (2013), 171–194.

42. Karen Barad, *Meeting the Universe Halfway: Quantum Physics and the Entanglement of Matter and Meaning* (Durham, N.C.: Duke University Press, 2007), 152–53.

43. Samantha Frost, "The Implications of New Materialisms for Feminist Epistemology," in *Feminist Epistemology and Philosophy of Science: Power in Knowledge*, ed. Heidi E. Grasswick (Dordrecht: Springer, 2011), 69–84.

44. Karen Barad, "Posthumanist Performativity: Toward an Understanding of How Matter Comes to Matter," *Signs* 38, no. 3 (2003): 808.

45. Barad, *Meeting the Universe Halfway*, 66–70.

46. Barclay, "New Materialism," 178.

47. Barad, "Posthumanist Performativity," 810; Barad, *Meeting the Universe Halfway*, 66 and 208.

48. "Body," Oxford Dictionaries, https://en.oxforddictionaries.com/definition/body.

49. Barclay, "New Materialism," 162.

50. Labanyi, "Doing Things," 223.

51. Bruno Latour, *Reassembling the Social: An Introduction to Actor-Network-Theory* (Oxford: Oxford University Press, 2007).

52. Barad, *Meeting the Universe Halfway*, 247.

53. Penny Summerfield, "Subjectivity, the Self and Historical Practice," in Handley, McWilliam, and Noakes, New Directions, 21–42.

54. Caroline Braunmühl, "Theorizing Emotions with Judith Butler: Within and beyond the Courtroom," *Rethinking History* 16, no. 2 (2012): 223. Original emphasis.

55. Ibid.

56. Rosenwein, *Emotional Communities*, 2.

57. María Rosón and Rosa María Medina-Doménech, "Emotional Resistances: Spaces and Presences of Intimacy in the Historic Archive," *Arenal* 24, no. 2 (2017): 407–39.

58. Nelson, *Argonauts*, 121.

59. On the history of the present, see Michel Foucault, *Discipline and Punish: The Birth of the Prison*, trans. Alan Sheridan (London: Penguin, 1991), 31; Colin Jones, "The Emotional Turn in the History of Medicine and the View from the Queen Mary University of London," *Social History of Medicine*, Virtual Issue, Emotions, Health, and Wellbeing, vol. 1 (2014): 1–2; and Ruth Leys and Marlene Goldman, "Navigating the Genealogies of Trauma, Guilt, and Affect: An Interview with Ruth Leys," *University of Toronto Quarterly* 79, no. 2 (2010): 656–79.

60. Recent works on the material culture of emotions include Alice Dolan and Sally Holloway, "Emotional Textiles: An Introduction," *Textile* 14, no. 2 (2016): 152–59; Anna Moran and Sorcha O'Brien, eds., *Love Objects: Emotion, Design and Material Culture* (London: Bloomsbury, 2014); and Stephanie Downes, Sally Holloway, and Sara Randles, *Feeling Things: Objects and Emotions through History* (Oxford: Oxford University Press, 2018).

61. Simone de Beauvoir, *Le deuxième sexe* (Paris: Gallimard, 1949), 2:5.

62. Carol Hanisch, "The Personal Is Political," in *Notes from the Second Year: Women's Liberation ; Major Writings of the Radical Feminists*, ed. Shulamith Firestone (New York: Radical Feminism, 1970), 85–86.

63. Donna Haraway, "Situated Knowledges: The Science Question in Feminism and the Privileged of Partial Perspective," *Feminist Studies* 14, no. 3 (1988): 575–93.

64. Judith Butler, Zeynep Gambetti, and Leticia Sabsay, eds., *Vulnerability in Resistance* (Durham, N.C.: Duke University Press, 2016).

65. Joseph Campbell, *The Hero with a Thousand Faces* (New York: Pantheon, 1949), 203–4.

66. Nelson, *Argonauts*, 5. See also Roland Barthes, *Roland Barthes by Roland Barthes* (Berkley: University of California Press, 1977), 114.

PART I

Diseased Bodies under Construction

The first section of this volume explores emotions from the point of view of the history of science and medicine. As chapters in this section reveal, physiologists, psychologists, and psychiatrists have conceptualized emotions and their effects on the body in diverse ways, and scientific and cultural understandings of emotions have influenced each other. Our contributors follow recent publications such as the special issues in *Isis* ("The Emotional Economy of Science") and *Osiris* ("History of Sciences and the Emotions"), which have argued that historians of medicine and science should pay attention to the history of emotions and vice versa, favoring an "integrated approach."[1] For instance, Otniel Dror has demonstrated that scientific definitions of emotions have historically depended on the technologies used in laboratory research and the conditions in which experiments were carried out.[2] But historians of science have examined not only the scientific theories of emotions. While the scientific ideal of mechanical objectivity as described by Lorraine Daston and Peter Galison presented the detached self as the greatest aspiration for scientists, Paul White has argued that emotions have been integral both to the construction of the scientific self and to scientific practice.[3]

One of the fields in which the scientific and the cultural elements of emotions has featured more prominently is the historical study of pain. Historians have dedicated themselves to understanding how people in the past have made sense of and expressed pain, once characterized by Elaine Showalter as a subjective experience that cannot be communicated to others.[4] In this line, Rob Boddice and Joanna Bourke, among others, have examined both the scientific definitions and the cultural practices that have shaped our experience and language of pain.[5] Bourke's focus on metaphors and Boddice's chapter in this book show that historical experiences of pain offer privileged points of entry to explore the entanglement of scientific theories and cultural practices of the past.

This integrated approach to the emotions and the sciences has been particularly important in the cultural history of medicine. As Fay Bound Alberti and Elena Carrera have argued, emotions have often been understood in relation to health and disease.[6] In particular, historians have frequently studied emotions in the context of pathologies—that is, when the presence of an emotion is a pathogen that makes the body (or the mind) sick. Anne Harrington has recently criticized that "most scholarship on the medicalization of emotions has focused on projects that locate emotions, one way or another, within individual brains and minds," proposing instead a relational model in which mother love is both "a pathology (for the mother) and a pathogen (for her vulnerable child)."[7]

All these approaches have favored the understanding of emotions as practices that do things in the world. Chapters in this section take up these debates, examining medical and cultural understandings of emotions, particularly in cases where the embodiment of emotions results in morbid or abnormal states. Either an unspeakable pain, a personality trait, or exaggerated excitability, emotions in these chapter produce particular kinds of bodies, providing examples of Scheer's "knowing body," bridging the mind and the body as two essential components of the emotions.[8]

In chapter 1, Rob Boddice's history of the gendered diagnosis of hysteria and tetanus shows how experiences of pain that were incommunicable under a particular emotional regime translated into bodily performances, which followed a cultural and medical script, that of hysterical attacks. Boddice reconstructs and analyzes the patients' emotional experiences from the point of view of their own bodily expressions and performances, rather than from the testimony of medical accounts. This approach offers new and productive insights into nineteenth-century hysteria and demonstrates that pain was a performative practice that turned patients into emotional bodies. How this practice manifested in bodily performances depended on the dominant emotional regimes of the context in which the attack took place.

Gian Marco Vidor approaches the concept of "emotional bodies" through the figure of the nineteenth-century "criminal of passion." Vidor's research on Italian psychiatry and criminology shows that in order to define who was really a "criminal of passion" (as opposed to other kinds of criminals), the medical and legal establishment engaged in a discussion about the nature and the effects of emotional phenomena. The main characteristic of the "criminal of passion," often illustrated by the literary figure of Othello, was the performative aspect of his or her emotions and passions, which made the criminal commit the offense but also led to feelings of remorse and, occasionally, even to suicide. Emotional bodies are here considered as liminal bodies, existing halfway between insanity and normality, only to be discovered through their criminal acts.

Patient's experience is also a key topic in Pilar León Sanz's contribution, focused on the emergence of psychosomatic research in the 1950s. For key theorists Seymour Fisher and Sidney E. Cleveland, emotions were personality forces that had an impact on the development of body image, which in turn played a fundamental role in the genesis of diseases such as cancer. The boundaries between emotional and physiological processes blurred in psychosomatic research, as the emotions felt by the patient in relation to the living experience of his or her own body affected the kind of disease he or she experienced. León Sanz demonstrates, therefore, that the idea of an "emotional body" that is the result of the performative work of emotions can already be found in twentieth-century psychological research.

Notes

1. Paul White, "Introduction," Focus: The Emotional Economy of Science, *Isis* 100, no. 4 (2009): 792–97; Otniel E. Dror, Bettina Hitzer, Anja Laukötter, and Pilar León-Sanz, "An Introduction to *History of Sciences and the Emotions*," *Osiris* 31, no. 1 (2016): 1–18. Fay Bound Alberti, *Matters of the Heart: History, Medicine and Emotion* (Oxford: Oxford University Press, 2010), 13.

2. Otniel E. Dror, "The Affect of Experiment: The Turn to Emotions in Anglo-American Physiology, 1900–1940," *Isis* 90, no. 2 (1999): 205–37, Otniel Dror, "The Scientific Image of Emotion: Experience and Technologies of Inscription," *Configurations* 7, no. 3 (1999): 355–401.

3. Lorraine Daston and Peter Galison, *Objectivity* (New York: Zone, 2007); White, "Introduction."

4. Elaine Scarry, *The Body in Pain: The Making and Unmaking of the World* (New York: Oxford University Press, 1985).

5. Joanna Bourke, *The Story of Pain: From Prayer to Painkillers* (Oxford: Oxford University Press, 2014); Rob Boddice, ed., *Pain and Emotion in Modern History* (Houndmills: Palgrave, 2014); Louise Hide, Joanna Bourke, and Carmen Mangion, "Perspectives on Pain: Introduction," *19: Interdisciplinary Studies in the Long Nineteenth Century* 15 (2012); Daniel S. Goldberg, "Pain, Objectivity and History: Understanding Pain Stigma," *Medical Humanities*, 43, no. 4 (2017): 238–43; Dolores Martín-Moruno, "Pain as Practice in Paolo Mantegazza's Science of Emotions," *Osiris* 31, no. 1 (2016): 137–62.

6. Alberti, *Medicine, Emotion and Disease*; Elena Carrera, ed., *Emotions and Health: 1200–1700* (Leiden: Brill, 2013). See also Penelope Gouk and Helen Hills, eds., *Representing Emotions: New Connections in the Histories of Art, Music and Medicine* (London: Routledge, 2005).

7. Anne Harrington, "Mother Love and Mental Illness: An Emotional History," *Osiris* 31, no. 1 (2016): 95.

8. Monique Scheer, "Are Emotions a Kind of Practice (And Is That What Makes Them Have a History?): A Bourdieuian Approach to Understanding Emotion," *History and Theory* 51, no. 2 (2012): 199.

1. Hysteria or Tetanus?

Ambivalent Embodiments and the Authenticity of Pain

ROB BODDICE

Hysterical Passage

On Friday, December 4, 1874, the emigrant ship *Earl Dalhousie* set sail from London, picking up passengers at Plymouth on her way to Adelaide, South Australia, where she arrived February 23, 1875. *The Times* of London had boasted on her departure of the superior berths for married couples "on a newly patented system" to "afford privacy and ventilation."[1] There were thirty-nine married couples aboard, as well as ninety-six single women, seventy-one single men, fifty-two children under age twelve, and ten infants. The report of her arrival in the *South Australian Chronicle* suggested all was well: "During the passage, the utmost good feeling has prevailed, and this due mainly to the attention bestowed by the captain and officers, Dr. J. Hudson, R.N., and the matron, Mrs. Thompson, a lady well qualified for the task entrusted to her."[2] It would be another eight months or so before the reasons for the particular mention of the staff surgeon and the ship's matron would become clear. In the doldrums and tropical heat, it had not all been plain sailing for the *Dalhousie*.

Things had gone awry around the twenty-fourth day of the journey, shortly after the *Dalhousie* crossed the equator. We know the details from John Hudson's report of the voyage to *The Lancet* in October 1875. Susan Bickford, age twenty-two, was described as being "of spare habit, intelligent, and healthy looking." She had given birth at age fifteen and since that time had endured "parental harshness and . . . restraint in a workhouse asylum." She was discovered lying prostrate and unconscious on December 5, one day into the voyage. Hudson found that Bickford was a "victim of nymphomania," with "long, strong, frequent" attacks brought on either by sudden shocks, such as loud noises or "flashes of light," or without due cause at night. The root cause was masturbation. If we trust the account of John Hudson, Susan Bickford masturbated intermittently from December 5 until February 7, that period being punctuated by "various remissions or intervals of calm, rational, and good behaviour, alternating with threats and feigned attempts to commit suicide." She was "peevish, quarrelsome, perverse, deceitful . . . pulling her hair and malingering, in order to excite sympathy." Under the effect of chloral hydrate, at the time a fashionable sedative, Bickford "would betray signs of good and evil training, such as bad language and pretty hymns."

"Intolerance of light," a symptom Bickford described as "fire in the head," combined with "hyperaesthesia of [the] left side of face, neuralgia, temporary paralysis and spasms of eyelids, face, neck, throat, &c., involving the muscles of expression, speech, deglutition, and voice, on one or both, but mostly on the left side." When seized by an attack, convulsions "extended to the chest, the arms, and more or less to the whole body, lasting from a few minutes to half an hour, and merging into complete and general rigidity (opisthotonos), the body being arched backwards, so as to rest on the head and heels, but rarely inclined to the right side." What could only be described as "tetanus" would last a few minutes or a few hours. In "a few instances the patient remained still and unconscious, as in a state of catalepsy, for twenty-four to thirty-six hours." In short, Susan Bickford, young mother, was cast as a sexually depraved hysteric. The serious symptoms with which she presented were undermined by her deceitfulness and the perception that she was a "malingerer," which is to say that she fabricated or exaggerated her symptoms in order to attract attention. That this took the form of tetanus did not seem to surprise John Hudson in the least. Its effects on the other passengers, however, were remarkable.

The outbreak of tetanus spread, on December 28, to the private, airy space of the married quarters. Maria Stevenson was twenty-six years old, "of spare habit, pale, epileptic aspect, and lively disposition." Her case was the tipping point for a widespread outbreak. There would be twelve cases on that day alone. She was "excited by jealousy," with attacks marked by violence and characterized by "delusions and vagaries, followed by . . . feigning and deception." Her body convulsed, with rigidity punctuated by muscle spasms. In a state of ecstasy, she thought herself "about to be buried at sea, . . . asking to be 'lowered gently.'" Hudson describes the detection of "the stage of imposture," the discovery of which caused her immediate recovery on January 16.

In the meantime, Anna M. Glasby, also married, succumbed. A "weak and delicate woman," her attack was brought on by the "sight of others" in duress. This was further explained by her long-standing "uterine weakness (abortions, &c.)." Hudson does not provide details about what might be subsumed under "&c." These cases were followed by that of Harriet Wickham, a domestic servant. Wickham, in her early twenties, was of "stout" build but "*apparently* listless and phlegmatic" [emphasis in original]. Wickham's attack did not result in tetanus, perhaps because of her "conspicuous ... moral and intellectual attainments." She fainted, then had a bout of "hysterical screaming, followed by singing and talking (soliloquy)." In her reverie she "disclosed evidences of a moral and cultivated mind," singing in German at one point and, at another, teaching singing lessons to an imaginary class of children. She instructed these phantasms on the Epistle of St. Paul to Philemon, impressing Hudson with her learning. In a calm state she announced, "We don't so readily get over broken hearts," but soon followed this with a bout of "disobedient and perverse conduct." On February 1, Wickham recovered, tendering a "becoming apology."

Three of the subsequent attacks affected "stout, robust, headstrong young women, of neglected training and education." The attacks were "strongly marked with a predominance of the animal spirits." The euphemistic tone of moral evaluation is unmistakable here. Overweight, unfeminine, impolite, and out of (emotional) control is the general picture. There were nine further cases in total, in young women both married and single, all of whom were "of excitable, hysterical constitutions," presenting with a range of symptoms from "vague fears and hallucinations to unconsciousness, extreme convulsions, and stiffness of the whole body." The cause in all cases, according to Hudson, "was probably emotional, and the nature of each apparently a reflex action of the nervous centres." There were no detrimental consequences to "uterine functions." Hudson, with the help of his matron, had treated the women with chloral hydrate, potassium bromide, henbane, valerian, aperients, bleeding (up to twenty ounces), cold compresses, and isolation on the deck (for safety).[3] When Adelaide port authorities boarded the *Dalhousie* in the early hours of February 23, they were met by a wide-awake assemblage of emigrants on deck who "cheered lustily" for their arrival.[4] Small wonder.

Presentation and Representation: Hysteria, Demons, and Tetanus

Hudson's report of the voyage to Adelaide appeared in *The Lancet* under the title "Epidemic of Hysterical Epilepsy and Tetanus." The setting and scale of the outbreak are, perhaps, extraordinary, but narrative accounts of hysterical tetanus were common enough. It is important to note that tetanus until the end of the nineteenth century, as with many diseases, was defined by its appearance, not by an understanding of its causes. Tetanus was descriptive of a bodily state—it literally means *taut*—not a specific pathogen. Nevertheless, physicians talked of the difference between "true" tetanus and imposters well before the development of the etiology of tetanus (*Clostridium tetani*) from the late 1880s. We have access to accounts of hysterical tetanus, more or less exclusively, through the male gaze of the physician. As such, we are left with a distinct picture of hysterical tetanus as bodily performance, by which is meant a conscious attempt to dissimulate a disease as a result of overwhelming emotional problems. Put another way, these performances, from the medical point of view, had no relation to the actual problem, which was not so much medical as *moral*.

There is a long narrative arc that explains this medical gaze, this politics of diagnosis. I will briefly survey it here because I want to emphasize the extent to which the historiographical focus has foregrounded the medical construction of hysteria, over and above the experience of the hysterical subject. In many instances this has taken the form of an analysis of the ways in which hysterical embodiments were transferences from medical personnel to their patients. This has been most effective in deconstructing the clinical encounter, demonstrating the extent to which patient behavior was *made* by and in such encounters. But this still raises the question of what it felt like to be hysterical in this period and also underplays the extent to which hysterical subjects were complicit in the making of hysterical bodily practices.

I refer to a politics of diagnosis as part of a wider interest in the way in which the institution of medicine has ascribed meaning or value to different states of pain and/or suffering and the ways in which the meaningful experiences of patients might be recovered and reconstructed. In contemporary medical studies of pain, old boundaries between physical and mental, or bodily and emotional, have been demolished.[5] Painful experience has been shown to arise through emotions.[6] There is nothing intrinsically painful about injury.[7] The historical record is littered with cases of the dreadfully wounded who nevertheless felt no pain.[8] Concomitantly, a painful experience does not require any kind of somatic derangement or lesion.[9] Pain is an *output* of the brain, not an *input* to the body.[10] Insofar as brains are in the world, plastic, socially constructed, as well as biologically bound, so meaningful pain is contextually situated.[11] This remains true regardless of whether the person in pain is merely experiencing pain rather than trying to communicate it, if indeed the two can be disentangled.[12] The major claim in this chapter, therefore, is that the hysterical subject was looking for an expression for pain during an era in which mere emotional *suffering* was not taken seriously by the medical profession. This pain had no visible sign and therefore no medical rationale. Following a scripted bodily practice to make a somatic representation of emotional pain was an attempt to express the experience of an emotional ordeal that could not otherwise be expressed. The script was provided by the world of medicine, empowered to search for the physiological roots of hysteria.[13] The attempt by hysterics to "read" that script can be understood as an "emotive" process. I am using a slight modification of William Reddy's original coinage of this term, as a "type of speech act different from both performative and constative utterances, which both describes . . . and changes . . . the world, because emotional expression has an exploratory and self-altering effect on the activated thought material of emotion."[14] The modification is to include nonverbal "utterances" in the practice of emotional expression. Facial expression and bodily gesture are as much a part of the emotive dynamic as trying to say how one feels.[15]

Let us turn to the writing of the script. Charles Bell, in his famous treatise on the anatomy and philosophy of emotional expression in the fine arts, construed hysterical tetanus as fraud. By placing his illustration of tetanus, based on three soldiers wounded in the head, in a section on the pain of the bodies of the demonically possessed, he showed his readers how to tell true tetanus from spurious "Demoniacs."[16] Since, for Bell, there is "no such thing in nature" as an "accidental and deranged action of the muscular frame" but only the "definable symptoms" of a disease, any deviance from a universal set of signs gave away the imposture. He marks the differences between true tetanus, associated with martial masculinity, and those spurious displays of the devil. In Domenichino's *Santo Nilo libera un ossesso* (1608–10) the painter represents "a lad possessed"—seized by convulsions, "rigidly bent back; the lower limbs spasmodically extended, so that his toes only rest on the ground." There are telltale signs, for Bell, of abuses of nature: "the hands spread abroad, the palms and fingers open, and the jaw fallen." All are implausible, according to Bell's insistence that a disease "will ever present itself with the same characters." There follows some further discussion of how to tell if someone is "feigning" illness. Bell highlights the convulsive possession of the moonstruck (literally, *lunatic*) boy in Raphael's *Transfiguration* (1516–20), pointing out that a physician would have been able to detect the boy's fraud, since "no child was ever so affected" by a real disease. Stiffened with contractions and with his eyes turned in their sockets, the image was far from verisimilitude. Bell was ostensibly employing his anatomical and physiological knowledge for the instruction of artists, but he was at the same time lending physicians a guide to differential diagnosis. If the Renaissance

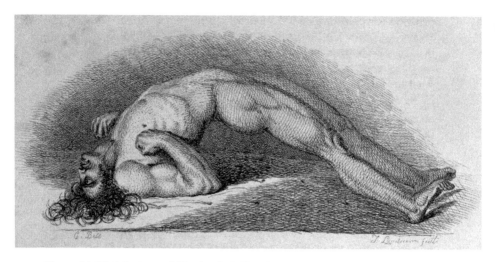

Figure 1.1: "Opisthotonos." Charles Bell, *The Anatomy and Philosophy of Expression as Connected with the Fine Arts* (London: Murray, 1844). Wellcome Library, London.

saw in these unconvincingly wracked boyish figures the work of the devil, nineteenth-century medicine until Charcot was at pains to show the varieties of hysteria and hysterical deception, to distinguish the possessed and the possessed by nerves from the veritable pain of the masculine diseased, which always presented in the same reliable way. Since the Renaissance at least, by this analysis, tetanic malingering had been used to gain attention.

Bell's careful distinctions would later be overridden by Charcot and Richer, who took the Renaissance demoniacs to be signs of universality in a long history of *grande hystérie*, despite their acknowledgement of Bell's essential truth that the representations of some artists did not correspond to anything real or known.[17] Charcot and Richer's encounters with hysterics at the *Salpêtrière* have become the classic example of the transference of medical expectations in the formation of somatic representations of hysterical conditions. They themselves influenced their patients to conform to their classical notion of how grande hystérie should look. The famous painting of Charcot's clinical lesson, demonstrating a woman falling into a hysterical contracture, shows Charcot's male staff transfixed on the patient, while the patient is the only one conscious of the hysterical form, which is neatly presented on the back wall of the theater. The patient, as Sander Gilman tells us, "knows how to be a patient" and strives to conform, while the medical men congratulate themselves on their insights.[18] Nowhere is this more clear than in Charcot's

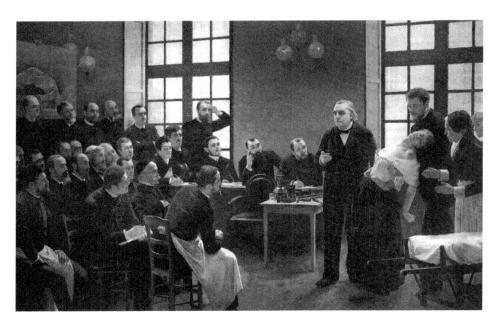

Figure 1.2: André Brouillet, "Une leçon clinique à la Salpêtrière" (1887).

work on hysterical men, who conformed to Charcot's idea of classic hysterical contractures within short periods of being admitted to his care, under the influence of Charcot's assistants, Charcot himself, and what Mikkel Borch-Jacobsen calls the "institutional ambience" of the hospital.[19] Through the work of men like Charcot, hysteria gained pathological authenticity: hysteria became "real," so to speak. The pains of hysteria, still categorically removed from the realm of pain caused by disease, were nevertheless elevated to the realm of medical scrutiny. If we focus on the patient here, then arguments about the degree to which Charcot transferred his expectations of the hysterical arch to his patients become irrelevant. In being able to understand and carry out the cultural script set by the medical establishment, hysterics themselves were able to find a permissible expression for their particular suffering. Treatment may not have been exactly what they required, but at the very least here was an outlet for emotional pain that otherwise was denied an expression in civil society. Hence, individuals with emotional trauma had a vested interest in being able to "read" the tetanus script. For patients at the Salpêtrière, the expectation that hysterics would assume the tetanic posture made the hospital itself an "emotional refuge."

The coinage is William Reddy's. He defines an "emotional refuge" as a "relationship, ritual, or organization [I would add "a place, or space"] . . . that provides safe release from prevailing emotional norms and allows relaxation of emotional effort."[20] I am modifying this definition somewhat, based on Reddy's own clarification of what is meant by an "emotional regime," which exists wherever "the sum of penalties and exclusions [I would add "and rewards"] adds up to a coherent structure, and the issue of conformity becomes defining for the individual."[21] We are always in an emotional regime, broadly defined, even within an emotional refuge. In the public and private spaces of late-nineteenth-century Paris, those suffering with emotional trauma would have employed great effort *not* to give expression to their pain. Such is the emotional regime that delimits acceptable behavior. Under the institutional gaze of Charcot and his staff, this effortful emotional restraint was released. But at the same time, Charcot himself was the authority of his own confined emotional regime. His patients, while liberated from the shackles of a broader, public emotional regime, had to employ "emotional effort" to meet Charcot's own prescriptions. Patients who had never before succumbed to what Charcot called the *arc de cercle* readily fell into this bodily practice on being admitted to his care. It was not only what Charcot was looking for but also what the patient was looking for. Recognition and diagnosis lead, at least to some degree, to relief. Under the medical gaze, hysterical tetanus had become *classical* and therefore acceptable. Outside the hospital, in public spaces and places of work, such gestures, with accompanying grimaces and ugly contortions, while no longer a sign of demonic possession, would still be seen as signs of madness, as well as moral transgression.

The Medical Gaze outside the Emotional Refuge

Outside such refuges, hysterical tetanus was a dangerous diagnostic problem. A brief examination of a few nineteenth-century case studies will show how the appearance of tetanus in women outside the clinical refuge was medically noteworthy only insofar as the cases transpired *not* to be true tetanus. Diagnosing the "fraud" depended, typically, on physicians' heavily gendered and dismissive accounts of hysterical maladies, which seemingly often carried greater weight than the evidence of disease before them. This will go some way toward affirming Mark Micale's evidence that the medical establishment had radically re-gendered hysteria in the nineteenth century to make it almost entirely feminine.[22] To show this, I am pursuing another of Micale's observations, that "we know almost nothing of the ideas and practices of the general mass of doctors" in making hysteria female in the nineteenth century.[23]

In Alfred Poland and J. S. Jewell's notes on the diagnosis of tetanus in the 1881 *System of Surgery*, hysterical tetanus only occurred "in females," and there were no instances of "fatal termination." The signs of tetanus, however, were "often so faithful, that many instances of reputed examples of successful treatment of tetanus have been merely conquest over hysterical spasms." Since most acute cases of tetanus ended in death, until a more certain test for tetanus came along diagnoses might hinge simply on the gender of the patient and whether he or she survived.[24] This zero-sum diagnostics is evident in a case from 1886. *The Lancet* documented the recovery process of a young woman who had been shot in the face at close range, her jaw filled with hundreds of pieces of lead shot. The doctor, having cleaned the wound to his satisfaction, noted the daily convulsions, stiffenings, and contortions of the afflicted woman, who presented a classic case of tetanus with well-marked opisthotonos. He pointed out en passant the patient was "fanciful and obstinate." Was this, he wondered, really tetanus or *only* hysteria? Plumping for the latter, he repeatedly dosed the patient with chloroform and watched her fully recover. Irrespective of the fact the woman had been shot in the head and of her "moaning with pain," her tetanic ordeal was written off as unreal.[25] The physician noted that had it been true tetanus, she surely would have died.

In another case in Washington, D.C., in 1879, a woman with a medical history of "lingering labour" and "adherent placenta" from her first pregnancy (out of wedlock) went into a convulsive state seven and a half months into her next pregnancy. In a condition brought on by "screeching noises in ears," she presented a "marked opisthotonos, the body being bowed until only the hand and heels touched the bed. Jaws clenched, eyes closed, unconscious during paroxysms, which lasted about four minutes. . . . She had two or three attacks, each with violent opisthotonos." She went on to recover. Her hysterical disorder was distinguished from "tetanus proper" by the presence of the noise, the closed eyes (they should really have been open), and the woman's ability to sleep before convalescence began. But the key to the case was that the patient had not died after becoming unconscious (if so, tetanus would have been ascribed as the cause). Since she had had waking spells, it was hysteria.[26]

In 1890 W. P. Munn put forward the unorthodox argument that death did not necessarily equate to evidence of traumatic tetanus, nor did it "absolutely exclude hysterical tetanus." If the spasms were severe enough and prolonged enough, the "vital powers" might be exhausted, no matter whether the cause were "a neuritis, a specific poison, shock following traumatism, or the neurasthenic condition of hysteria." Should "mental anxiety" remove the "restraining influence which regulates the nervous impulses proceeding from the spinal and cerebral centers," the motor centers might, he argued, "go mad." To demonstrate this, he presented a case of hysterical tetanus in a woman with "an extremely retroflexed uterus, firmly adherent and projecting well into the rectum." During profuse menstruation, combined with a regular bout of dysentery, the patient became convulsive: "[A]ll the extensor muscles of the limbs and back went into a state of clonic spasm. She assumed the arched position characteristic of opisthotonos, maintained it for a moment, then was drawn sideways and fell on the floor. She cried out with pain at the onset of the spasm but in a few moments became unconscious." The unconsciousness, during which the spasms did not relent, lasted half an hour, despite the administration of half a grain of morphia. It was, said Munn, "not feigned, but real." The spasms returned after a further two hours and were relieved only by the "free administration of chloroform." The "opisthotonic convulsions and spasmodic tossings" went on for fourteen hours. She recovered slowly, Munn tells us, convalescing for three months, "as in true traumatic tetanus," and would "certainly have died if morphia and chloroform had not been administered so heroically." Given his case notes, why did he diagnose hysteria and not tetanus? His final analysis explains his diagnostic difficulties:

> Hysterical tetanus may occur in men as well as in women, but is of rarer occurrence. We are likely to err in diagnosis in such cases, for hysteria is not immediately thought of when we have a man to do with. On the other hand, hysteria is about the first thing one thinks of when called to attend a woman for any nervous or convulsive disorder.[27]

Thus, outside the clinical refuge, women with tetanus were predetermined to be hysterical. For men, the reverse was likely the case. Even as the possibilities of emotional trauma opened up in World War I, and even as tetanus had been isolated as a specific pathology, men with hysterical tetanus were still more likely to be taken at face value as actually suffering from the disease. An article in the *British Journal of Surgery* in 1918, for example, noted the difficulty that war surgeons had had with cases of apparently localized tetanus in patients who had already been vaccinated with antitetanic serum. In many cases it was concluded that this was a new presentation of tetanic disease. Such cases ought to have been "curable at a single sitting by psychotherapy," according to one physician, but they were often allowed to go on unchecked by credulous medical authorities.[28]

The classic lines of inquiry about hysteria, and in particular the ways in which it was gendered, center on such medical luminaries as Charcot and, later, Freud. The bodily effects of the emotionally traumatized were, through medical universalization, ultimately directed away from the field of mainstream medicine toward psychoanalysis. Acceptance of hysterical embodiments was closely tied to those institutions or "refuges" where hysterical embodiments were expected or could at least be tolerated. As the language of emotional trauma developed in the twentieth century, from hysteria to shell shock to PTSD, the acknowledgement of the medical establishment that emotional pain is real pain, penetrating beyond the embodied sign to its neuropsychological causes, was slow in coming. Throughout the nineteenth century, and even for much of the twentieth century, bodily representations of emotional pain could easily be medically overlooked or downplayed as so much chicanery or malingering, signs of weakness of character and suspect morality. Such signs were intrinsic to being female and, where they appeared in men, were effeminacy revealed.[29]

Emotional Pain and Authentic Embodiments

In 1993 Louise Bourgeois first presented *The Arch of Hysteria*. The piece is well known for its subversion of the typical gendering of the hysteric, placing a curved, taut human frame associated with Charcot's Salpêtrière female patients into a male form. Bourgeois smooths away any sign of genitalia, emasculating the form, and removes the head, indicating the absence of reason. The piece hangs from the ceiling, appearing to float in the air. But if this hanging form—a literal and figurative *suspension* of a normative historical discourse of female madness—serves to question how emotional disturbance or mental illness is read, it nevertheless does so through the physical presence of a pained body. Hysteria, however subsumed in the language of the unreal or the imaginary, has an embodied sign. The cause of "illness" may be in the head (wherever that may have gone), but that notwithstanding, the pain is real.

Bourgeois asks us to take seriously the pain experience of the hysteric's wracked body, against the combined historical voices of medical history, which tell us this bodily sign is a deception. Bourgeois references a long-standing confusion concerning the hysterical arch and the reading of pain signs. Since the arch of hysteria could be diagnostically indistinguishable from that of tetanus, the degree to which the condition was taken seriously by the medical profession hinged on gendered notions of who was more likely to suffer each complaint. By the time Bourgeois presented her *Arch*, this bodily form had lost its power as a recognized embodiment of emotional trauma and is "hardly ever seen today."[30] The work serves as medico-historical critique, for at the height of its fame in the nineteenth century the hysterical arch was a medical paradox: opisthotonos in the hysteric was as much tetanus as opisthotonos in tetanus suffers, because the sign of tetanus *was* tetanus. But patients with real tetanus tended to die, whereas patients with hysteria tended not to. The obvious conclusion, the conclusion that Bourgeois rejects, was that hysterical opisthotonos was *performance*.

Metaphors of performance are problematic if we are to take seriously the emotional trauma of nineteenth-century hysterics and those in emotional pain in general. They risk endorsing the situated medical gaze of physicians who rejected the reality of this kind of pain. The acquired bodily practices of hysterics were not *conscious* performances but biocultural attempts at emotional expression: they were efforts to emote pain. Contemporary insights from the neurosciences about the centrality of emotions to the experience of pain, and the constructedness of situated expressions of painful experience, are enough of a clue for us to take seriously that what these women *said*, in the context of what they *did*, were accurate portrayals of how they felt.[31]

The cases of hysterical tetanus and epilepsy on board the *Dalhousie* can be reread from the point of view of the women in question. Most were single. All were among the laboring classes, heading to Australia for opportunities denied to them, for a host of reasons, at home. Most were in the line of domestic service. We can assume a degree of socioeconomic precariousness in many of the cases. Hudson's case notes on Sarah Bickford, for example, suggest a childhood marked by hardship and cruelty, including having been taken to sea at age ten and having spent time in the workhouse asylum. Although she gave birth at fifteen, she was traveling alone. The child, either dead or given up, must have been a source of great sorrow to her. Listed as "housemaid," she would have had the promise of work in Adelaide, but not without great uncertainty.[32] Doubtless the voyage itself was reason for fear and anxiety. It is not necessary, however, to assign emotional labels to whatever Bickford was going through, but only to enter into the historical particularities of her plight: boarding an emigrant ship alone, leaving difficulties but heading for uncertainties, and carrying the weight of past trauma. Bickford had a breakdown—an emotional crisis—and gave expression to it in the available gestural scripts to which she then had access. The discourse of female sexual weakness combined with emotional instability was so prevalent that probably anybody had vernacular knowledge of it, but Bickford's background may well have given her direct access to the cultural script of hysteria. As Bickford was overcome by her situation, it is unsurprising that her pain manifested in the way it did. I see this as an emotive process. Bickford strove to find expression, within the cultural limits available to her, for the way she felt. Since this gained traction with the ship's surgeon, her behavior acted as a modifier for the way she felt. Diagnosis—nymphomania—was in this case more moral than medical but nevertheless provided Bickford with a map for emotional navigation. Her emotional trauma was ascribed to her bodily practice of masturbation, which, when ceased, allowed her a release from the initial trauma. The circle—feeling, expression according to feeling rule or cultural script, modified expression, modified feeling—is easy in this case to trace.

Importantly, Bickford's ordeal and the medical response to it were taking place in a public space. In late-nineteenth-century terms, the epidemic that occurred on the back of Bickford's hysteria was a case of sympathetic contagion. The medical view was that women of already unstable physiological constitution naturally succumbed to the *sight* of emotional trauma. Stepping back from the medical gaze, it is more productive to imagine the emigrant ship becoming an emotional refuge. Though morally transgressive, Bickford's behavior was diagnostically identifiable: the sign of her nymphomania was tetanus. Back in Plymouth, or London, such a diagnosis may have had dire institutional and employment consequences. But as the reports of the *Earl Dalhousie*'s arrival in Adelaide testify, what happened aboard ship stayed aboard ship. The only note of circumspection related to the quality and character of the emigrants' work skills. The local newspaper observed that "several of the immigrants, per Earl Dalhousie, have found employment, but it is full early to form an opinion how far good judgment has been used in their selection."[33]

Other women on board who were carrying their own emotional pain recognized, at some level, that the risk of giving vent to such behavior in that environment was not the same as it might have been at home in the community. Again, I do not want to ascribe conscious agency here. The outbreak of hysteria was not contrived and not consciously performed. But the afflicted were surely aware that the emotional atmosphere aboard ship was isolated from the normal social implications of hysterical transgression. Put another way, the self-contained world of the colonists on board was out of reach of both the emotional regime of the place they had left behind and the place to which they were headed.

Hudson, in his report to *The Lancet*, attributed the outbreak to "emotional" causes, which in turn had an impact on nervous reflexes. This was to describe nothing more, in the language of the time, than the sex of the afflicted. The condition of being female, with fragile emotions, undeveloped moral characters, and attendant uterine and sexual mysteries, was sufficient to predetermine hysteria. Being female constituted a telling medical history in and of itself. The real emotional trauma of these women was not really taken seriously. Wickham calmly declared her broken heart to Hudson, but this was mentioned as part of a narrative of delirium, *not* a contributing factor to her apparent illness. Yet armed with the knowledge that a "broken heart" can genuinely be experienced as pain, I see no reason why we shouldn't take Wickham at her word. For a single domestic servant resorting to free passage on an emigrant ship, her words have more than a ring of truth about them: "We don't so readily get over broken hearts." Her own recovery again involved a *moral* diagnosis. The nadir of her behavior was "disobedient" and "perverse." Being confronted with the social transgression, her improvement was linked directly to her own apology. Again, the emotive process is easy to trace: emotional trauma, expression according to cultural script, modified expression, modified feeling.

A new vista has opened up in exploration of the history of bodily gestures and bodily practices situated within contexts of emotional prescription. This is what despair, sexual frustration, grief, or unrequited love *looks* like at a specific time and place. The medical establishment *expected* to see recognizable symptoms of tetanus and epilepsy in hysterics with "emotional problems." In some contexts this could be readily dismissed; in others it focused the attention. This cultural script, made known through prominent cases and reports, was unwittingly transferred from doctor to patient, and from patient to patient, so that the patient strove to meet the acknowledged posture that would gain recognition from the doctor for her plight. Recognition might also have meant dismissal from the realms of medicine proper and displacement into the realms of moral transgression. Nevertheless, the availability of an expression—a bodily practice—for hysteria afforded women and later men who were suffering emotional pain a categorical refuge in which their plight could be seen, recognized, and, perhaps, treated. If this were combined with an emotional refuge—a place where bundles of traumatic feelings could be emoted without inhibition—the chances of a diagnostic salve for emotional pain were all the greater.

Notes

1. See http://www.theshipslist.com/ships/australia/earldalhousie1875.shtml; "Emigration," *The Times*, December 9, 1874.

2. "Shipping News," *South Australian Chronicle and Weekly Mail*, February 27, 1875.

3. All quotations from John Hudson in "Epidemic of Hysterical Epilepsy and Tetanus," *Lancet*, October 9, 1875, 525–26.

4. "Shipping News," *South Australian Chronicle and Weekly Mail*, February 27, 1875.

5. For an overview, see Rob Boddice, "Introduction: Hurt Feelings?," *Pain and Emotion in Modern History*, ed. Rob Boddice (Houndmills: Palgrave, 2014): 1–15; Rob Boddice, *Pain: A Very Short Introduction* (Oxford: Oxford University Press, 2016).

6. For a compelling account of this, see Nikola Grahek, *Feeling Pain and Being in Pain*, 2nd ed. (Cambridge, Mass.: MIT Press, 2007).

7. Ronald Melzack, "Pain: Past, Present and Future," *Canadian Journal of Experimental Psychology* 4 (1992): 623.

8. Patrick Wall, *Pain: The Science of Suffering* (New York: Columbia University Press, 2002), 3–12.

9. Daniel Goldberg, "Pain without Lesion: Debate among American Neurologists, 1850–1900," *19: Interdisciplinary Studies in the Long Nineteenth Century* 15 (2012): none.

10. Ronald Melzack, "Evolution of the Neuromatrix Theory of Pain," *Pain Practice* 5 (2005): 85–94.

11. See the paradigm-shifting work of Lisa Feldman Barrett, *How Emotions Are Made: The Secret Life of the Brain* (New York: Houghton Mifflin Harcourt, 2017), which adds weight to a number of studies from within the world of pain science. See Robert J. Gatchel, Yuan Bo Peng, Madelon L. Peters, Perry N. Fuchs, and Dennis C. Turk, "The Biopsychosocial Approach to Chronic Pain: Scientific Advances and Future Directions," *Psychological Bulletin* 133 (2007): 581–624; Geoff MacDonald and Lauri A. Jensen-Campbell, eds., *Social Pain: Neuropsychological and Health Implications of Loss and Exclusion* (Washington, D.C.: American Psychological Association, 2011). The turn to the neurosciences in history offers great potential for the exploration of these claims. See Daniel Lord Smail, *On Deep History and the Brain* (Berkeley: University of California Press, 2008), 112–56; Jeremy Trevelyan Burman, "History from Within? Contextualizing the New Neurohistory and Seeking Its Methods," *History of Psychology* 15 (2012): 84–99; Lynn Hunt, "The Experience of Revolution," *French Historical Studies*, 32 (2009): 671–78.

12. From a cultural historical point of view, the contextual experience of pain has already been extensively explored: Esther Cohen, *The Modulated Scream: Pain in Late Medieval Culture* (Chicago: University of Chicago Press, 2010); Joanna Bourke, *The Story of Pain: From Prayer to Painkillers* (Oxford: Oxford University Press, 2014); Javier Moscoso, *Pain: A Cultural History* (Basingstoke: Palgrave, 2012).

13. The pre-Freudian physiological focus in studies of hysteria and related disorders has been documented by, among others, Lilian R. Furst, *Before Freud: Hysteria and Hypnosis in Later Nineteenth-Century Psychiatric Cases* (Lewisburg, Penn.: Bucknell University Press, 2008). A notable case in point is the essay (45–53) by George Miller Beard, "Neurasthenia, or Nervous Exhaustion," which appeared in the *Boston Medical and Surgical Journal* in 1869. Neurasthenia is defined as an entirely somatic disorder, subject to physiological inquiry, but it was caused by the close relationship of body and mind, being brought about by "bereavement, business and family cares, parturition and abortion, sexual excesses, the abuse of stimulants and narcotics, and civilized starvation" (47). Even an entirely physiological understanding of the manifestation of the disorder nevertheless had to take account of the possibility of emotional trauma when considering its aetiology. The *Boston Medical and Surgical Journal*, for example, noted in 1831 that "hysteria clothes herself in the garb of so many diseases," and

John Forbes's *Cyclopaedia of Practical Medicine* (1833) tried carefully to distinguish between tetanus and hysteria under the same heading of "convulsions." T. N. Smith, "Observations on Hysteria," *Boston Medical and Surgical Journal* 3 (1831): 541; Adair Crawford, "Convulsions," *The Cyclopaedia of Practical Medicine: Comprising Treatises on the Nature and Treatment of Disease, Materia Medica and Therapeutics, Medical Jurisprudence*, vol. 1, ed. John Forbes (London: Sherwood, Gilbert, and Piper, and Baldwin and Craddock, 1833–35), 466.

14. William Reddy, *The Navigation of Feeling: A Framework for the History of Emotions* (Cambridge: Cambridge University Press, 2001), 128.

15. Methodologically, I see no difference between a bodily posture as an utterance and a written or spoken statement. Insofar as the historian does analytical work, there is always a process of translation from primary source to historical text, such that the reading of and speaking for the body is not an act of ventriloquism any more than is the interpretation of a text so as to establish its true meaning in context. I am not speaking for these women, for their bodies spoke for themselves. By rebuilding the context—the script—we can find out what they said.

16. Charles Bell, *Essays on the Anatomy and Philosophy of Expression* (London: Murray, 1824). Other accounts of tetanic presentations of possession can be found in Jeannette Stirling, *Representing Epilepsy: Myth and Matter* (Liverpool: Liverpool University Press, 2010), chapter 2. See also the account of Mary Glover's demonic possession, manifested as circular contraction, in 1602, in Andrew Scull, *Hysteria: The Biography* (Oxford: Oxford University Press, 2009), 4.

17. Jean-Martin Charcot and Paul Richer, *Les Démoniaques dans l'art* (Paris, 1887), xi. Incidentally, they rejected Bell's criticism of Domenichino on the grounds that hysterics do indeed look like this (50–51).

18. Sander L. Gilman, "The Image of the Hysteric," in *Hysteria beyond Freud*, ed. Sander L. Gilman, Helen King, Roy Porter, G. S. Rousseau, and Elaine Showalter (Berkeley: University of California Press, 1993): 345–452, esp. 345–46, 353.

19. Mikkel Borch-Jacobsen, *Making Minds and Madness: From Hysteria to Depression* (Cambridge: Cambridge University Press, 2009), 26+.

20. Reddy, *Navigation of Feeling*, 129.

21. Qtd. in Jan Plamper, "The History of Emotions: An Interview with William Reddy, Barbara Rosenwein, and Peter Stearns," *History and Theory* 49 (2010): 243.

22. Mark Micale, *Hysterical Men: The Hidden History of Male Nervous Illness* (Cambridge, Mass.: Harvard University Press, 2008); see also Elaine Showalter's classic, *The Female Malady: Women, Madness and English Culture, 1830–1980* (London: Virago, 1985).

23. Mark Micale, *Approaching Hysteria: Disease and Its Interpretations* (Princeton, N.J.: Princeton University Press, 1995), 119.

24. Timothy Holmes, ed., *A System of Surgery, Theoretical and Practical*, 3 vols. (Philadelphia: Lea's, 1881), 1:571.

25. James Laffan, "Hysteria or Tetanus?" *Lancet*, 128 (3287), August 28, 1886, 397–98.

26. D. Webster Prentiss, "Case of Hysterical Tetanus," *American Journal of the*

Medical Sciences 78, no. 156 (1879): 451–52. See also the debate on tetanus recorded in the *Confederate States Medical and Surgical Journal* 1 (1864): 44–46, esp. 45.

27. W. P. Munn, "Tetanoid Manifestations in Hysterical Patients," *Pittsburgh Medical Review* 4 (1890): 247–9.

28. Arthur F. Hurst, "War Contractures—Localized Tetanus, Reflex Disorder, or Hysteria," *British Journal of Surgery* 6, no. 24 (1918): 579–605, esp. 581.

29. See, for example, Joanna Bourke, "Phantom Suffering: Amputees, Stump Pain and Phantom Sensations in Modern Britain," *Pain and Emotion in Modern History*, ed. Rob Boddice (Houndmills: Palgrave, 2014), 66–89.

30. See Gilbert H. Glaser, "Epilepsy, Hysteria and 'Possession': A Historical Essay," *Journal of Nervous and Mental Disease* 166, no.: 4 (1978): 268–74. Glaser states that "the style of hysterical phenomena has changed over the years, a circumstance of great interest and not adequately explained. Muscular manifestations have given way to visceral phenomena. The sexually suggestive *Arc de Cercle* [opisthotonos], a suspension bridge posture . . . is hardly ever seen today, while it was common previously" (271). By 1986 Edward Shorter could assert that "the underlying incidence of the disorder may well be constant across the ages but its form changeable, in accordance with . . . cultural influences." See Edward Shorter, "Paralysis: The Rise and Fall of a 'Hysterical' Symptom," *Journal of Social History* 19 (1986): 549–82, esp. 549. See also Nicholas P. Spanos and Jack Gottlieb, "Demonic Possession, Mesmerism, and Hysteria: A Social Psychological Perspective on Their Historical Interrelations," *Journal of Abnormal Psychology* 88, no. 5 (1979): 527–46, esp. 540–41. In R. Douglas Collins's recent *Algorithmic Diagnosis of Symptoms and Signs: A Cost-Effective Approach*, 3rd ed. (Philadelphia: Lippincott Williams and Wilkins, 2013), it is still apparently possible to fail to distinguish between hysteria and tetanus from opisthotonos (348).

31. See notes 5–11. In addition, certain insights about emotional labour and emotional practice are further clues to the relationship of effortful gesture to felt experience. See Monique Scheer, "Are Emotions a Kind of Practice (and Is That What Makes Them Have a History?): A Bourdieuian Approach to Understanding Emotion," *History and Theory* 51, no. 2 (2012): 193–220; A. R. Hochschild, "Emotion Work, Feeling Rules, and Social Structure," *American Journal of Sociology* 85 (1979): 551–75.

32. *South Australian Chronicle and Weekly Mail*, February 13, 1875.

33. *South Australian Chronicle and Weekly Mail*, February 27, 1875.

2. The Criminal of Passion

Its Construction in Italian Legal and Medical Discourses, 1860s–1920s

GIAN MARCO VIDOR

IN THE SECOND HALF of the nineteenth century, in several European countries, legal and medical scholars switched the focus of the criminological debate from the crime to the criminal, from what had been a purely philosophical and juridical entity to a social and physiological being.[1] These new forms of knowledge regarding offenders emerged in the long path carved out by (popular) physiognomy and phrenology, enhancing but also deeply rethinking the interrelation of the body—especially the face and the skull—and un/moral and il/legal behavior. They reinforced and reshaped the view of the body as an "avowal of one's interiority."[2] Yet aside from some general similarities to older forms of knowledge, the new forms of deciphering the (criminal) body, their purposes and methods, as well as the role of those who applied them and those subjected to them were quite different.[3]

In Italy, the publication in 1876 of Cesare Lombroso's first edition of his "Criminal Man" marked this shift, giving rise to a new disciplinary field that focused—as the title suggests—on (criminal) human beings and not the (criminal) law. "Criminal anthropology," with its theories and methods, rapidly attracted a large following of students and supporters. Among these were the jurists Enrico Ferri (1856–1929) and Raffaele Garofalo (1851–1934), who, together with the physician Cesare Lombroso, became the three pillars of what became known as the "Positivist School" or simply the "Italian School." The highly polemical confrontation with other streams of medical and psychological thought and especially with the so-called "classic school" of legal thought often generated an oversimplification, sometimes also reproduced in historiography. There was a complex intellectual dynamism within the field and the substantial theoretical and methodological differences among the three generations of followers of what I shall refer to as positivist criminology.[4]

Cesare Lombroso (1835–1909) and his colleagues suggested that crime had a multiple causality, extensively analyzing the role of social, economic, cultural, and demographic factors. Yet biological determinism was for many a fundamental key in the etiology of crime. Consequently, criminals were perceived as literally embodying fundamental data for empirical research.[5] The body of male and female criminals, both adults and children, could be measured by new methods and instruments. Their moral qualities and mental capacities could be assessed together with the social dangerousness of these individuals. Their presence and geographic distribution in Italian society could be quantified through statistical analysis, providing data considered to be reliable and useful in new—and science-backed—state politics concerning the repression of criminals, the prevention of crime, and the protection of society.[6]

Influenced by the theories and methodologies of earlier "criminologists," like Prosper Lucas (1808–1885), Henry Mayhew (1812–1887), and, especially, the psychiatrist Bénédict Augustine Morel (1809–1873), Lombroso (re-)formulated and (re-)elaborated—with several contradictions and a certain amount of confusion—the notions of atavism, degeneration, and moral insanity, working on what was regarded as the connection in the etiology of both mental pathogenesis and criminogenesis.[7] Strictly linked to the elaboration of these notions and empirically supported by a thorough collection and prolific production of data, positivist criminologists channeled a great deal of their intellectual efforts in classifying the different "types" of criminal. Expanding on Lombroso's classification, which was characterized by frequent adjustments, a certain approximation, and many incongruities, Enrico Ferri formulated a more stable, but not much more successful, categorization, based on Lombroso's research, but rejecting most of his anatomical components and other aspects of biological determinism.[8]

In this context, the physiology, anatomy, and psychology of those who self-reported or were thought to have committed a crime under the influence of emotional phenomena also became the object of a new and more systematic scientific approach. The body of these supposed criminals was scrutinized by positivist criminologists with the hope of detecting measurable and stable characteristics that could enable them to inscribe them in a fixed criminological category: the criminal of passion. Contested by many, these specific categorization attempts dovetailed in a century-old debate about emotional phenomena, their classification, and their impact on human (criminal) behavior. Before the second half of the nineteenth century the behavior and the body of those who were tried for committing an, often, violent crime in the heat of passion were scrutinized in search of evidence of guilt or innocence. In fact, as Enrico Ferri stated, the problem of "the juridical and moral relationship between passion and crime" was as "old as humankind."[9] But since "this problem" had not been solved by the "classic school" of legal thought due to a methodological deficiency, the positivists—as Ferri put it—had the feeling that they could finally offer a science-backed solution on a theoretical and practical level.[10]

Compared with other positivist criminological categories such as the "born criminal" or notions like atavism, which dominated the debate in Italy and in Europe, attracting both enthusiasm and harsh criticism, the "criminal of passion" was somehow a minor category within the intellectual debate. In a way, it lacked the constructed intellectual boldness and the sensationalistic flavor associated with other positivist criminological categories. It was an old legal and cultural category viewed from a new, "more scientific" perspective. Nevertheless, for a certain period it was the topic of a specific *querelle*, led by two of the most renowned jurists, Enrico Ferri on the Positivist School side and Giovanni Battista Impallomeni (1846–1907) on the side of the "classic school" of legal thought.[11] According to Impallomeni, there was no specific criminological category of "the criminal of passion."[12] Furthermore, the scholars' contributions to the (re-)definition of this cultural category was amplified and reshaped by the constant interest of the press in crimes and criminals of passion.[13]

The Role of the Body in Defining the Criminal of Passion

The (non-)existence of a "criminal of passion" with detectable psychological, moral, and physical features came to enrich the debate on the three main areas of enquiry that often overlapped. The first area is represented by a specific legal inquiry concerning which emotions should be taken into consideration by criminal law and by judicial authorities, how, and with what legal consequences. Second, the debate about the "criminal of passion" influenced and was influenced by the sciences of the mind and the ongoing (re-)categorization of different mental illnesses: Who was mentally ill and who was not—consequently, who was responsible, or not, for his or her actions? Third, the debate about the "criminal of passion" enriched and was enriched by research in the fields of philosophy and physiology on emotional phenomena in humans and other animals. This research aimed to answer questions regarding the nature of emotional phenomena, how they functioned, how they should be classified, their impact on the body and the mind, and how they related to questions of morality and cognition.

In the classification established by positivist criminology the "criminal of passion" occupied an almost liminal position, near the threshold to normal individuals. This category was much more nuanced and complex than it may seem to twenty-first-century readers. It was not limited to those who committed violent acts, often homicides, against those with whom the criminal had a preexisting emotional connection, usually a lover or family member (particularly involving female victims and issues of love, sexual intercourse, and male honor). The category also included those who committed crimes under the influence of political and religious passions.[14] A "criminal of passion" might be someone who had killed his wife or attempted to assassinate a king.

Positivist criminologists scrutinized the bodies of crime of passion perpetrators, applying the same methodology used for other criminological categories. This expertise "functioned as a kind of magic lantern, through which could be seen to pass and pass again the image of the criminal or the madman, an image that was shattered into fragments only to be reassembled, first the physical, then the psychic aspect, in every detail."[15] A cranial anthropometry was performed and their general and tactile sensitivity was measured, together with their reaction to physical pain. Their visual capacity was evaluated and other physiological functions and physical features were described and assessed. Personal and family medical histories were also taken, listing all hereditary, congenital, or acquired diseases. Together with these data, some of which was meticulously recorded in numbers and percentages, the positivistic anthropological observation was often supplemented by descriptions of facial expressions. For Mario Carrara, professor of forensic medicine, Francesco Salvatore C., age twenty-six, who had killed his victim with nine stab wounds, had "a numb face, always with a fixed expression like a mask."[16]

Despite the frequently reported difficulty of collecting data on such offenders due to their rareness, Lombroso and his followers looked for those characteristics among the data collected that seemed to better enable them to categorize the "criminals of passion."[17] Interestingly, their anatomical features were assessed as normal or quasi-normal. In both Ferri's and Lombroso's opinion, the bodies of "criminals of passion had no particular characteristics that would distinguish them from an 'honest man,'" and sometimes such criminals even had "a delightful and pleasing physiognomy."[18] According to Ferri, the "regularity of their lineaments" could have a positive influence on the verdict contributing greatly to an acquittal or a lenient sentence. Therefore, "criminals of passion" were very rare among prisoners.[19]

As explained by the alienist Giuseppe Bonanno, there was very little to say about the "anthropological characteristics" of "criminals of passion." As he explained in his 1896 *Criminal for Passion* (the first monograph produced by the Positivist School on these criminals), these offenders were not born criminals; therefore, their anatomy lacked any "specific degenerate features."[20] Moreover, their physiology was only partially of any particular significance. From a "functional point of view" the "criminals of passion" did not show any anomaly: in general their senses were normally developed and the diseases that may have afflicted them in the past or present lacked any "hereditary character." The only specificity of their physiology—at least in most of them—was what was seen as an overall exaggerated sensitivity, especially to physical pain.[21]

In the second half of the nineteenth century, physical (human) pain was the focus of a great deal of research activity. In Italy the work of the physiologist Angelo Mosso (1846–1910) and the physician and anthropologist Paolo Mantegazza (1831–1910) on the experience and expression of pain represented an important chapter in the rich positivist science of emotions, and these two scholars were among the most prominent figures in this field.[22] In physiological research on humans and animals, several different methods and technical devices were developed for performing an "electro-diagnosis." These came to be used as contemporary diagnostic tools in psychiatry as can be seen, for example, in the *Guide for the Diagnosis of Madness*, first published in 1885 by one of the most eminent Italian alienists, Professor Enrico Morselli (1852–1929).[23] In Morselli's opinion, in measuring the "skin sensibility" faradization was easier and more accurate than other methods, allowing extreme levels of sensitivity to be determined, even if only roughly and empirically.[24] Presumably, Bonanno was aware of this famous manual. In fact, the measurements Bonanno quoted or took directly on nine of the nineteen cases studied were obtained by faradization, mainly on both hands, using a machine designed by the German physiologist Emil du Bois-Reymond (1818–1896).[25]

But why was this specific characteristic significant in identifying a criminal of passion? From a criminological as well as from a psychiatric perspective—which in the historical period in question often overlapped—measuring general sensitivity and sensitivity to pain was regarded by many scholars as a significant indicator of emotional sensibility. In Lombroso's words, "criminals of passion" had both an emotional "exaggerated excitability" and an "excessive affectivity," which were seen to differ greatly from the apathy and the coldness of other types of criminals, especially the "born criminals."[26] Bonanno emphasized the importance of a greater physiological sensitivity, since it provoked what he metaphorically defined as "an acceleration of the emotional element." And "modifying the mind deeply," this acceleration contributed, in his opinion, to "the mental derangement" that could lead to committing a crime.[27] Moreover, in Ferri's opinion, "criminals of passion" showed both a "sensitivity higher and more intense than the normal one" and a "great emotionality." According to Ferri, the work of Angelo Mosso and Carl Georg Lange on human physiology of emotions revealed that both bodily sensitivity and emotional sensibility "seemed to move from the cardiac centers."[28]

Furthermore, without dismissing the social-cultural elements, the Positivist School took into consideration psycho-physiological elements intrinsically linked to age and gender. Those who could be classified as "criminals of passion" were mostly between twenty and thirty years old, an age group in which bodily vigor was at its peak and the psychological capacity to resist "the tyranny of passion" was considered to be at its weakest.[29] Also in this context Lombroso claimed to have observed a peculiar result of sexual desire in puberty, which he attributed essentially to boys. In this period of life, he stated, the desire for a woman and, specifically, the denial of sexual intercourse or the interruption of a sexual relationship could produce a sudden removal of any "moral sense," leading to a violent crime.[30]

Performativity of Emotions in Defining a Criminal of Passion

Placed in a liminal position, near the threshold of normality, the body of a "criminal of passion" was of little use for the positivistic criminological categorization that was based on pathological markers and organicist formulas. While criminological categories such as the "born criminal" were heavily anchored in the body, Lombroso and his followers gained nothing by looking at the anatomy and little by looking at the physiology of those who were supposed to have committed a crime in the heat of an emotion or passion. Instead, their scientific gaze focused on what could be defined as the performative dimensions of emotional phenomena. They examined not only the nature of passions and emotions but also how they made people behave and act. Criminologists of the Positivist School aimed to distinguish with an almost "scientific" certainty a real "criminal of passion" from someone who pretended to be one. In order to achieve this, they documented what could be defined as a sort of "emotional anamnesis," taking into consideration the role of emotions in the lives of the defendants before, during, and after a criminal deed. The work of Enrico Ferri—who was a university professor, an active lawyer, and a member of the parliament—offers a good insight into the characteristics attributed to "criminals of passion" by the Positivist School.

Building on his personal experience and on a critical analysis of the studies produced by the Positivist School, Enrico Ferri grouped criminals in five main categories:[31] the criminal madmen, the born criminals, the criminals by contracted habits, the occasional criminals, and the criminals of passion.[32] According to Ferri, "criminals of passion" were a specific subcategory of "occasional criminals."[33] Ferri felt that in order to distinguish "criminals of passion" from other criminals, it was not sufficient to establish that they had acted—or were said to have acted—primarily under the influence of passions. Moreover, the intensity of an emotion alone was not a reliable identifying parameter.[34] Ferri, in fact, dismissed the classification established by Francesco Carrara (the jurist of the "classic school" of legal thought, 1805–1888) between "blind passions" (*passioni cieche*), which influence, with their high intensity, people's will and actions, and "reasonable passions" (*passioni ragionatrici*), which leave all mental capacities untouched.[35] Instead, Ferri divided passions into two groups (from a criminological point of view): the "anti-social passions" and the "social passions." The "anti-social passions," such as greed, revenge, and hatred, tended to disrupt the normal conditions of social life. The "social passions," by contrast, were perceived as having the function of fostering and strengthening a fraternal social life (Lombroso characterized them as "generous and sublime" passions.)[36] These passions were love, honor, political passion, and religious passion. Ferri regarded the crimes committed under the influence of these passions as an expression of what he termed as "social egoism," since perpetrators were somehow not entirely detached from the norms of social life.[37] In his opinion, these passions usually had a useful function in society, and only under particular circumstances linked to the social environment or to an "individual anthropological state" did they become dangerous, leading to a crime. For him, this was true, for example when it came to sexual desire, maternal love, or a political passion.[38]

According to the Positivist School, individuals who committed a crime—like homicide—spurred by a social passion, still had to be punished, but less severely than those who committed the same act under the influence of an anti-social passion.

In order to establish whether a person really had committed a crime under the influence of these social passions, both the (criminal) actions caused by emotional phenomena and the emotional phenomena generated by (criminal) actions had to be systematically scrutinized by an expert, according to the methods of the Positivist School. With the exception of some minor disagreements, both Ferri and Lombroso agreed on the notion that "criminals of passion" shared several clearly distinguishing characteristics that were all directly or indirectly linked to the performative dimensions of emotional phenomena.[39] In their opinion, these characteristics could easily help to distinguish faux "criminals of passion" from real ones, therefore enabling a fair and correct application of the criminal law.

The passions that spurred these persons often drove them to commit a crime openly, in public, during the day, in front of witnesses, and without any accomplices. With other people usually as targets, such crimes were often committed with ill-chosen methods, using the first tool at hand.

As mentioned earlier, scholars of the Positivist School observed that "criminals of passion" were thought to possess an excessive physical sensibility and were emotionally agitated before, during, and after the crime: they did not show what Lombroso called the "marble apathy" typical of common criminals. But, unlike Lombroso, Ferri states that in some cases a crime of passion could be premeditated: passion in these cases was seen as a "slow fire." Ferri makes a distinction between an "emotional criminal" (*delinquente emotivo*), driven by a sudden, unforeseen, and temporary "psychological hurricane," and a "criminal of passion" (*delinquente per passione*), permanently possessed by a passion that manifested itself through different levels of resistance in performing a criminal action.

Other characteristics were more directly linked to emotions and their performative dimensions. First of all, their emotional landscape after the criminal deed was dominated by remorse. According to the Positivist School, these offenders immediately acknowledged their crime with such a deep remorse that they often felt the impulse to commit suicide.[40] Furthermore, when convicted they were always repentant prisoners.

Even when acquitted, their emotional reactions were peculiar. Ferri highlighted that although "criminals of passion" showed a certain relief when acquitted or given a lenient sentence, they did not feel and express that cynical and cheerful joy usually displayed by "born criminals." The joy of a "criminal of passion" was described as more moderate and melancholic. The two scholars pointed out that the moral compass of a real "criminal of passion" was intact and only paralyzed by a slow or sudden emotional fire. For both Lombroso and Ferri, the real "criminals of passion" amended their lives. In contrast to "born criminals" or "mad criminals," they were not perceived as a threat to the public, and they could successfully be reintegrated into society.

Genuine "criminals of passion" were considered to be very rare. Basing his analysis on criminal statistics from Italy and several other European countries, presented in an atlas, Ferri stated that the crimes committed under the impulse of a passion represented around 5 percent of all violent crimes.

For both Lombroso and Ferri, most of the supposed "criminals of passion" were impostors who used passion as a simple and easy excuse to hide their real motives. Ferri specified, for example, how sexual love in "born criminals" (especially in urban murderers and thieves) was antisocial, since it was simply a wild lust. In "born criminals" sexual love was fed by pride and led to brutal jealousy.

The two scholars were confident that their scientific approach would help to unmask all those impostors. Furthermore, it must be clarified that both scholars did not include among the "crimes of passion" those homicides—clearly indicated in the 1889 Italian criminal code (article 377)—in which a family member had caught another member of the family in the act of adultery or illicit sexual intercourse (*concubito*). In such cases the penalties (time of imprisonment) normally given for manslaughter, homicide, or physical injuries were reduced to less than one-sixth, and in cases normally punished with life imprisonment, the penalty was reduced to imprisonment of one to five years.[41] In Ferri's opinion the clause concerning mitigating circumstances established by article 377 was synonymous with "a barbaric right to kill." These crimes, he claimed, were not the result of a strong passion like love. These offenders—mainly men—simply had what he defined as "possessive egoism." In contemporary society, Ferri argued, this right to kill was barbaric, a relic of the past, in which a husband ruled over his wife as he did over the animals that belonged to him. It was simply a matter of possession. For Ferri, these cases were in no sense "crimes of passion." Ferri underlined that in contemporary society no one should have the right to kill. He pointed to how Italy had taken away the right of the state to kill (the death penalty was formally abolished in 1889) but tolerated the murder of adulterers.[42] According to both Ferri and Lombroso, the solution was divorce.[43] Ferri was confident that the contemporary industrial society would abolish the mitigating circumstances clause, although this was only achieved a hundred years later, in 1981, a few years after the legalization of divorce.

Fictional Characters and the Scientific Construction of the Criminal of Passion

The criminological debate in Italy was supported and framed by vast academic and professional editorial activity, particularly in journals.[44] Fundamental elements of this constantly reshaped body of knowledge were legal and medical cases. As shown, for example, by Bonanno's work on "criminals of passion," some cases were directly observed and described firsthand by a scholar, and some were reported on indirectly from other sources, especially from periodicals collecting clinical cases or commenting on the most recent legal sentences.

But this vast literature was also disseminated by frequent references to criminals and criminal deeds from national and international visual arts, poetry, popular tradition, and especially theater and literature. The psycho-criminological analysis of fictional characters—often complemented by quotations from literary texts—could fill paragraphs, chapters, or be the subject of entire treatises.[45] This was also relevant for the so-called "criminals of passion."

As pointed out by Enrico Ferri, who dedicated a whole book to the representation of offenders in the arts, "criminals of passion" had always attracted the attention of artists, particularly writers and playwrights, whose best works often included portraits of "the murderer out of furious jealousy" or the "avenger of the family honor."[46] Ferri, who defined himself as a "criminal psychologist,"[47] attributed to these fictional characters the same characteristics that positivist criminology found in genuine "criminals of passion": youth, a good-natured character, strong sentimentality, being under the influence of burning passions, and an intact "moral sense." Ferri saw the success of these characters in the fact that the public could easily identify itself with them because, although having committed a criminal act, these characters did not differ much from the average honest man.[48]

Othello, an archetype of the "criminal of passion," was obviously a common reference in crime and court news, as demonstrated, for example, by an overview of the Italian newspaper *La Stampa*.[49] Furthermore, if we believe Nicola Ratti, a judge at the court of Palermo in the early twentieth century, there was no defense lawyer in trials about jealousy and love who did not refer to "the Moorish prince" as the most prominent "criminal of passion."[50]

But in addition to these general and vague references in texts dealing with emotions and crime, Othello, together with other fictional characters, was subjected to an often sophisticated psycho-criminological study, which, as in real legal and medical cases, analyzed the performative dimensions of the relationship between emotional phenomena and crime. Every author had his own views regarding the primary emotional drive that led Othello to kill Desdemona and then himself, the role of Othello's racial origins and character, and the role of Iago. Such discourses were often lengthy and contributed to shaping each author's legal and psychological theory about those who committed a crime in the heat of passion and the legal consequences of their actions.

Ludovico Fulci (1850–1934), a legal scholar and member of the Italian parliament, provides a good example in his analysis. In his view, Shakespeare, in Othello, "glimpsed a truth" of what can be called the phenomenology of emotions leading to a criminal act. Fulci thought that the transformation of a passion into "an irresistible force" was directly influenced by individual character and (biological) heredity.[51] In the jurist's opinion, Othello, of Arabic origin, had "a superior intelligence" and, at the same time, felt greatly the impetus of passions, since "he carries in his veins a savage nature that the crossbreed of races could only abate but did not destroy completely." Analyzing Othello's drama as a legal case, Fulci showed how his actions were shaped by the co-presence of different passions. The jealousy that the infamous Iago nourished led him to kill Desdemona. Yet before striking her body, although "intoxicated by vengeance," he stopped; his eyes looked at her breast: "before taking her life, he wanted to smell her one more time." In interpreting Fulci's analysis, we surmise that these hesitations of the body and these sensorial rapid experiences indicated the persistent presence of a deep feeling of love, which had not been neutralized by the wish for vengeance and the sense of having been dishonored and betrayed. Othello did not "deserve disdain but compassion" since he was a man "who loved too much"; a man, whose violent sensibility easily led him to become the victim of Iago's deception. Therefore, Fulci agreed with Shakespeare in acquitting "the Moorish prince."[52]

But what was the role of these literary references? As it has been shown, they were often used in order to illustrate certain principles, to dismiss certain theories or to reinforce a particular legal or medical discourse. This held true also for the perpetrators of crimes of passion. As the scholar Graham Frankland pointed out in relation to Freud's abundant use of literature, references to literary characters in studies on human behavior "helped to establish a deeper literary communion" between an author and his reader,[53] no doubt enhancing the effectiveness of analysis of the relationship between emotions and criminal actions in legal and medical literature.

Abundantly present in Lombroso's work, for instance, literary references had a specific epistemological place in the intellectual and political enterprise of Italian positivist criminology (as it was the case, especially as far as Lombroso was concerned, references to common knowledge, popular stereotypes, and proverbs).[54] As clearly explained by Enrico Ferri, arts were important from a criminological perspective since they had anticipated, sometimes with the "clairvoyance of the genius," the most recent and crucial achievements in modern Italian criminology. He stressed that, with an "accurate intuition of the truth," artists had often portrayed those physiological and psychological characteristics of the criminal man that the Positivist School only recently had succeeded in systematizing.[55]

The role of the arts in anticipating the scientific gaze was also relevant for other modern sciences, like ethnography or psychiatry. In Ferri's opinion, the

French neurologist Jean-Martin Charcot, for instance, could find similarities between the facial expressions of patients affected by serious hysteria and artistic depictions of possessed people.[56] Ferri evaluated Shakespeare's plays as the artistic works that offer the "most ingenious and still unsurpassed" psychological description of three main types of criminal as theorized by the Positivist School: the 'born criminal' (Macbeth); the 'criminal madman' (Hamlet) and the 'criminal of passion' (Othello). Although the last was the type most recognizable in common experience and by "common psychology," in Ferri's view, Othello could be understood with an "anthropological precision" only by adding to this "common gaze" the knowledge produced by a "veritable criminal psychology," i.e. by positivist criminology.

As Jonathan Hiller masterfully points out with reference to Lombroso, positivist criminologists not only used art as an epistemological and legitimizing factor, but their theories and concepts would also have an influence on late nineteenth century Italian literature, theatre, and opera, an influence that would persist well into the twentieth century.[57] Verdi and Arrigo Boito's 1887 *Othello* as well as Leoncavallo's *Pagliacci* staged crime of passion characters whose emotional performances were imbued with elements borrowed from Italian criminal positivism.[58]

Conclusion

The attempts of the Positivist School and its critics to understand and define crime of passion perpetrators fostered and furthered the analysis of the physiology and psychology of human emotional phenomena far beyond questions of legal responsibility and mitigating circumstances in criminal trials.

Although these attempts, like many other theories and methodologies formulated by the Positivist School, barely had an impact on legal norms established in the criminal codes of 1889 and 1930, they shaped, and at the same time were shaped by, cultural and social representations and perceptions of the criminal of passion, in reality as much as in fiction. The influence of fiction on the construction of the new criminological category was not a generic one. Perceived as significant (arche)-types of the criminal of passion, fictional characters were included in the corpus of numerous scholars' cases studies, in addition to numerous legal and medical examples observed in the real world.

Finally, the focus on this specific criminological category confirmed what the historian Patrizia Guarnieri has already highlighted: there has been "a certain tendency to disparage and exaggerate (even to sensationalize) the quantifying and somaticist elements in the Italian culture of Lombroso's time, and to underestimate another important element, the one related to a chiefly psychological approach."[59] Certainly, the body played a role in shaping the criminal of passion according to the Positivist School, but it was limited to a specific physiological phenomenon, bridging, in a way, the soma and the psyche. Newly emerged electrophysiological techniques allowed Positivist criminologists to establish what was regarded as a meaningful link between high physiological sensitivity and excessive emotional sensibility. It was this emotional sensibility and the performative dimensions of emotions that came under close scrutiny in order to distinguish a genuine 'criminal of passion' from someone who pretended to be one. In fact, by examining the criminal of passion, a category at the margins of its main area of criminological debate, the Positivist School developed a sort of phenomenology of passions and emotions that switched its focus from the body to the psyche, highlighting the complex link between the soma, the psyche, and emotions.

Notes

1. Renzo Villa, *Il deviante e i suoi segni: Lombroso e la nascita dell'antropolgia criminale* (Milan: Franco Angeli, 1985), 78–86.

2. Jean-Michel Labadie, *Les mots du crime: Approche épistémologique de quelques discours sur le criminel* (Brussels: De Boeck-Wesmael, 1995), 160.

3. Mary Gibson, *Born to Crime: Cesare Lombroso and the Origins of Biological Criminology* (Westport Conn.: Praeger, 2002), 9–52. Jean-Jacques Courtine and Claudine Haroche, *Histoire du visage: Exprimer et taire ses émotions (XVIe—début XIXe siècle)* (Paris: Payot, 2007), 227; Dina Siegel, "The Methods of Lombroso and Cultural Criminology," in *The Cesare Lombroso Handbook*, ed. Paul Knepper and P. J Ystehede (London: Routledge 2013).

4. Ettore Dezza, "Zanardelli: Un Codice Positivista?" in *Il codice penale per il Regno d'Italia (1889)*, ed. Sergio Vinciguerra (Padua: Cedam, 2009); Mario Sbriccoli, "Caratteri originari e tratti permanenti del sistema penale italiano (1860–1990)," in *Storia del diritto penale e della giustizia: Scritti editi e inediti (1927–2007)* (Milan: Giuffrè, 2009). On the relationship between the "positive school" and psychological disciplines see Patrizia Guarnieri, "Alienists on Trial: Conflict and Convergence between Psychiatry and Law (1876–1913)," *History of Science* 29, no. 86 (1991). Valeria Babini, *Il caso Murri: Una storia italiana*, Biblioteca storica (Bologna: Il Mulino, 2004), 159–86.

5. Gibson, *Born to Crime*, 1–8; Mary Gibson, "La criminologia prima e dopo Lombroso," in Silvano Montaldo, ed. *Cesare Lombroso: Gli scienziati e la nuova Italia* (Bologna: Mulino, 2011).

6. Guarnieri, "Alienists on Trial: Conflict and Convergence between Psychiatry and Law (1876–1913)."

7. Villa, *Il deviante e i suoi segni*; Antonello La Vergata, "Lombroso e la degenerazione," in Montaldo, *Cesare Lombroso*; Nicole Hahn Rafter and Mary Gibson, "Editors' Introduction," in *Criminal Woman, the Prostitute, and the Normal Woman.* ed. Cesare Lombroso and Guglielmo Ferrero, trans. Nicole Hahn Rafter and Mary Gibson (Durham, N.C.: Duke University Press, 2004), 31.

8. On the incongruities and contradictions in Lombroso's classification, beside the literature quote in the previous footnote, see also Daniele Velo Dalbrenta, "In Search of the Lombrosian Type of Delinquent," in Knepper and Ystehede, *Cesare Lombroso Handbook*. On Enrico Ferri, see Roberta Bisi, *Enrico Ferri e gli studi sulla criminalità* (Milan: FrancoAngeli, 2004), 20–28.

9. Enrico Ferri, "Il delitto passionale nella civiltà contemporanea," in *Arringhe e discorsi: A cura di Bruno Cassinelli* (Milan: Dall'Oglio, 1979), 318.

10. Ibid., 318.

11. Emilia Musumeci, *Emozioni, crimine, giustizia: Un'indagine storico-giuridica tra Otto e Novecento.* (Milan: Franco Angeli, 2015), 181–87.

12. Gianbattista Impallomeni, "A proposito di delinquenti passionali," in *Per 50° Anno d´insegnamento di Enrico Pessina* (Naples: Studii diritto penale, 1899). See also Emmanuele Lasserre, *I delinquenti passionali e il ciminalista Impallomeni*, trans. Laura Impallomeni (Palermo: Stabilimento Tipografico Virzì 1910).

13. Gian Marco Vidor, "The Press, the Audience, and Emotions in Italian Courtrooms (1860s—1910s)" *Journal of Social History* 52 no. 2 (2017): 231–54. Guido Panico, *L´artista e la sciantosa: Il delitto Cifariello, un dramma della gelosia nella Napoli della Belle Époque* (Naples: Liguori, 2011); Paola Daniela Giovanelli, "Teatro in aula: Due processi famosi (il caso 'Murri'e il caso 'Nigrisoli') sulle pagine del 'Carlino," in *Il Resto del Carlino in un secolo di storia: Tra cronaca e cultura*, ed. Maria Luisa Altieri Biagi (Bologna: Pátron, 1985).

14. On political crimes, emotions, and criminological theories in nineteenth-century Italy see Daphne Rozenblatt, "Scientific Expertise and the Politics of Emotions in the 1902 Trial of Giuseppe Musolino," *History of the Human Sciences* 30, no. 3 (2017): 25–49.

15. Guarnieri, "Alienists on Trial."

16. "Ha la faccia un po' intontita, con un'espressione sempre uniforme come una maschera," Mario Carrara, "Contributo allo studio dei delinquenti per passione," *Archivio di psichiatria, scienze penali ed antropologia criminale per servire allo studio dell´uomo alienato e delinquente*, no. 18 (1897). For another example see Francesco Carrara, "Omicidio in passionale," in *La perizia psichiatrico-legale con metodi per eseguirla e la casuistica penale classificata antropologicamente* ed. Cesare Lombroso (Turin: Fratelli Bocca, 1905).

17. Giuseppe Bonanno, *Il delinquente per passione: Studio di psicologia criminale* (Turin: Fratelli Bocca, 1896), 52–54; Carrara, "Contributo allo studio"; Cesare Lombroso, *L´uomo delinquente*, 4th ed., vol. 2 (Turin: Fratelli Bocca, 1896), 204. Ferri, "Il delitto passionale."

18. Cesare Lombroso, *L'amore nel suicidio: E nel delitto* (Turin: Ermanno Loescher, 1881), 18. The idea that there was a link between beauty and morality was shared by many positivist scholars—and even those who were opponents of Positivist School theories. See, for example, Giuseppe Ziino, *Compendio di medicina legale e giurisprudenza medica [. . .] ad uso de' medici e de' giuristi: Volume Primo. Quarta Edizione* (Milan: Società Editrice Libraria, 1906), 217. On this link in Paolo Mantegazza see Nicoletta Pireddu, "Introduction—Paolo Mantegazza: A Scientist and His Ecstasies," in *The Physiology of Love and other Writings*, ed. Paolo Mantegazza (Toronto: University of Toronto Press, 2007).

19. Enrico Ferri, *L'omicido: Nell'antropologia criminale* (Turin: Fratelli Bocca, 1895), 234–35.

20. Bonanno, *Il delinquente per passione*.

21. Ibid., 53–54. Ferri, "Il delitto passionale," 325. Enrico Ferri, *Sociologia criminale*, 3rd ed. (Turin: Fratelli Bocca, 1892), 181. Lombroso, *L'uomo delinquente*, 2:206.

22. On Paolo Mantegazza and Angelo Mosso see Dolores Martín Moruno, "Pain as Practice in Paolo Mantegazza's Science of Emotions," *Osiris* 31 (2016): 137–62; Dolores Martín Moruno, "Love in the Time of Darwinism: Paolo Mantegazza and the Emergence of Sexuality," *Medicina and Storia* 10, nos. 19–20 (2010): 147–64; Danny Rees, "Down in the Mouth: Faces of Pain," in *Pain and Emotion in Modern History*, ed. Rob Boddice (Houndmills: Palgrave, 2014), 164–86.

23. Enrico Morselli, *Manuale di semejotica delle malattie mentali: Guida alla diagnosi della pazzia per i medici, i medico-legisti e gli studenti; Esame anamnestico, antropologico e fisiologico degli alienati*, vol. 1 (Naples: Vallardi 1885), 293–428. On Morselli see Daphne Rozenblatt, "Madness and Method: Enrico Morselli and the Social Politics of Psychiatry, 1852–1929" (PhD diss., University of California, 2014).

24. Morselli, *Manuale di semejotica*, 1:376–77.

25. Bonanno, *Il delinquente per passione*. See the chart summing up the analysis of the cases at the end of the book.

26. Lombroso, *L'uomo delinquente*, 2:208; Cesare Lombroso, *Delitti di Libidine*, 2nd ed. (Turin: Fratelli Bocca, 1886), 21; Lombroso, *L'amore nel suicidio*, 20.

27. Bonanno, *Il delinquente per passione*, 53–54.

28. Ferri, "Il delitto passionale."

29. Bonanno, *Il delinquente per passione*, 2:204–5;

30. Lombroso, *L'uomo delinquente*, 2:218–19. The link between "bodily vigor" and criminal behavior in general—in other words, not specifically linked to passion—was a shared opinion also outside "positivist criminology." As the legal scholar and professor Bernardino Alimena (1861–1915) stated, "It seems that crime is like all the other phenomena of life tied to our age, and follows as a shadow the development of our body; it grows as our body grows, it grows stronger when one enters puberty, it reaches the maximum in the age when one is stronger and decreases as the forces decrease." (Pare che la criminalità sia come tutti gli altri fenomeni della vita legata alla nostra età, e segua come un'ombra lo sviluppo del nostro corpo; cresce come cresce il nostro organismo cresce più fortemente quando si entra nella pubertà,

raggiunge il massimo nell'età in cui si è più forti, diminuisce come diminuiscono le forze.) Bernardino Alimena, *I limiti e i modificatori dell'imputabilità*, vol. 3 (Turin: Fratelli Bocca 1899).

31. Ferri, *Sociologia criminale*. This edition was translated into English in 1898: *Criminal Sociology* (New York: Appleton). For the analysis I have used the original Italian version, but the English terminology used in this article is often taken from the 1898 English edition.

32. Ferri, *Sociologia criminale*, 163.

33. Ibid., 196.

34. Ferri, "Il delitto passionale."

35. Francesco Carrara, *Programma del corso di diritto criminale, dettato nella R. Università di Pisa: Parte Generale* (Lucca: Giusti, 1867), 184–85. On Carrara's view on emotions and their influence on the Italian legal thinking see Musumeci, *Emozioni, crimine, giustizia. Un'indagine storico-giuridica tra Otto e Novecento*, 30–33.

36. Lombroso, *L´uomo delinquente*, 2:214. Jurist Ferdinando Puglia (1853–1909) also used a similar categorization: see "Passioni ed emozioni: Loro influenza sulla responsabilità dei delinquenti," *Archivio di psichiatria, scienze penali ed antropologia criminale per servire allo studio dell´uomo alienato e delinquente* 3 (1882).

37. Ferri, "Il delitto passionale"; Ferri, *Sociologia criminale*, 573.

38. Ferri, "Il delitto passionale."

39. All the characteristics illustrated in the part that follows come from the detailed analysis of both Lombroso's and Ferri's work. For Lombroso see *L´uomo delinquente*, 2:204–65; *Delitti di Libidine*, 20–32; *L´amore nel suicidio: E nel delitto*, 11–32. For Ferri see "Il delitto passionale."

40. In Lombroso's opinion there were some exceptions. Some "criminals of passion," like those who committed the deeds under the influence of a political or a religious passion, did not feel and show any regret or remorse. Lombroso, *L´uomo delinquente*, vol. 2. Lombroso wrote also a specific work on anarchists, *Gli anarchici* (Turin: Bocca, 1895). For a critical view on this aspect of Lombroso's theories see Trevor Calafato, "*Gli Anarchici* and Lombroso's theory of political crime," in Knepper and Ystehede, *Cesare Lombroso Handbook*.

41. Luigi Franchi, *Codice penale e di procedura penale*, Terza edizione, Codici e leggi del Regno d´Italia (Milan: Hoepli 1908).

42. Ferri, "Il delitto passionale nella civiltà contemporanea."

43. On divorce and family violence in Italy see Mark Seymour, "Debating Divorce in Italy: Marriage and the Making of modern Italians, 1860–1974" (New York: Palgrave Macmillan, 2006).

44. Mario Sbriccoli, "Il diritto penale liberale: La rivista penale di Luigi Lucchini," in *Storia del diritto penale e della giustizia: Scritti editi ed inediti (1927–2007)* ed. Mario Sbriccoli (Milan: Giuffré 2009); Angela Santangelo Cordani, *Alla vigilia del codice Zanardelli: Antonio Buccellati e la riforma penale* (Milan: Giuffré 2008), 1–10; Antonella Meniconi, *Storia della magistratura italiana*, Saggi (Bologna: Mulino, 2012), 47–57; 99–112. The number of legal journals reached the amount of 170 in 1921.

45. Ludovico Fulci, *L'evoluzione nel diritto penale: La forza irresistibile*, 2nd ed. (Messina: Capra, 1891), 254–76. Enrico Ferri, *I delinquenti nell'arte* (Genoa: Libreria editrice ligure, 1896).

46. Ferri, *I delinquenti nell'arte*, 26, 29.

47. Ibid., 7.

48. Ibid., 26–27.

49. Founded in 1867 in Turin and published as *Gazzetta Piemontese* until 1895, *La Stampa* has become one of the most important national newspapers since the beginning of the twentieth century. References to Othello in cases of criminal offences and of criminal trials could be found, for example, in the following issues: July 26, 1869, 3; August 15, 1875, 2; April 15, 1876, 1; August 13, 1876, 1; August 18, 1876, 3; June 1, 1878, 3; March 13, 1883, 3; March 21, 1883, 3; October 22, 1885, 3; April 18, 1886, 2; April 19, 1887, 2; September 2, 1887, 3; December 1, 1887, 2; February 3, 1888, 2; March 14, 1890, 2; November 13, 1895, 2; November 15, 1895, 2; August 4, 1905, 3; April 13, 1905; July 12, 1905, 3; September 14, 1905, 2.

50. Nicola Ratti, "Passione e Delitto Capo 2: Le passioni nella scienza," *Il circolo giuridico: Rivista di legislazione e giurisprudenza* 34 (1903).

51. Fulci, *L'evoluzione nel diritto penale*, 262–65. As highlighted by Mary Gibson, the importance of hereditary elements in the etiology of criminal acts remained unchanged also in the positivist criminological theory after Lombroso. Gibson, *Born to Crime: Cesare Lombroso and the Origins of Biological Criminology*, 211.

52. Fulci, *L'evoluzione nel diritto penale*, 262–65.

53. Graham Frankland, *Freud's Literary Culture* (Cambridge: Cambridge University Press, 2000), 9.

54. Jonathan Hiller, "Lombroso and the Science of Literature and Opera," in Knepper and Ystehede, *Cesare Lombroso Handbook*.

55. Ferri, *I delinquenti nell'arte*, 15, 28.

56. Ferri gave the example of the "possessed girl" portrayed in the Raphael painting *The Transfiguration*. In reality it is a clearly a boy, as correctly reported by Charcot and Richer. Ferri was Probably biased by the fact that most famous Charcot's patients diagnosed as hysteric were women. Among other works, Ferri refers to Jean-Martin Charcot and Paul Richer, *Les demoniaques dans l'art* (Paris: Delahaye et Lecrosnier, 1887), 31.

57. Hiller, "Lombroso."

58. Ibid., 244–49.

59. Guarnieri, "Alienists on Trial, 402.

3. Locating Cancer

Body Image and Emotions from a Psychosomatic Perspective (1950–1959)

PILAR LEÓN-SANZ

> The history of emotions is where the history of ideas meets the history of the body.
> —Thomas Dixon, "History in British Tears," 2015

IN 1986 SEYMOUR FISHER, in the introduction to his comprehensive *Development and Structure of the Body Image*, predicted: "I firmly believe we will eventually find that measures of body perception are among our most versatile predictors of how people will interpret and react to life situations."[1] This chapter, which analyzes research on body image and emotions in the frame of the practice of American Psychosomatic Medicine, echoes Fischer's idea, which aimed to provide a more comprehensive vision of the significance of the human body in medicine. The American Psychosomatic Medicine School, it is important to note, emerged in the context of the development of holistic medical theories in the beginning of the twentieth century in several countries, mainly from 1920 to 1960.[2]

As Charles E. Rosenberg pointed out, medical holism implied an emphasis on inclusiveness and integration, and it included a variety of styles that should be distinguished.[3] In the case of the American Psychosomatic Medicine, medical holism attempted to explain how some of the personal aspects could contribute to the diseases and ill-health.[4]

The leading figures in psychosomatic medicine in the United States (1940 to 1960), such as Franz Alexander (1891–1964), one of the founders of this school, had a predominantly psychoanalytical perspective. They studied the role of depth-psychological factors in the pathogenesis of physical diseases.[5]

Their interests lay in physical disorders and disabilities preceded or aggravated by psychological factors, in which some aspects of the person, such as personality or unconscious conflicts, and not just a diseased organ, was the center of the physician's concern.[6]

Underlining the role of emotional factors in somatic illnesses gave a more general and holistic view of the patient. For example, from the 1950s, Harold Wolff (1898–1962) and his collaborators at Cornell University Medical College studied how the effects of life "situations" and emotions altered the function of virtually every bodily system.[7] They found that personal topics meaningful to each subject elicited emotional responses and short-term changes in bodily function.

The doctors from this school emphasized the importance of individual psychology in the so-called "organic neuroses" that gave rise to a "biographical pathology." They explained the genesis and shaping of the morbid process from the perspective of the "meaning" they have in the patient's biography. Psychosomatic school attempted to comprehend human illness scientifically, but from the viewpoint of the patient's "human" or "personal" condition. They tried to extend its scientific knowledge to the corporal and mental dimensions of human nature. Later on, one's social environment also acquired a great importance in the etiology of diseases because "many emotions due to the complications of our social life cannot be freely expressed and relieved, through voluntary activities, but remain repressed and then are diverted into wrong channels."[8]

By the 1960s, the focus of psychosomatic observation and research shifted to the role of stressful experiences, which emanated from the environment and were individually interpreted, altering bodily functions and impairing health.[9]

We can assume that the concept of the "body" was a central issue in holistic medical movements in the mid-twentieth century and particularly in the American Psychosomatic School, where the term "body" acquired specific connotations.[10] Scientists and physicians offered alternative notions regarding the function of emotions and their effect on body and mind as well as on the interplay of both.[11]

As antecedent of this movement, Freud both implicitly and explicitly emphasized body image, because he argued that body image was basic to the development of the total ego structure and becomes a substantial nucleus of later ego elaborations. Freud's conception of the development of sexuality is in many ways a body-image-oriented theory.[12] We find also allusions to body-image phenomena in the different psychoanalytic groups derived from Freud. For example, Alfred Adler (1870–1937), although he did not explicitly consider the body-image phenomena, nonetheless linked his descriptions of personality dynamics with implicit body-image references.[13]

American psychosomatic physicians such as Franz Alexander or Harold Wolff sought to reveal meaningful links between emotions, personality, and patterns of symptoms associated with certain types of body malfunction. But, regarding body image, in the opinion of Fisher and Cleveland, although Alexander and Wolff tried to reduce the gap between personality concepts and body notions, their interest on body as a psychological phenomenon was limited because they paid scarce attention to the study of "normal" bodies—that is to say, bodies that did not develop clinical symptomatology.[14]

Conversely, others psychosomatic physicians such as Seymour Fisher and Sidney F. Cleveland apprehended body image as a representation of the body learned through experiencing the body.[15] Notably, in the 1950s, these American researchers explained that the exterior body or the different internal parts or organs of the body were psychologically significant. They presented the connections between body-image types and different personalities and diverse ways of experiencing emotions. As a result, these scientists explored body image predictors of how people could understand and react to life situations.

Their studies are not a mere analytic tool. They aimed to show how personality forces may distort the physiological processes and produce physical illness. Here we have the performative interest of this subject: the framework of the body is part of disease construction and of the development of illness symptoms. As the introduction in this volume has explained, "emotional bodies" can be a particularly useful category of analysis to understand the creation of new systems of symbolic relations as a result of the repetition of certain emotional practices, whether they are gestures or linguistic acts.

To discuss this, I present first the key theorists, the psychologists Seymour Fisher (1922–1996) and Sidney E. Cleveland (1919–), who built a concept of body image at that time. Their work continues to shape our understanding of this field. In the second section I will focus on the bases of the theory on body image, emotions, and illness that Fisher and Cleveland developed in the 1950s because these were the beginnings of important theories on body image that developed in the subsequent decades. In their work, one sees what might be gained by introducing methodological tools and hypotheses generated for the study of emotions and body image in the recent past. I will also contextualize their theories with the research on body image published by other scientists, such as Paul Schilder or Lawrence S. Kubie. Third, I propose to shed new light on the production of knowledge about the emotion-body-disease connection (the cancerous body, in this case). I will consider the measures and also the links between feeling of body and its spatial dimension, and the topography of cancer. In the final part I will comment on some critiques raised by these psychological techniques and research tools. I will also highlight how Fisher and Cleveland's theories allow us to adopt the notion of performativity Martín-Moruno and Pichel included as they understand it as the "doing of a certain action" that has material results by means of its very recurrence.[16] From a performative point of view this research explained, on the one hand, the transformative character of emotions in the body and, on the other, the impact of body image in the genesis of diseases, such as cancer, and the symptoms associated with them.

The Key Theorists

At the beginning of the twentieth century we find two traditions in research on body perception.[17] One is inspired by the British neurologist Henry Head (1861–1940), who studied the body schema and the perception of body parts in neurological patients. From this perspective, the recognition of "body image" was initiated as clinical attempts to understand such phenomena as "phantom limb," "autotopagnosia," "hemiasomatognosia," or "anosognosia." The other body-image tradition explored "the value of body-image constructs in the area of normal behavior."[18] Paul Schilder, for example, combined the concept of the somatopsyche (the postural model of the body) and Freud's idea that the ego is primarily a body ego to arrive at his own formulation of the fundamental role of the body image in a human being's relationship to himself, to others, and to the world.[19] Seymour Fisher and Sidney E. Cleveland develop their ideas from these premises.

Seymour Fisher earned his doctorate in psychology at the University in Chicago (1948), one of the most renowned centers on psychosomatic medicine at that time. Much of Fisher's early work on body image was done with Sidney E. Cleveland when both worked at the Veterans Administration Hospital (Houston, Texas) and Baylor University College of Medicine. Until 1960 they published many articles, which were included in their volume *Body Image and Personality* (1958, 1968). The book develops a theory regarding the connection among body image, body boundaries, body reactivity, and the behavioral variations. The impact of this research was evidenced by the number of book reviews published at that time, although, as we will observe below, some of them criticized Fisher and Cleveland's methodologies.[20]

From 1961 onward Fisher worked in Syracuse as head of the Psychology Research Division at the State University of New York Health Science Center. He helped to make "body image" an active area of psychology research, even to the present day.[21] He assembled his publications in the volume *Body Experience in Fantasy and Behavior* (New York: Appleton-Century-Crofts, 1970), a comprehensive text on the psychological significance of the body: the adaptation of attitudes of the person's concept about its size, its strength, its attractiveness, its sexual potency, aspects of cleanliness, plasticity, concepts such as masculinity and femininity, and vulnerability to external intrusion. The last two-volume work on the subject was published in 1986: *Development and Structure of the Body Image* (Hillsdale, N.J.: Erlbaum). In more than one thousand pages, Fisher reviewed his body-image research from 1969 to 1985 and returned to topics such as the organization of the body-image boundary, assignment of meaning to specific body areas, or the distortions in body perception.

Building a Body-Image Concept

The studies on body image were connected with the importance of the body for the holistic medical theories. For Fisher and Cleveland, the influence of body image involved "all phases of an individual's functioning, whether 'physiological' or 'psychological' or 'biochemical.' [They are] intimately linked and can be meaningfully conceptualized as exerting mutually determining types of effects."[22]

In their theory, body image was focused on the individual's feelings and attitudes toward his or her own body. In this vision, emotions were part of the body-image concept. Specifically, they assumed that, as each individual develops, he or she has the difficult task of significantly organizing the feelings and the sensations from his or her body, one of the most important and complex phenomena in a person's total perceptual field.

Fisher and Cleveland distinguished their theory from that of others who had also explored the body-image concept, such as Schilder, because, for them, body image implied a reference to conscious and unconscious attitudes of self-corporeality. Methodologically, Fisher and Cleveland's work exemplifies both the research strategies of the American School of Psychosomatic Medicine, on the one hand, and the field of empirical psychology, in increasing development at that time, on the other.[23]

Fisher and Cleveland analyzed the meaning of body image using parameters such as the "Barrier score," the "Boundary limit," and "Body reactivity." These indicators were obtained through the Rorschach test responses, looking for objective and clinically useful data. They relied on statistical tools, mainly the chi-square formula. They understood body reactivity as the way in which the body image, and in other cases the body-image fantasies, were reflected in the physical body and in the healthy, vulnerable, or diseased organs. And, vice versa, physiological reactivity led to the creation of a concrete body image. Body reactivity reflected the association between the psychological aspects, the three-dimensional estimation of the body, and physiological reactivity parameters such as blood pressure, heart rate, finger temperature, saliva output, Galvanic skin response (GSR), respiration rate, and the like.[24]

Throughout these parameters, Fisher and Cleveland explained that the body surface can be sorted into psychologically meaningful divisions and that it was possible that changes in the reactivity of these divisions may provide valuable information about the emotional state of the individual: "Studies are now underway to determine whether there are characteristic alterations in the skin resistance levels of various body sectors that accompany specific emotional responses (e.g., anxiety, anger, relaxation, and depression)."[25] They assumed that if one pattern of symptoms was the outcome of a given sequence of physiological events and that if a second symptom pattern was the result of still another physiological sequence, it would follow that any variable that distinguished the two symptom patterns would, at the same time, demonstrate a relationship to the underlying events. Therefore, "since the Barrier score significantly distinguished subjects relative to their susceptibility to body-exterior symptoms versus body-interior symptoms, it seemed logical to speculate that degree of boundary definiteness was somehow tied up with associated differential physiological response patterns which might be presumed to exist."[26]

Fisher and Cleveland concluded that one should also consider the possibility that the correlation between organ awareness and organ activation may be potentially useful in detecting organ malfunction.[27] For instance, they inferred that the occurrence of psychosomatic symptoms in the exterior body layers (for example, neurodermatitis) was linked with a definite body boundary concept, whereas the occurrence of symptoms in the body's interior (for example, stomach ulcers) was linked with indefinite boundaries. As a result, they distinguished between exterior and interior body reactivity, and they observed the repercussions of the body spatial axis.[28]

For them, the manner in which the individual deals with angry impulses, for instance, can tell a great deal about his/her ability to be self-steering. It was usually in situations of stress and frustration that anger was aroused; and often in such situations there was a conflict between wanting to express the anger in an aggressive, self-determined fashion and fearing of the consequences of being aggressive.[29] This explanation allowed them to propose a psychological model analysis related with physiological models and to measure the interrelationship between emotional and corporeality. It was an exciting possibility due to the difficulties encountered when seeking these forms of association between the physiological and psychological spheres. In the case of arthritics, for example, they explained that "we were struck by how much difficulty [the patients] had in expressing anger. It seemed as if they were afraid to express anger and felt it necessary to contain it inwardly in a tightly controlled fashion."[30] This confirms the role of the body boundary concept expressed above.

Measuring the Influence of Emotions and Body Image in Cancer Patients

In the 1950s, when cancer began to acquire more medical and social visibility,[31] psychosomatic studies pointed to a series of connections between cancer and personality factors. As more research was produced, it gradually became clear that certain cancer phenomena were linked to psychological variables.[32] Fisher's studies coincided with other numerous research studies on the psychogenic aspects of cancer published in this period in the United States.[33]

We can observe the sort of experimental work Fisher and Cleveland employed by reviewing the study they carried out to link body image and cancer.[34] In 1956 these scientists, using blind sorting of Rorschach protocols, studied the body-image fantasies of patients whose cancer involved the exterior of the body (such as skin cancer, melanoma, or breast cancer) and compared them with the body-image fantasies of patients with cancer affecting internal organs (for example, cancer of the colon, lung, stomach, or cervix). The study included fifty-nine "exterior" cases and thirty "interior" cases.[35] A chi-square was made between the number of "barrier" and "penetration" scores for the two groups on the assumption that such scores indicated body-image concepts. Their control group included patients previously tested with the Rorschach over ten years after colostomies performed because of cancer.[36]

The results showed that the exterior group gave more barrier responses and the interior group more penetration scores. And they concluded that "formal scores and impressionistic sorting procedures both indicate that to a statistically significant degree the patient with body-exterior cancer has a greater tendency to conceive of his body as enclosed by an impenetrable boundary than does the patient with interior cancer."[37] They also affirmed that "the differences in body-image scores between the body-exterior cancer group and the body-interior cancer group seem to reflect basic differences in personality orientation."[38]

Apparently, then, emotion and personality variables may play a significant role in the total complex of factors that determined the site of development of cancer in an individual. The link between emotional body and the topography of cancer reinforced the idea that the organism acted as a psychophysical unity—an idea, as noted observed at the beginning of the chapter, that corresponds with the American Psychosomatic approach.

The Body Spatial Axis

Cleveland and Fisher's body reactivity theory also took into account the question of body spatial axis. This notion was not new. Elida Evans, a disciple of Carl Jung, published, as early as 1926, the groundbreaking *A Psychological Study of Cancer*, wherein she specifically referred to which side of the body the cancer was located.[39] Fisher and Cleveland's experiments demonstrated characteristic patterns of response such that either one side tended to be more reactive than the other or that the gradient does not manifest definite directionality. Body reactivity—or, better, the ratio of reactivity—also was useful for studying the differences between upper-body site and lower site, which was significantly linked with the relative size attributed to each in body-schema judgments.[40]

Further, it was shown that in right-handed persons there was an optimum norm gradient that involved greater reactivity on the left than on the right side, and vice versa. A more important point raised involves the connections between the body spatial axis with weakness, sexual maturity, and gender. For example, Fisher explains that the left directional gradient was significantly more frequent among those with a mature body image than among those with a poorly defined body image.

Analyzing the Emotional Bodies Measures: A Theory of Suspicion

Fisher and Cleveland's research took place in the midst of a boom in technological assessment of psychological processes, especially personality tests, through MMPI tests and the Rorschach, among others.[41] Doctors gave numerous recommendations about the need to measure the influence of the personal body image or how emotions affect the body perception.[42] The empiricism of the studies on emotional bodies coincided with the process of control of emotions Frank Biess and Daniel M. Gross described.[43]

Fisher and Cleveland's studies took into account the symptoms described by patients. These subjective descriptions were classified by professionals, following procedures supposedly objective and valid, such as the test of Rorschach. As a result, patients and doctors alike played a function in the building of the image and the emotional bodies. In the process, patient's observations of his or her own body provided moderately accurate information about its reactivity. The degree of awareness of a given part of the body surface in the total body scheme was linked with its degree of activation. The fact that self-reports of body experiences offered valid observations about the body's physiological or pathological functioning had important theoretical significance with regard to the use of introspection as a method for obtaining data, although Fisher was aware that introspection and self-observation had fallen into disrepute.[44]

But obtaining data for a formulation of general rules on body image was not easy, because of the simultaneous role of the body as both participant and object of the perceptual process and because the results were based not merely on memory associations and emotional experiences, but also on intentions, will, and aims. Continual testing was needed to find out what parts fit the plan and fit the whole.

Moreover, in the cases of patients, the perception of one's own body image was not static, due in part to the performative character of emotions. Consequently, the psychologists had to explain how to model something that is continually changing into a structure.[45] For example, they quoted the analysis of biographical material that indicated that "the low Barrier men are in general very friendly and enjoy social interaction" and that, at the same time, "low Barrier people are more oriented toward things than people and that they were relatively poor in their ability to empathize with others."[46]

Fisher and Cleveland's empirical work received both positive and negative criticism. The major criticism was their persistence in emphasizing the exploratory nature of their work, with a resulting tendency to speak as though they had indeed made a major discovery regarding the degree to which the emotional was an influence over or a determinant to personality development.[47] Besides, at least in cancer, their methodology—as Patricia Jasen affirms—was clearly designed to secure the results they sought and provided confirmation of their belief that breast cancers were associated with a higher tendency to perceive the body "as enclosed by an impenetrable boundary."[48] Fisher and Cleveland's research, although stimulating and suggestive, was very difficult to replicate.[49] They were also censured because of the indiscriminate application of their three main parameters ("Barrier score," "Boundary limit," and "Body reactivity") to multiple situations. H. J. Wahler, for example, said that the B (Barrier) score seems to have a Midas-like quality.[50] And Joseph Masling (State University of New York in Buffalo) commented that their choice of statistics limited their experiments to the analysis of a single variable at a time.[51]

George M. Perrin and Irene R. Pierce, both members of the American Psychosomatic Association, included the work by Fisher and Cleveland in the stern critical review over the empirical methods used by several Psychosomatic School members in studies that linked emotions, personality factors, and cancer.[52] In their opinion, the chi-square analysis Fisher and Cleveland used "did not yield a significant difference between the 2 groups" (exterior-interior cancer sites) examined.[53] And they disapproved of the criteria of classifying cancer as "internal" and "external" because each group included different types of cancer.[54] However, the exterior-interior classification for illnesses was not new. Schilder had applied it,[55] and the psychoanalyst Lawrence S. Kubie (1896–1973) had also used this distinction in 1944.[56]

Other critics disapproved of the importance the researchers attached to emotional issues as etiology factor of illness, which they and the contemporary psychosomatic research, in general, considered. The question was criticized as a cause of "disconnection" with physicians working on cancer[57] and because it led to a delay in the development of studies that explored both medical and psychological perspectives and an integrated approach to patient care.[58]

In short, and as Pope suggested, there was no convincing evidence of the measures of the influence of emotions and personality in the body or of the central causal role for the body-image boundary in behavior.

Emotional Bodies' Performativity and Disease

Despite the criticism expressed above, Joseph Masling noted that, until Fisher and Cleveland, no one had ever combined ideas on body-image influence as they did, and no one had ever shown such energy, novelty, and discipline in collecting data that illustrated their theses. "They looked for relations between variables that previously had appeared to have nothing in common."[59] We can summarize their contributions regarding emotional bodies' performativity in the following points:

a) They proposed a new concept of body image that included the emotional element.

As we have observed, these psychologists' body-image theory differed from the paradigm Cannon established and from Selye's contributions, and it was also different from the neuropathological explanations developed by the neuroscience of the time.[60] Fisher's idea of "reactivity" implied "a distinct departure from the usual frame of reference utilized in viewing physiological reactivity"[61] or measuring visceral emotions.[62] For Fisher and Cleveland, "it was not based on the typical distinction involving sympathetic versus parasympathetic response or on the classical 'emotion' categories (e.g., anger, anxiety). Rather, implicit in the formulation was that there is another universe of physiological reactivity events that has to do with the psychologically important spatial aspects of the body."[63] In sum, they attempted to show that body image and body-image fantasies were expressions of the basic attitudes that an individual adopts toward his or her body.

Their experiments on body image in the 1950s support Dror's perception about the development of several parallel paradigms (modern psychological, Freudian, Jamesian, Darwinian, and so on) to establish physiological models and logic of emotions.[64]

b) From a performative approach, Fisher and Cleveland studies demonstrated, with creativity and originality, the relationships between participants' life stories or socialization processes and the body-image responses.

In this context, we note that an individual's expectations, emotions, and wishes may selectively influence the reactivity of various elements of his or her body system. For instance, high Barrier people data suggested that the subjects were more likely to gratify themselves when the opportunity presented itself and more likely to express anger outwardly than inwardly when frustrated. For Fisher and Cleveland, it was quite possible that the need for an excitation landmark in a given body area could give rise to some form of physiological response in that sector. "We feel," Fisher noted, "that certain patterns of attitudes about the body played a part in determining in a gross manner the site of development of various physical symptoms."[65]

These psychologists raised the idea that experiences of socialization could be transformed into body-image attitudes and that certain social roles learned by an individual could also be translated into a body-spatial representation. They further asked themselves if, for an individual, social experiences could be duplicated terms of body topography. In effect, one of the most important results that emerged from studying both the body boundary and right-left dimensions was that, throughout the differential reactivity of the body sectors, researchers could trace the manner in which the individual had experienced or learned important social roles (in other words, how he or she had experienced his or her parents as standing for definite values and a well-articulated way of life). This point connected with the "biographical pathology" of the American Psychosomatic Medicine School mentioned at the beginning of the chapter. These attitudinal patterns, conceptualized under the term "body image," were probably developed very early in life and exert a significant influence over a long period.[66]

Fisher and Cleveland also described how fantasies grow out of the individual's experiences with others and in some ways reflect one's lifestyle. One may conceive of the body image as partially defining the way in which an individual pictures his or her relationship to the world. Thus, a patient with rheumatoid arthritis or the patient with neurodermatitis who conceives of his or her body as sheathed by a heavy, protective boundary seems to have evolved a system of personality defense based on entrenching oneself behind thick barriers. In contrast, the patient with spastic colitis or stomach disturbances who visualizes his or her body exterior as thin and easily penetrated has evolved quite a different style or personality defense. In the case of cancer: "We take the view that the 'choice' of an exterior vs. an interior cancer site can represent the final, extreme result of adherence to a certain style of life."[67]

And, in some "as yet unexplained manner, this influence may include a tendency toward sensitizing or rendering more susceptible certain general areas of the body to physical illness in times of stress and trauma" or strong emotions.[68] Following Roy Porter, historian of medicine, we appreciate that their idea about the human body was, in a wide sense, as "an expressive medium" in which "the boundaries and crossings of self and society" are negotiated.[69] Moreover, among the effects of emotions in shaping the identity of both individual and collective bodies, Fisher and Cleveland highlighted the connections between body image, sexuality, and disease. For these scholars, there was evidence of significantly higher Barrier scores in females than males, in both adult and child populations.[70] Later on, Fisher conceptualized this difference, in the context of other body-image data and indicated that the female in Western culture is more directly in communication with her body than the male and also has a greater sense of security about it.[71] There was also converging evidence that women may have a more clearly articulated and stable body concept than men.[72] Consequently, we can observe, as Frevert has shown, that although science has changed, some ideas about the diversity of emotions between men and women have not.[73] And "cultural modes, patterns of socialization and self-perception are still deeply gendered."[74] In the 1950s genre distinction in medical knowledge and professional practices was maintained.[75]

These scientists also proposed a gendering of the cancer pathogenesis that had already been described in medical literature. As Patricia Jasen also pointed out, the link between sexuality and cancer continued to be focused on women—even when male patients were included in the studies.[76] And this constitutively shapes psychosomatic theory, connected with psychoanalysis.

c) Cleveland and Fisher's theory that linked body image, emotion, and disease evolved in the frame of the medical theories.

Thus, subsequent Western psychiatric publications have highlighted the importance of "physical appearance" for the clinical evolution and the efficacy of the treatment of patients before experiencing cancer and after the application of therapeutical strategies, especially with regard to the body image one developed.[77] The emotional impact of one's "physical appearance" was present in Fisher and Cleveland, but, for these scientists, body image and the role of emotion was more radical: feeling the body was connected with the awareness of the vulnerability of certain organs.[78] As well, they considered body image as a pathogenesis factor, and not only as something concomitant to the disease. Furthermore, as Fisher and Cleveland stated, "the data do, however, support the assertion that the body-image boundary was a more accurate reflection of central personality attitudes than of actual body structure." Such an assertion was consistent with the clinical hunch that body image could be used as a diagnostic index of personality structure, if one were able to evaluate it reliably. "We have assumed that it is this position of the body, intermediate between 'outside' and 'inside,' which makes it a unique projection screen for patterns of attitudes; and we have concluded that the body image is formed of these projected attitudes."[79]

Conclusion

Fisher, Cleveland, and their disciples pointed to the body as a unique and important determinant of behavior and as a mirror of the interpersonal climate surrounding it. What began as a new, somewhat curious method of treating responses to inkblots had later become an important and common research tool.[80] And it led to ways and means of examining the influence of the emotions and psychology on somatic illnesses.

Reading this material more than fifty years after it was written provides an insight into psychological research in an earlier stage. Fisher and Cleveland's theory intended to reduce the gap between personalities and body concepts. In their thought, the body, this primary structure of the self, could crystallize into clinical changes. It represented part of the experience of the unit of the self. And from the perspective of performativity, emotional body image results from the individual's subjective existences with his or her body and the manner in which he or she has organized these experiences.

Notes

I thank my colleagues and co-editors of this volume, Pedro Gil-Sotres and Rocío G. Davis for their comments and suggestions. This chapter is part of the Emotional Culture and Identity Project of the Institute for Culture and Society (University of Navarra).

The chapter's epigraph is from The History of Emotions blog, September 10, 2015, https://emotionsblog.history.qmul.ac.uk/2015/09/weeping-britannia.

1. Seymour Fisher, *Development and Structure of the Body Image* (Hillsdale, N.J.: Erlbaum, 1986) 1:xiii.

2. Abundant bibliography on this subject exists. See Christopher Lawrence and George Weisz, eds., *Greater than the Parts: Holism in Biomedicine, 1920–1950* (Oxford: Oxford University Press, 1998); about American Psychosomatic Medicine, see Herbert Weiner, "The Concept of Psychosomatic Medicine" and "Psychosomatic Medicine and the Mind-Body Relation: Historical, Philosophical, Scientific, and Clinical Perspectives" in *History of Psychiatry and Medical Psychology: With an Epilogue on Psychiatry and the Mind-Body Relation*, ed. Edwin R. Wallace IV and John Gach (New York: Springer, 2008), 485–516 and 781–834; Dorothy Levenson, *Mind, Body, and Medicine: A History of the American Psychosomatic Society* (Baltimore, Md.: Williams and Wilkins, 1994).

3. Rosenberg emphasized that twentieth-century notions of holistic integration were different from their classical and early modern predecessors. Meanwhile, historical holism focused on conceptions of the body in time; organismic holism turned on the body understood as functioning unit. Charles Rosenberg, "Holism in Twentieth-Century Medicine" in Lawrence and Weisz, *Greater than the Parts*, 335–355, 335 and 339.

4. Weiner, "Psychosomatic Medicine and the Mind-Body Relation," 785.

5. As Alexander announced programmatically in the first issue of the journal *Psychosomatic Medicine*, thanks to Freud, psychiatry, taken as the study of the morbid personality, would become the gateway for a more synthetic medical perspective. Franz Alexander, "Psychological Aspects of Medicine" *Psychosomatic Medicine* 1 (1939): 7–18, 12.

6. Weiner, "Concept of Psychosomatic Medicine," 488. About this approach, see also Pilar León Sanz, "El carácter terapéutico de la relación médico-paciente" in *Emociones y estilos de vida: Radiografía de nuestro tiempo*, ed. Lourdes Flamarique and Madalena D'Oliveira (Madrid: Biblioteca Nueva, 2013), 101–30, 102–8.

7. William J. Grace, David T. Graham, Lawrence E. Hinkle, Thomas H. Holmes, Adrian Ostfeld, and Stewart Wolf all worked with him. H. G. Wolff, *Stress and Disease* (Springfield, Ill.: Thomas, 1953); H. G. Wolff, S. G. Wolf Jr., and C. C. Hare, eds., *Life Stress and Bodily Disease* (Baltimore, Md.: Williams and Wilkins, 1950).

8. Alexander, "Psychological Aspects of Medicine," 14.

9. Weiner, "Psychosomatic Medicine and the Mind-Body Relation," 789.

10. Bettina Hitzer, "Healing Emotions" in *Emotional Lexicons: Continuity and*

Change in the Vocabulary of Feeling, 1700–2000, ed. Ute Frevert (Oxford: Oxford University Press, 2014), 142.

11. A review of the body concept in psychiatry in Sonu Shamdasani, "Psychoanalytical Body," and Mark Micale, "Psychiatric Body," both in *Medicine in the Twentieth Century*, ed. Roger Cooter and John Pickstone (Amsterdam: Harwood Academic, 2000). 307–22, 323–46, respectively.

12. Seymour Fisher and Sidney F. Cleveland in *Body image and Personality* (Oxford: Van Nostrand, 1958; New York: Dover Publications, 1968), 3–53, 42.

13. Ibid., 46.

14. Ibid., x.

15. Sidney E. Cleveland, "The Place of the Head in the Body Image Concept," *Research and Clinical Studies in Headache* 4 (1976): 1–17.

16. Following Butler's approach, Martín-Moruno and Pichel explain that performativity is "linked to the formation of the subject but also to the production of the matter of bodies." Judith Butler, *Bodies that Matter: On the Discursive Limits of Sex* (New York: Routledge, 1993); regarding "performativity and science," see Hans Rudolf Velten, "Performativity and Performance" in *Travelling Concepts for the Study of Culture*, ed. Birgit Neumann, Ansgar Nünning (Berlin: De Gruyter, 2012), 249–66, esp. 263.

17. Fisher and Cleveland analyzed previous research on body image in *Body Image and Personality*, 3–53. See also Thomas F. Cash and Thomas Pruzinsky, *Body Image: A Handbook of Theory, Research, and Clinical Practice* (New York: Guilford, 2002), 2.

18. Fisher and Cleveland, *Body Image and Personality*, 6

19. Paul Schilder, *The Image and Appearance of the Human Body: Studies in the Constructive Energies of the Psyche* [1935] (Oxon: Routledge, 2000), 304. Paul Schilder (1886–1940), Austrian psychoanalyst and psychiatrist, moved to the United States in 1928. He was one of the initiators of group psychotherapy. See Isidore Ziferstein, "Psychoanalysis and Psychiatry: Paul Ferdinand Schilder 1886–1940" in *Psychoanalytic Pioneers*, ed. Franz Alexander, Samuel Eisenstein, and Martin Grotjahn (New York: Basic 1966), 458.

20. Bernard Lubin, "Body Image and Personality," *Psychosomatic Medicine* 20, no. 5 (1958): 425–25; Benjamin Pope, "Body Image and Personality," *Journal of Nervous and Mental Disease* 127, no. 6 (1958): 561–64; H. J. Wahler, "Book review," *American Journal Orthopsychiatry* 30, no. 2 (1960): 433–436; Sarnoff A. Mednick, "Book Review," *Contemporary Psychology: A Journal of Reviews* 5, no. 3 (1960): 109.

21. Fisher's son wrote in 2004 that the study of body image was his father's life's passion. The Annual Body Image Dissertation Award was organized by Drs. Cash and Pruzinsky, colleagues and disciples of Fisher, in his honor. Jerid M. Fisher, "Announcement," *Body Image* 1 (2004): 221–24.

22. Seymour Fisher and Sidney E. Cleveland, "Relationship of Body Image to Site of Cancer," *Psychosomatic Medicine* 18 (1956): 304–9, esp. 9.

23. Thomson, "Psychological Body," 295.

24. Fisher and Cleveland, *Body Image*, 307–41. Body reactivity factor was developed in Seymour Fisher and Sidney E. Cleveland, "An Approach to Physiological Reactivity in Terms of a Body Image Schema," *Psychological Reviews* 64 (1957), 26; Seymour Fisher, "Body Image and Asymmetry of Body Reactivity," *Journal of Abnormal and Social Psychology* 57 (1958): 292; Seymour Fisher, "Body Reactivity Gradients and Figure Drawing Variables," *Journal of Consulting Psychology* 23, no. 1 (1959): 54–59; Seymour Fisher and Joseph Abercrombie, "The Relationship of Body Image Distortions to Body Reactivity Gradients," *Journal of Personality* 26, no. 3 (1958): 320–29; Seymour Fisher, "Head-Body Differentiations in Body Image and Skin Resistance Level," *Journal of Abnormal and Social Psychology* 60 (1960): 283.

25. Seymour Fisher, "Body Image and Upper in Relation to Lower Body Sector Reactivity," *Psychosomatic Medicine* 23 no. 5 (1961): 400–402.

26. Seymour Fisher, "Extensions of Theory Concerning Body Image and Body Reactivity," *Psychosomatic Medicine* 21, no. 2 (1959): 142–49. Fisher and Cleveland, *Body Image*, 307.

27. Seymour Fisher, "Sex Differences in Body Perception" *Psychological Monographs: General and Applied* 78 no. 14 (1964): 1–22; Seymour Fisher, "Body Attention Patterns and Personality Defences." *Psychology Monographs* 80 no. 9 (1966): 1–31.

28. The first time these authors applied the "Barrier score" and the "Boundary limit" factors occurred in patients with rheumatoid arthritis and neurodermatitis. Seymour Fisher and Sidney E. Cleveland, "Behavior and Unconscious Fantasies of Patients with Rheumatoid Arthritis," *Psychosomatic Medicine* 16 (1954): 327–33; Sidney E. Cleveland and Seymour Fisher, "Psychological Factors in the Neurodermatoses," *Psychosomatic Medicine* 18 (1956): 209–20.

29. Fisher and Cleveland, *Body Image*, 172.

30. Ibid., 55.

31. For a review of the evolution of knowledge on cancer, see David Cantor, "Cancer," in *Companion Encyclopedia of the History of Medicine*, ed. William F. Bynum and Roy Porter (London: Routledge, 1997), 537–61; David Cantor, "Diseased Body" in Cooter and Pickstone, *Medicine in the Twentieth Century*, 347–66, esp. 349.

32. Hitzer and León-Sanz, "The Feeling Body and its Diseases: How Cancer Went Psychosomatic in Twentieth-Century Germany," *Osiris* 31, *History of Science and the Emotions* (2016), ed. Otniel E. Dror, Bettina Hitzer, Anja Laukötter, and Pilar León-Sanz.

33. See Fred Brown, "The Relationship between Cancer and Personality," *Annals of New York Academy of Sciences* 125 (1966): 865–73; Jimmie C. Holland, "History of Psycho-Oncology: Overcoming Attitudinal and Conceptual Barriers," *Psychosomatic Medicine* 64 (2002): 206–21; Patricia Jasen, "Malignant Histories: Psychosomatic Medicine and the Female Cancer Patient in the Postwar Era." *Canadian Bulletin of Medical History* 20 no. 2 (2003): 265–97; Bettina Hitzer, "Oncomotions: Experience and Debates in West Germany and United States after 1945," in *Science and Emotions after 1945: A Transatlantic Perspective*, ed. Frank Biess and Donald M. Gross (Chicago: University of Chicago Press, 2014), 157–78.

34. Fisher and Cleveland, "Relationship of Body Image."

35. First, they included a small group of patients (six melanoma patients as exterior group and eleven patients with cancer of the cervix as interior group). The completed exterior group consisted of one man with skin cancer, six women with melanomas, and fifty-two women with breast cancer. The interior group involved one woman and two men with cancer of the colon, two men with cancer of the lung, one man with cancer of the stomach, and twenty-four women with cancer of the cervix. The median age of the groups was fifty-two and fifty, respectively. Fisher and Cleveland, "Relationship of Body Image," 306.

36. As Patricia Jasen points out, "the fact that the subjects' Rorschach test results were already on file at the Anderson Hospital and Tumor Center indicates that psychological testing was commonplace among cancer patients at that institution." Jasen, "Malignant Histories," 278.

37. Fisher and Cleveland, "Relationship of Body Image," 309. See also Fisher, "Extensions of Theory."

38. Fisher and Cleveland, "Relationship of Body Image," 309.

39. Elida Evans, *A Psychological Study of Cancer* (New York: Dodd, Mead, 1926), 19.

40. Fisher, "Body Image and Upper."

41. Rebecca Schilling and Stephen T. Casper, "Of Psychometric Means: Starke R. Hathaway and the Popularization of the Minnesota Multiphasic Personality Inventory," *Science in Context* 28 (2015): 77–98. About the social opposition against this movement (because of the determinism and classification of people, healthy or sick), see Thomson, "Psychological Body," 298, 301.

42. As Schilder said at that time, "the empirical method was preferable to mere speculation." Schilder, *Image and appearance*, 286. And Dror affirms that "various psychoanalytically oriented psychosomatic clinicians incorporated instruments for seeing emotions into their therapeutic interactions," although the opposition took issue with the psychoanalytic method. Otniel Dror, "Seeing the Blush: Feeling Emotions," in *Histories of Scientific Observation*, ed. Lorraine Daston and Elizabeth Lunbeck (Chicago: The University of Chicago Press, 2011), 326–348, 338.

43. Biess and Gross, *Science and Emotions*, 1–5.

44. Seymour Fisher, "Organ Awareness and Organ Activation," *Psychosomatic Medicine* 29 no. 6 (1967): 643–47. Dror analyzes the question of the introspection and the self-observation in "Seeing the Blush," 341.

45. Schilder, *Image and Appearance*, 288, 297.

46. Fisher and Cleveland, *Body Image*, 204.

47. Pope (Institute of the University of Maryland) said that their proposal was based on a study of a small and heterogeneous number of cases. "Book Review."

48. Jasen, "Malignant Histories," 278.

49. Pope, "Book review."

50. Wahler, "Book Review," 433–36. Pope made a similar observation and reflected the "amazement and incredulity that such a wide range of behavior phenomena could be successfully predicted from a single measure." Pope, "Book Review," 561.

51. Joseph Masling, "Bodies under Investigation: Body Image and Personality by S. Fisher and S. E. Cleveland (1958)," *Journal of Personality Assessment* 72 no. 1 (1999): 164–74, esp. 171.

52. George M. Perrin and Irene R. Pierce, "Psychosomatic Aspects of Cancer: A Review," *Psychosomatic Medicine* 21 (1959): 397–421. This publication had significant influence in the course of the research of the American Psychosomatic School. See Hitzer and León-Sanz, "Feeling Body."

53. Perrin and Pierce, "Psychosomatic Aspects of Cancer," 413.

54. Ibid. 414.

55. For him, "the topography of the postural model of the body was the basis of emotional attitudes towards the body." Schilder, *Image and Appearance*, 15.

56. Lawrence S. Kubie, "The Basis of a Classification of Disorders from the Psychosomatic Standpoint," *Bulletin of the New York Academy of Medicine* (1944): 46–65.

57. Thomas Hackett, "The Psychiatrist: In the Mainstream or on the Banks of Medicine?," *American Journal of Psychiatry* 134 (1977): 432–34. Hackett (1928–1988), psychiatrist at Massachusetts General Hospital, was also president of the American Academy of Psychosomatic Medicine.

58. Holland, "History of Psycho-Oncology," 211.

59. Masling, "Bodies under Investigation," 164. Perrin and Pierce also underlined the original approach of Fisher and Cleveland in "Psychosomatic Aspects of Cancer," 413.

60. Following the theories by Walter B. Cannon and Hans Selye, "emotional stress" was linked to a new humoral conception of body and mind. Feelings had an effect on the body through hormones contained in the blood, not through the nerves. Hitzer, "Healing Emotions," 118–50. Dror affirms that feelings and emotions were "reconceptualized in terms of 'emotional excitement' and its embodied essence of adrenaline." Dror, "Seeing the Blush," 328.

61. Fisher, "Extensions of Theory," 142.

62. About this question, see Dror, "Seeing the Blush."

63. Fisher, "Extensions of Theory," 142.

64. Otniel Dror, "What Is Excitement?," 121–34.

65. Fisher and Cleveland, "Relationship of Body Image," 308.

66. About this question, see Pilar León Sanz, "El carácter terapéutico," 101–30.

67. Fisher and Cleveland, "Relationship of Body Image," 309.

68. Ibid., 308.

69. Porter, *Bodies Politic*, 35. Thomson affirms that, in the second half of the century, a "psychological society" that had a great influence with regard to people imagining themselves as psychological bodies was created. Thomson, "Psychological Body," 303.

70. Fisher and Cleveland, *Body Image*, 391.

71. The question was being studied in several laboratories, which shows the popularity of the field: Ronald Hartley, *A Homonym Word Association Measure of the Barrier Variable and Its Comparison with the Inkblot Barrier Measure* (Seattle: University of Washington, 1964); George R. Jacobson, "Effect of brief sensory deprivation on

field dependence," *Journal Abnormal Psychological* 71 (1966): 115–18; Joyce Constance Morton, *The Relationship between Inkblot Barrier Scores and Sociometric Status in Adolescents* (Vancouver: University of British Columbia, 1964); Cail Cordon, *Developmental Changes in Responses on the Holtzman Ink Blot Technique* (Austin: University of Texas, 1966). See Fisher, *Development and Structure*.

72. Fisher, "Sex Differences."

73. Frevert studies particularly the evolution of the gendering of rage and the historical changes in self-control, question linked with the Fisher and Cleveland's body-image theory. Ute Frevert, "Gendering Emotions," in *Emotions in History: Lost and Found* (Budapest: Central European University Press, 2011), 87–147.

74. Ibid., 145.

75. About this question, see also Lesley A. Hall, "The Sexual Body" in Cooter and Pickstone, *Medicine in the Twentieth Century*, 261–75; Dror, "Seeing the Blush."

76. Jasen, "Malignant Histories," 265–297.

77. For instance, one relatively recent article concludes: "People who are greatly concerned about either aspect of their body image are vulnerable to poorer psychosocial adjustment when confronting treatment for breast cancer." Charles S. Carver, Christina Pozo-Kaderman, Alicia A. Price, Victoria Noriega, Suzanne D. Harris, Robert P. Derhagopian, David S. Robinson, and Frederick L. Moffatt, "Concern about Aspects of Body Image and Adjustment to Early Stage Breast Cancer." *Psychosomatic Medicine* 60 no. 2 (1998): 168–74, esp. 174.

78. Fisher and Cleveland, "Relationship of Body Image."

79. Fisher and Cleveland, *Body image*, 367.

80. For Masling and Ganellen, Fisher and Cleveland's method provided predictions as good, and sometimes even better, than other standard tests as the MMPI. Masling, "Bodies under Investigation," 165; Ronald J. Ganelle, "Comparing the Diagnostic Efficiency of the MMPI, MCMI-II, and Rorschach: A Review," *Journal of Personality Assessment* 67 no. 2 (1996): 219–43. And Jasen adds that "Fisher and Cleveland asked more important and far more interesting questions than is true for much of what is found in today's journals." Jasen, "Malignant Histories," 280.

PART II

Performing Emotional Bodies

This section moves from the history of medicine to the history of photography, examining how bodies performing in front of a camera have turned into emotional bodies. Authors in these chapters explore the performativity of emotions from different points of view: the authority figure of doctors who project ideas on children's bodies in pain, the bodily reactions to photographic technologies such as the magnesium flash, and the family memories raised by a photographic exhibition.

Authors such as Roland Barthes and Susan Sontag have articulated their relationship to photography in emotional terms. In *Camera Lucida*, Barthes's exploration of grief after the death of his mother leads him to understand the essence of photography, the now renowned *ça-a-été* (this-has-been).[1] Sontag also identifies emotions at the core of her first proper meeting with photography. She remembers:

> One's first encounter with the photographic inventory of ultimate horror is a kind of revelation, the prototypically modern revelation: a negative epiphany. For me, it was photographs of Bergen-Belsen and Dachau which I came across by chance in a bookstore in Santa Monica in July 1945. Nothing I have seen—in photographs or in real life—ever cut me as sharply, deeply, instantaneously.... When I looked at those photographs, something broke. Some limit had been reached, and not only that of horror; I felt irrevocably grieved, wounded, but a part of my feelings started to tighten; something went dead, something is still crying.[2]

Sontag has not been the only one to describe the emotional impact that photographs of the Holocaust can have. Marianne Hirsch makes an emotive defense of looking at the horror images of the Holocaust precisely because they "resist the work of mourning."[3] In Hirsch's words, these photographs "can only be confronted again and again, with the same pain, the same incomprehension, the same distortion of the look, the same mortification. And thus, in their repetition, they no longer *represent* Nazi genocide, but they *provoke* the traumatic effect that this history has had on all those who grew up under its shadow."[4] The ways in which photographs provoke emotions in the viewer has been explored in the collective volume *Feeling Photography*, edited by Elspeth Brown and Thy Pu.[5] A central concern in this work, as in chapter 6 of this book, is the question of the creation of photographic meaning by the spectator and the role of affect in this process. Chapters 4 and 5 take a different approach to the analysis of emotions and photography. Following the work of Elizabeth Edwards, among others, the focus of these chapters is not on the image but on the materiality of photography: photographs, cameras, and what people do with them.[6] This perspective allows for an analysis of photographic practices as emotional practices in which emotions are performed in particular contexts and produce particular bodies.

This part continues to examine theories and experiences of emotions, focusing on the means through which embodied emotions are performed. With this aim, the following chapters explore different photographic practices from the nineteenth century to the present day. Underlying is the idea that taking, circulating, sharing, exhibiting, and looking at photographs mobilize emotions through the actions of the body. The emphasis on the history of medicine, while still present, slowly disappears to allow for a comprehensive analysis of how individual bodies perform emotions and emotional expressions through different practices. As a result, these chapters introduce different articulations of the concept "emotional body," from sick children to actors and even academic authors.

In chapter 4, Leticia Fernández-Fontecha explores how competing scientific and medical fields turned children in pain into different kinds of emotional bodies during the late nineteenth century. As in Boddice's case, pain was performative, although in a different sense. While for scientists such as Alfred Genzme and Paul Emil Flechsig, children's insensitivity to pain turned them into an index of evolutionary development, for the emergent pediatrics children's pain turned them into subjects of care. With this aim, hospitals such as Great Ormond Street sold cartes de visite portraying the patients in order to raise funds. During the photographic sessions, children in pain became role models of disciplined behavior. Playing with toys while posing as subjects of good care changed the emotional experience of the sick children and, at least for a while, embodied a different body—that of the playful child.

In chapter 5 Beatriz Pichel further explores the performativity of the photographic act, examining how new theories of the bodily nature of emotions were confirmed by experiments performed on hysterical patients at the Parisian hospital La Salpêtrière and how these findings communicated to nonmedical spheres such as theater through photographic practices. To this end, Pichel traces the production of Albert Londe, medical photographer at the Salpêtrière and pioneer of theatrical photography and artificial lighting. This contribution focuses on the material aspects of emotional bodies, discussing how making gestures in photography became a way to understand the bodily nature of emotions in the late nineteenth century.

Finally, María Rosón explores the relationship between individual and collective bodies in her analysis of the construction of memories through vernacular and artistic photographic practices. The analysis of the photobook *Yolanda* by Spanish photographer Ignacio Navas leads Rosón to examine the performativity of photography in constructing a social type, the "*yonki*" (drug addicts during the 1980s and 1990s), as well as the performativity of emotions. In this chapter, the author becomes an emotional body, as the emotions and memories aroused in her by *Yolanda* made her write this piece of research. In this case, individual emotional bodies (Yolanda, the artist, the author) intertwine with collective bodies (the yonkis and their descendants).

Notes

1. Roland Barthes, *Camera Lucida: Reflections on Photography*, trans. Richard Howard (London: Vintage, 1993). More on this in the conclusion of this volume.

2. Susan Sontag, *On Photography* (New York: Anchor Doubleday, 1989), 19–20.

3. Marianne Hirsch, "Surviving Images: Holocaust Photographs and the Work of Postmemory," *Yale Journal of Criticism* 14, no. 1 (2001): 5–37.

4. Hirsch, "Surviving Images," 28. Original emphasis.

5. Elspeth H. Brown and Thy Pu, eds., *Feeling Photography* (Durham, N.C.: Duke University Press, 2014).

6. Elizabeth Edwards and Jane Hart, eds., *Photographs, Objects, Histories: On the Materiality of Images* (London: Routledge, 2004).

4. The Language of Children's Pain (1870–1900)

LETICIA FERNÁNDEZ-FONTECHA

MENTIONING THE WORDS "children" and "pain" together will evoke for some people Oscar Rejlander's photographs of children crying that Charles Darwin used in *The Expression of the Emotions in Man and Animals* (1872). One of these images—captioned "Mental Distress" in the book but widely known as "Ginx's Baby"—proved very popular, and Rejlander sold 250,000 cartes de visite based on it.[1] The photograph shows what Darwin claimed was the characteristic physiognomy of a baby "weeping or crying": eyes closed "so that the skin round them is wrinkled, and the forehead contracted into a frown," the mouth open with the lips "retracted in a peculiar manner," and the teeth "being more or less exposed." For Darwin, the "violent and prolonged screams" of children were emotional expressions associated with "pain, moderate hunger, or discomfort."[2] But how, in fact, can we know *why* this particular child is crying? Is "Ginx's Baby" a representation of pain, hunger, frustration, or Darwin's "mental distress"? Does this photograph tell us anything from a medical point of view? Many late-nineteenth-century medical professionals would certainly have said that it does.

As a research subject, the child in pain—which combines the previously separate fields of the history of childhood and the history of medicine—has been little investigated by historians.[3] Works that have reviewed the history of childhood pain—written mostly by psychologists—suggest that beliefs about the sensitivity of children and infants underwent huge changes during the second half of the nineteenth century.[4] This article develops Joanna Bourke's argument in *The Story of Pain* that children's pain was subject to a reevaluation that concluded in the first half of the twentieth century with "many scientists and clinicians claiming that infants were almost totally insensible to pain."[5] By developing this line of argument and extending it to the field of the history of pediatrics, this chapter explores how the emotional expression of children's suffering (mainly cries and screams) was interpreted differently by the various professional bodies with the power to shape its meaning.

Two key questions emerge about the *communication of children's pain*. First, are children's expressions of pain and suffering capable of communicating certain states, conditions, and emotions? And, if so, is there a univocal correspondence between expressions and their internal referents that justifies a scientific program of description, classification, and analysis? Anthropologists (or *proto-anthropologists*) tended to frame childhood within an evolutionary perspective—interpreting infant emotions as stages of development in a linear notion of progress—while pediatricians tried to decode the language of children to treat and heal them. The second—more radical—question emerged from the widespread belief that infants are *mechanically programmed* to cry: beyond the communicational use of screams and cries to relate to adults nonverbally, are children capable of *feeling* pain?

This article explores how the nonverbal expression of children's suffering was framed by different research programs, understood from varying theoretical angles, and interpreted differently, depending on which professional body was shaping its meaning. The emerging life sciences, such as embryology and psychology, often claimed children were essentially insensitive to pain, while pediatricians—who faced the practical challenge of diagnosing and treating children—saw screams and cries as proof of the existence of pain and used such expressions to diagnose children's illnesses or injuries. Darwin tried to connect children's expressions to their emotions, while physiologists linked pain to the nervous system. Thus, the child's scream and cry created significantly different "emotional bodies" in pediatric and experimental contexts. To shed light on this issue, it is important to investigate what physiologists, psychologists, doctors, and pediatricians considered to be the causes of pain in children and, where appropriate, to explore their reasons for believing that such pain did not exist.

In addition to scientific sources previously analyzed in published works about infant-pain experiments, this chapter involved an extensive literature search for medical and pediatric publications on infant pain, which began with the Institute of Child Health (University College London) Library Historical Collections on the History of Paediatrics and also included vernacular medical texts. The study of pediatrics textbooks and journal articles can illustrate changes in medical ideas about children's pain and show how these shifts affected popular understanding of the body. With this aim in mind, this chapter examines Great Ormond Street Hospital's cartes de visite that were used in fundraising. Photographs of children in pain—in the laboratory, the sickbed, and the fundraising photograph—are useful tools to unravel the complex social and political meanings of pain.

The Insensible Body

In 1842 Charles Darwin posed for a camera for the first time in an intimate portrait with his eldest son, William—the only known photograph of the naturalist with a member of his family. Five years before this photograph was taken, Darwin had started to make notes about William's development in his "M" and "N" notebooks,[6] later published as "A Biographical Sketch of an Infant" in the journal *Mind*. With the aim of evaluating the child's distinct behaviors and reactions, Darwin differentiated the innate from the acquired, showing that development implied a process of hierarchy, with a gradual increase in behavioral complexity. Darwin—who considered childhood to be the only natural, rather than cultural, stage of life—wove together the polarities of the child as an adult-in-training and the adult as a man of will.

The child's emotional body became pivotal to Darwin's investigations of the universality of expression,[7] and his observations on his son's physical and mental development led to his 1872 publication *The Expression of the Emotions in Man and Animals*. Darwin believed that the child lacked the (adult) human attribute of free will but possessed the instinctive expressions of human beings and the traits they shared with animals.[8] The child's emotional expressions thus illustrated human history. Darwin considered a child's crying or screaming to be central to the expression of human emotions, as it was one of the first expressions to appear and one of the most common. While other habits, such as laughing and weeping, were acquired gradually, "the art of screaming . . . from being of service to infants, has become finely developed from the earliest days."[9] Considered an innate expression, screaming proved ideal for studying the similarities between human and animal behavior. The first photographs of the chapter "Special Expressions of Man: Suffering and Weeping"—which marks the narrative's transition from animals to humans—are of babies screaming and crying, among which the most notable is "Mental Distress" ("Ginx's Baby"), used to illustrate what Darwin claimed was the characteristic physiognomy of a baby "weeping or crying."[10] According to the naturalist, the "violent and prolonged screams" of children were emotional expressions associated with "pain, moderate hunger, or discomfort."[11] Within the context of the evolutionary process, these expressions were seen as reflex actions strengthened by custom and were considered unreliable as indicators of pain.[12] "A Biographical Sketch of an Infant" launched a new field of

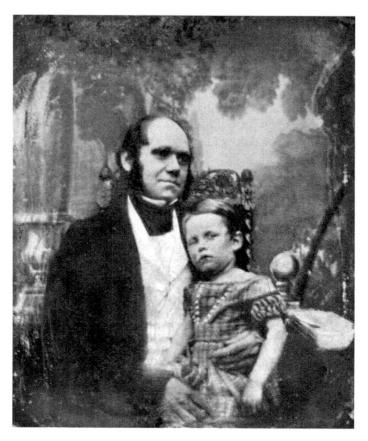

Figure 4.1: "Charles Darwin and William Darwin." Unknown photographer, 1842.

observation and experimentation—the child in his early months—and would ultimately allow a naturalization of experiments involving childhood pain during the so-called "century of the child."[13]

Darwin was one of various authors who saw children's pain (or children's expressions of pain) as a representation of something else—whether the primitive past of the species or the confirmation of a "common sense" superstition. Many nineteenth-century contributions to what would later become infant-pain denial came from Germany, where the growth of university science programs coincided with an interest in the psychophysical and the emergence of experimental physiology. This new physiology sought to understand the nature of the nervous system with an approach based on methodological skepticism and experimental caution.[14] German internist Adolf Kussmaul

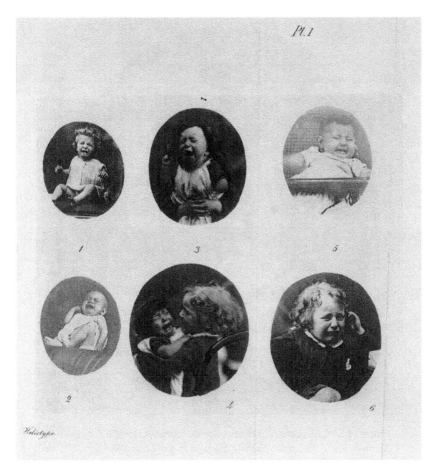

Figure 4.2: "Fold-out plate of weeping children and babies from Chapter VI, Expression of Suffering," photographs by Oscar Reijlander and Herr Kindermann. Charles Darwin, *The Expression of the Emotions in Man and Animals* (London: Murray, 1872). Facing page 148, pl. 1. Wellcome Library, London, General Collections.

(1822–1902) conducted experiments on child behavior, which he wrote up and published as *Untersuchungen über das Seelenleben des Neugeborenen Menschen* (Investigations of the Mental Life of the Newborn Child) in 1859. Kussmaul analyzed the "normal" development of childhood to understand the constitution of the adult mind, and his report on the behavior and sensory repertoire of the newly born can be considered as a work of experimental psychiatry wherein children became a privileged subject for laboratory research.[15] While Darwin's discussions were based on observations that were

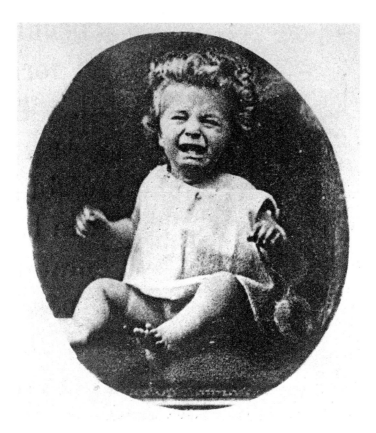

Figure 4.3: "Child crying," photograph by Oscar Reijlander. Charles Darwin, *The Expression of the Emotions in Man and Animals* (London: Murray, 1872). Facing page 148, tab. I, fig. 1. Wellcome Library, London, General Collections.

more incidental than experimental, Kussmaul conducted experiments on the function of the senses, including touch, sensitivity to temperature, smell, vision, hearing, pain, muscular sensitivity, and "air hunger."[16] Unlike the rest of the book, the section on sensitivity to pain did not include experimental results—the children's cries during initial experiments with tartaric acid led him to abandon this approach.

The first to combine Darwin's and Kussmaul's lines of research in an experimental test of infants' pain sensitivity was Alfred Genzmer (1851–1912), who, as a doctoral candidate in medicine and surgery at Halle-Wittenberg University, published *Investigations on the Psychic Function of the Newborn*—a critical study of Kussmaul's work—in 1873.[17] Genzmer deliberately produced pain in children, pricking them with pins in the nose, upper lip, and hands. Even though "small drops of blood oozed from these openings," Genzmer claimed that the children "gave no evidence of discomfort—not even a slight quivering,"[18] although "the wetness of their eyes" increased when the pins were placed in their faces. He concluded that pain was "exceptionally poorly developed in the neonate."[19] Genzmer presented pain as a tool of the experimental method and children as objects of experimentation linked to the investigation of the development of organic functions. His work was continued by disciples, including Traugott Kroner (1854–1899), who in 1882 delivered an inaugural lecture at the University of Breslau on the same subject,[20] and Silvio Calnestrini, whose 1913 experiments on seventy children concluded that infantile touch showed a surprisingly light reaction to painful stimuli and a limited electrical excitability of the nervous system.[21]

This theoretical framework was strengthened by the development of experimental embryology. In 1872 an investigation of children's brains by University of Leipzig psychiatry professor Paul Emil Flechsig found that the myelination of nerve fibers was produced at different rhythms during development, and that while the newly born had both myelinated and unmyelinated fibers, only the former were completely functional. Flechsig concluded that the demyelination of the neonate ensured that sensory stimuli, such as pain, were not completely functional.[22] Genzmer's work remained obscure until it was cited by William Thierry Preyer in an 1889 work that explicitly merged Genzmer's research program with Darwin's theories. The English physiologist William Thierry Preyer's *The Soul of the Child* (1882) drew both on Genzmer's empirical work in physiology and on the baby biographies. Strongly influenced by the theory of evolution, Preyer understood development as a trajectory in which language and assertive action gradually replaced instinct and reflex. Preyer took issue with Genzmer, writing: "It is an error to maintain that the very young child is not yet capable of having the genuine feeling of pain or even a high degree of unpleasant feeling."[23] Noting that his infant son Axel "reacted by movements upon the slightest touches of his face,"[24] Preyer thought that babies showed indications of experiencing pain and declared that it was something "unmistakable for every diligent observer. Above all, crying is characteristic: it is piercing and persistent in pain."[25] Preyer concluded that infants do experience pain (although to a lesser degree than adults), but he shared Darwin's view that their emotional expressions were reflex actions reinforced by habit and were therefore not reliable as markers of pain. Preyer's view of pleasure and pain as a child's basic instincts and his comparison of infants and animals was common currency in the late nineteenth and early twentieth centuries. Originating in Darwinism, this perspective view sought to explain behavior in adaptive terms—attaining pleasure and avoiding pain were assumed to motivate action. Millicent Washburn Shinn wrote, in her 1900 book *The Biography of a Baby*, that her baby "had no experience of skin pain in her early days, and being kept at an equable temperature, probably received no definite sensations either of heat or of cold."[26] Pain was presented as a sensation learned through experience and tied to the evolutionary process and that of self-consciousness. As Claudia Castañeda has indicated, the underlying theme of the baby biographies is not only the individual self but also human nature.[27] The child in pain thus becomes an emotional bodily theater through which human history could be observed. Following the publication of Darwin's *On the Origins of Species* (1859) and the emergence of evolutionary psychology and psychiatry, there were pronounced displacements in the construction of childhood. The enduring popular notion of the child as an animal or savage received an apparent scientific validation in the "recapitulation" theories, which saw in the child a mirror of ancestral forms—both human and animal.

The belief that a child's external features reveal its inner qualities—moral character and intellectual capacity, in particular—emerged during the Enlightenment, and it became possible to consider the child as more than "an object of aesthetic contemplation" and see it also from the perspective of scientific curiosity.[28] During the nineteenth century, evolutionary theories showing the link between humans and animals provoked a change in concepts of human development, which was now seen as a dynamic process rather than a series of static events.[29] From this perspective, children embodied a primitive past and a link to the natural world that could be studied to reveal the processes behind the formation of adult capacities. This approach was notably advocated by George Romanes (1848–1894), a prominent Darwinist and pioneer of comparative psychology. In *Mental Evolution in Man*, Romanes wrote: "The emotional life of animals is so strikingly similar to the emotional life of man—and especially young children—that I think the similarity ought to be taken as direct evidence of a genetic continuity between them."[30] He argued that by studying the "psycho-genesis of a child" it was possible to ascertain if there were a difference in kind between human self-consciousness and the emotions displayed by animals. The child was considered as the perfect embodiment of the concept that "ontology repeats phylogeny"—that each living organism goes through the evolutionary stages of its genus.[31] In the manner of the baby biographies, he took an incident where his own child knocked his head against a table.[32] On asking where he was hurt, the child "immediately touched the part of his head in question—i.e. indicated the painful spot." Now, Romanes asks, "will it be said that in doing this the child was predicating the seat of injury?"[33] If so, he continues, "all the distinctive meaning which belongs to the term predicating . . . is discharged."[34] The "gesture-signs" that are "abundantly employed" by animals would have to be regarded in a similar way because "they differ in no respect from those of the still speechless infant."[35]

The clinical and academic interest in the functioning of reflex actions and the nervous system, the development of the scientific method, and the Darwinist vision of the infant as an inferior primitive being and the child as an adult in training contributed to the development of a mechanistic vision of childhood. Nonetheless, it is surprising how quickly science seemed to abandon its interest in children (and their pain). But all these detailed scientific annotations about the child's first movements and expressions, related to sensation and to pain, did not stem from an interest in the child itself. Instead, the focus was on the child as an index of evolutionary development and as the key to understanding the adult mind and the appearance of self-consciousness. By suggesting that the child's body embodied the animal and the savage, Preyer and Darwin contributed to the naturalization of experiments on children's pain and to its subsequent denial. While these two approaches converged, there is a marked contrast between Darwin's account of the child as the embodiment of the long-lost savage and the scientific practices of Genzmer and Canestrini. By deliberately producing pain in the laboratory—pricking infants with pins in the nose, lips, and hands, for instance—as part of an experimental method that led to infant pain denial, these two scientists ended up creating a very different kind of body: that of the child in pain, with its performative dimension.[36]

The Sick Body

The children's hospitals that emerged in Great Britain in the mid-nineteenth century soon became the primary location of observation and clinical practice involving ill children and the primary source of specialist research that was published in respected journals throughout Europe. The construction of the sick child as an object of study ran parallel to decoding the meaning of infants' gestural language of pain as—in contrast to adults or older children, who could speak—gestures that were all that physicians could rely on. Joanna Bourke has suggested that infantile physiological responses, facial expressions, and paralinguistic vocalizations are a "gestural language"—a form of language that is invaluable for assessing pain.

In 1833, in a review of a pioneering French text about childhood illness, a contributor to *The Lancet* recognized that, despite medicine's general progress, children's illnesses had been ignored or attributed to teething, the presence of worms, or a vague notion of "growth."[37] Although earlier doctors had recognized illnesses that were either very common during childhood or considered exclusive to children, the study of pathologies proper to this period of life developed as a medical specialty—pediatrics—only in the second half of the nineteenth century.[38] The interest of physiology and evolutionary psychology in child development coincided with the aspirations for legitimacy of another professional group: children's doctors. This medical specialism, based on the scientific construction of the child/adult dichotomy, started to organize the care of childhood in more scientific ways, and the first hospitals dedicated exclusively to the care of sick children were created in different European cities. In London, the Royal Hospital for Sick Children, also known as the Great Ormond Street Hospital (GOSH), opened in February 1852 as the first specialist hospital for children in England. Although treated at first with suspicion, the hospital's fame soon began to spread across the whole city.

Five years before Great Ormond Street opened, its founder Charles West delivered a series of lectures to students at the Middlesex Hospital about the illnesses of infants and children,[39] which contained the seeds of his future pediatric practice. West argued that children showed their pain behaviorally and physiologically, providing sufficient proof to be correctly recognized by any decent doctor whose praxis was not based on folklore or ancient forms of diagnosis. Doctors needed to obtain information from the child's expression and behavior, said West, who advised young doctors that while a child might not yet be able to talk, "yet it has a language of its own, and that language must be your object to learn."[40] West compared the children's doctor to an explorer in a country surrounded by inhabitants speaking a foreign language, a metaphor also used by Thomas Rotch, the first chair in pediatrics at Harvard, who told the American Pediatric Society in 1891: "We have entered upon the especial investigation of and research in this branch of anthropology with the keen interests of explorers in an almost unknown country."[41]

West and Rotch were writing as pediatrics consolidated itself as a specialism. With high levels of infant mortality in the cities, it was gradually accepted that the hospitals were an acceptable place for sick children.[42] Their defenders believed that children's hospitals had beneficial effects, both physical and moral. Hospital wards were seen as extensions of middle-class homes, promoting good behavior and making working-class children more respectable,[43] and the pediatrician came to be seen as a healer of the body and trainer of the spirit. By the end of the nineteenth century, pain—seen within the scientific community as little more than a symptom of a disease or injury—was reclaimed for its diagnostic value.[44] In the middle of the century, the Irish doctor Richard Tonson Evanson argued that pain and the expressive gestures that accompanied it were the most direct manner of accessing childhood illness.[45] Doctors such as West and Evanson encouraged the screams and cries of the children because they believed that in promoting the abundance of such signs, they could arrive at a more accurate diagnosis.

This semiotic effort was a specific epistemological tool adopted by the new discipline of pediatrics, and it marked a differentiated approach to the inclusion of pain in a body of scientific knowledge. Toward the end of the nineteenth century, pediatricians embraced the anatomo-clinical tradition and tried to connect signs of pain with organic injuries. Hence, a search for the most systematic tests for pain in children began expanding observations about childhood crying and examining the changes in children's facial expressions or sleeping habits under the effects of illness. The semantics of pain encountered many of the same problems that any scientific analysis of natural language needs to tackle, mainly homonymy (the same sounds having different meanings) and polysemy (the inability to connect each term to a single meaning, and a single meaning to each term), beginning with the polysemy of tears. "Crying is the chief, if not the only means that the young infant possesses of indicating his displeasure, discomfort or suffering," declared the American doctor Louis Starr, who believed that healthy children rarely cried.[46] Although crying seems to be the behavior most often associated with pain, there were debates over whether crying always indicated discomfort, pain, or illness in a child. For this reason, doctors sought to develop a scheme for evaluating children's pain based on different kinds of crying, trying to distinguish cries of pain from those caused by boredom, frustration, or exercising the lungs. Evanson thought that crying that came from acute suffering "is clear, loud, sounding and continuous," belonging more to exhalation than inhalation.[47] The pediatrician also included complementary gestures, such as the position of the eyebrows and the hands, in an attempt to construct an invariable connection between the sign and the anatomic injury. For Starr, the first professor of pediatrics at the University of Pennsylvania Medical School, a direct relationship could be established between different kinds of crying and specific illnesses and degrees of pain. While hydrocephalic crying consisted of a sudden, paroxysmal, and loud crying that implied headache, "loud brazen crying" was a precursor of spasmodic croup, and a child who cried during a coughing fit or soon afterwards was suffering from pneumonia.[48]

The American pediatrician Luther Holt, who was particularly concerned that the pain of infants under two months of age should not be ignored, argued in 1899 that the absence of tears before this time should not be taken as an indication that the young baby did not feel pain. Holt divided children's cries into several functional groups according to whether the cause was hunger, indigestion, temper, weakness, exhaustion, discomfort, pain, or habit. Holt suggested that children suffering extreme pain cried in a sharp and penetrating way, contracting their facial features, raising their legs, and sometimes falling into an exhausted sleep.[49] In his opinion, crying that resulted from less severe pain was more like moaning and less sharp in tone. Ralph Vincent, who founded The Infants' Hospital in Westminster in 1907, also affirmed that crying produced by an intense pain had clear characteristics: "It is sharp and penetrating and is united with the contraction of the extremities and the features." Some lines later he adds: "One of the cries which is often misinterpreted is that which results from the pain of indigestion. The cry itself is not as sharp as in the case of those that result from more intense pains and is closer to that of the cry of hunger."[50] Just as Darwin saw a direct relationship between emotions and their expression, Starr believed that pain was expressed always through the same gestures and expressions. He described the facial expression of childhood pain and indicated how to infer the origin of the pain from these expressions—for instance, "the contraction of the frown denotes headache," the stretching of the nasal cavities indicated chest pain, and "the raising of the upper lip pointed to abdominal pain."[51]

The Performance of Children's Pain

Although Darwin had used photography to support his claim of the universality of most expressions, subsequent pediatric treatises contained few photographs. However, this does not imply that photography was not being used in the field of children's health. It was used in fundraising and other campaigns for specialist children's hospitals and as a support for medical practice. In the early 1870s, GOSH started to use photography in its fundraising, selling cartes de visite featuring photographs of patients.[52] Two well-respected photographic companies—the Stereoscopic Company and Faulkner—were hired to take these images, which presented the hospital as a welcoming place for children, with little indication of medical technology or illness. These photographs show happy children posing for the photographer despite their illnesses and physical limitations. One such photograph portrays Annie Kennet, age three, admitted to the hospital with a diseased knee in spring 1872. She spent more than two months in the hospital before being sent to convalesce but returned to the hospital in the autumn of the same year and had her right leg amputated up to the thigh.[53] Another photograph shows Sydney Jones, admitted on June 13, 1873, whose diseased right

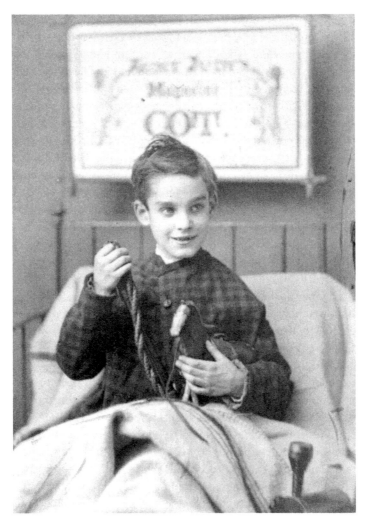

Figure 4.4: *Sidney Jones* (c.1875), Hospital for Sick Children. Photograph by Robert Faulkner and Co. Fundraising Album, Great Ormond Street Hospital for Children NHS Foundation Trust.

knee led doctors to perform a similar amputation.[54] A third image shows Sarah Coulson, who spent a whole year at the hospital, being admitted at six years old, in August 1875, suffering from burns.[55] Although all three children suffered from painful conditions and two of them underwent surgery, there is little visible sign of the pain of their illnesses and the procedures they went through.

The representation of the body in pain had to follow certain codes.[56] As fundraising tools, these images sought to convey a sense of hope to the people who viewed them, especially those who were potential donors. At a time before the expansion of state sponsorship and national healthcare coverage, hospitals and other medical institutions depended on patronage.[57] These images also needed to provide a positive image of recovery, hence the emphasis on the presence of donated toys and their beneficial effect on the child patients.[58] Sydney's portrait presents all these features: the bed suggests a painful condition, while the presence of toys underlines the role of distraction as a coping mechanism in dealing with illness and treatment. The boy's smile transforms the hospital ward from a terrifying place of disease and death into an everyday environment typical of a happy childhood. In a photograph clearly designed to appeal to a middle-class audience, the boy wears a check smock and adopts a pose that echoes Victorian studio portraits of gentlemen. These children came from poor families, and their physical recovery was presented as also involving moral betterment.[59] The photograph—which presents Sydney as the living embodiment of the hospital's civilizing influence—showed how children in pain *should* behave when in pain.

These images were made by Robert Faulkner, known as a specialist in two fields: children's photography and backgrounds. Faulkner's use of graduated backgrounds—a technique he patented and one that was praised by the *British Journal of Photography*—meant that his portraits of sick children resembled his earlier portraits for bourgeois clients, facilitating the identification between patients and potential donors. In addition to the impact of these two techniques in the achievement of the images, there is another important element at play in these photographs by Faulkner: the performance by the children themselves. As other accounts published in the photographic press relate, the best way to photograph children involved playing with them and allowing them to adopt the most comfortable poses.[60] In this context, the toys become not only signs to the viewers of the facilities at the hospital but also traces of the prior play between the photographer and the children. Play adds another layer of meaning to these photographs. It suggests that these pictures were important not only because of their effect on the public but also because of the very act of photography. These photographic sessions were spaces in which children who had not moved from their beds in months could receive attention by engaging with toys and play. In this way, the moment of taking the picture could provide a momentary relief thanks to the privileges it involved. This interpretation of the photographic act is consistent with Faulkner's method. As many articles in the photographic press pointed out, having a portrait taken caused anxiety to many sitters. Hiding the shutter not only avoided distractions but also allowed a more comfortable experience and an easier relationship between the photographer and the photographed person. These photographs thus allow us to reconstruct how photography engaged with medical and scientific debates on the nature of expressions of pain in children. Photographs helped communicate the hospital's aims and construct social meanings of pain through their publication in journals. But besides the photographs, the very act of taking pictures also shaped the child patients' experiences of pain by introducing moments of relief.

Conclusion

The debate about childhood pain highlights an important issue at the place where the history of science and the history of childhood meet: the lack of scientific unity and scientists' reflections on the definition, conceptualization, and treatment of pain. The diversification of knowledge about the human body and its treatment that took place during the nineteenth century and was consolidated in the twentieth century turned pain into an unstable object that was invested with different properties and meanings in each discipline: as the sign of illness, as a symptom of an organic lesion, as a necessary element in the process of learning. The central argument of this chapter is that each of these disciplines used the same symptoms or expressive signs to construct its own figuration of childhood: the savage child, the child without pain, the sick child, the innocent child. The infant-pain research discussed here highlights the importance of thinking of emotions as practices and of pain as kind of political practice.[61] If, as Lucy Bending has shown in *The Representation of Bodily Pain in Late Nineteenth-Century English Culture*, the appropriation of physical pain by different interpretations opens the door to potential abuse by the authorities, then pain is subject not only to cultural conditioning; it is also susceptible to being represented or distorted by those power groups. The infant-pain research presented in this chapter may be seen as a paradigm for the ways in which pain can be manipulated and defined by those in power.

The scientific and pediatric texts used in this chapter demonstrate the lack of unity among scientists at the end of the nineteenth century and the varied renderings of the child emotional body. By understanding development as a trajectory in which language and assertive action gradually replaced instinct and reflex, the scientific texts by Darwin and Romanes show the story of human development. In biographical portraits, the child is presented as a developing body, an example of the "human" that illustrates the history of humanity. In other words, the application of Darwinism to the interpretation of human development throughout each individual's lifespan contributed to the construction of a scientific concept: the idea that children and natural emotions represented earlier stages of human development. In addition, scientific practices not only construct notions, they also constitute pragmatic devices for the generation of knowledge and experimental realities that include bodies. While the textual rendering of the child body produced the instinctual and emotional body, the practices of Gezmer and his followers generated the body of the child in pain.

The application of the scientific method in the late nineteenth century by natural scientists transformed the child into a mechanistic object, an instrument for the discovery of medical and scientific truths. In relation to adults, the mechanistic, natural, and instinctive nature of children often seemed to give permission to suspend the complex philosophical and moral questions related to experimentation with human subjects. The most obvious manifestation of this reduction "ad infantiam" was none other than the recurrent denial of infant pain. While Darwin and Preyer did not subscribe to this belief, their attention to children as a sign of human evolution—rather than as self-sufficient objects of knowledge—and their understanding of crying as a *natural* expression paved the way for later treatment of children as beings incapable of authentic suffering. This, combined with the extreme experimental caution that treated infant expressions of suffering through the skeptical interpretation of reflex actions, provided the conditions for the consolidation of infant-pain denial in scientific practice during the twentieth century.

But while the scientific method transformed the child into a scientific and mechanistic object, pediatricians saw children from the perspective of disease and treated pain communication as the main source of access to the roots of medical problems. In contrast to scientists and psychologists—who saw the child as a fledgling adult—children's doctors recognized the existence of a language of pain specific to childhood. They therefore thus emphasized the gulf between real children and the idea that they were merely men and women in miniature. Doubts about the existence of a "natural language" of gestures that anyone could read were not sufficient to deter the effort to find such a language in the field of pediatrics. Thus, the rights of children in the pediatric world are not based on the right to be treated as future adults but are rather a form of insulation: the child hospital institutionalized and imparted in a physically constructed way the right to be a child and to exist in a space separated from the adult world. Additionally, we cannot forget that healthy children were considered to be a national asset and their health to be that of the country itself.[62] In the Great Ormond Street Hospital photographs the sick child became a discursive category, an object of institutional efforts to return children both to health and to the values of innocence and goodness belonging to the Romantic conception of childhood. But photography did more than record the sick body: the very act of taking pictures, and the performances of courage and play that were enacted during the photographic sessions, also shaped the children's experiences of pain and relief, creating a very different emotional body, that of the playful child.

Notes

1. Jonathan Smith, *Charles Darwin and Victorian Culture* (Cambridge: Cambridge University Press, 2006), 226; Phillip Prodger, "Rejlander, Darwin, and the Evolution of 'Ginx's Baby,'" *History of Photography* 23, no. 3 (1999): 260–68.

2. Charles Darwin, *The Expression of Emotions in Man and Animals* (London: Murray, 1872), 147.

3. Scholars across various disciplines have written numerous works that provide a cultural perspective on pain, of which the following key texts are noteworthy: David Biro, *The Language of Pain: Finding Words, Compassion, and Relief* (New York: Norton, 2010); Sarah Coakley and Kay Kaufman Shelemay, eds., *Pain and Its Transformations: The Interface of Biology and Culture* (Cambridge, Mass.: Harvard University Press, 2007); Esther Cohen, *The Modulated Scream: Pain in Late Medieval Culture* (Chicago: University of Chicago Press, 2010); David B. Morris, *The Culture of Pain* (Berkeley: University of California Press, 1991); Elaine Scarry, *The Body in Pain: The Making and Unmaking of the World* (Oxford: Oxford University Press, 1985); Joanna Bourke, *The Story of Pain: From Prayers to Painkillers* (Oxford: Oxford University Press, 2014); Rod Boddice, ed., *Pain and Emotions in Modern History* (Basingstoke: Palgrave Macmillan, 2014). For a recent literary review on the subject of the sick child, see Hannah Newton, *The Sick Child in Early Modern England, 1580–1720* (Oxford: Oxford University Press, 2012), 1–30.

4. David B. Chamberlain, "Babies Don't Feel Pain: A Century of Denial in Medicine," *Journal of Prenatal and Perinatal Psychology and Health* 14 (1999): 145–68; Patrick McGrath, "Science Is Not Enough: The Modern History of Pediatric Pain," *Journal of Pain*, 152 (2011): 2457–59; E. Pabis, M. Kowalczyk, T. B. Kulik, *Anestezjol Intens Ter* 42 (2010); Anita Unruh, "Voices from the Past: Ancient Views of Pain in Childhood," *Clinical Journal of Pain* 8 (1992): 247–54; Elissa Rodkey and Pillai Riddell, "The Infancy of Infant Pain Research: The Experimental Origins of Infant Pain Denial," *Journal of Pain* 14 (2013): 343.

5. Bourke, *Story of Pain*, 214.

6. Marjorie Lorch and Paula Hellal, "Darwin's 'Natural Science of Babies,'" *Journal of the History of the Neurosciences* 19, no. 2 (2010): 140.

7. Phillip Prodger, *Darwin's Camera* (Oxford: Oxford University Press, 2009), 105; Jonathan Smith, *Charles Darwin and Victorian Culture* (Cambridge: Cambridge University Press, 2006), 226; Prodger, "Rejlander, Darwin."

8. Prodger, *Darwin's Camera*, 105; Jonathan Smith, *Charles Darwin and Victorian*

Culture (Cambridge: Cambridge University Press, 2006), 226; Prodger, "Rejlander, Darwin," 260–68.

9. Charles Darwin, *The Expression of Emotions in Man and Animals* (London: Murray, 1872), 210.

10. Darwin, *Expression of Emotions*, 147.

11. Ibid., 147.

12. Rodkey and Riddell, "Infancy of Infant Pain Research," 343.

13. Ellen Key, *The Century of the Child* (New York: Putnam's, 1909). On theories about children's pain in the first half of the twentieth century, see Leticia Fernández-Fontecha, "Signos, legibilidad y diagnóstico: El problema del dolor en la infancia, 1870–1920," *Cuadernos de Historia Contemporánea* 36 (2014): 89–112.

14. Moscoso, *Pain*, 122.

15. Alfred Kussmaul, *Untersuchungenuber das Seelenleben des Neugeborenen Menschen* (Leipzig: Winter, 1859), cited in Rodkey and Riddell, "Infancy of Infant Pain," 343.

16. Wolfgang G. Bringmann, Norma J. Bringmann, and William D. G. Ballance, "Experimental Approaches to Developmental Psychology before William Preyer," in *Contributions to a History of Developmental Psychology: International William T. Preyer Symposium*, ed. G. Eckardt, W. G. Bringmann, and L. Sprung (Berlin: Mouton, 1985), 159–60.

17. Alfred Genzmer, *Untersuchugen Ueber die Sinneswahrhehumugen des Neugeborenen Menschen, Inaugural Dissertation* (Halle: Plötzche, 1873).

18. Ibid., 12. Cited in Rodkey and Riddell, "Infancy of Infant Pain," 344.

19. Ibid., 22. Cited in Rodkey and Riddell, "Infancy of Infant Pain," 344.

20. Kroner, Traugott, "Uber die sinnesempfindungen der neugeborenen," Separat-Abzug aus der Breslauer arztl. Zt., No. 4 (1882): 14. Cited in Florence Maater, *Child Behavior: A Critical and Experimental Study of Young Children by the Method of Conditioned Reflexes* (Boston: Gorham, 1918), 20.

21. Maater, *Child Behavior*, 20.

22. Paul Flechsig's work, summarized by Frederick W. Mott, can be found in "Cerebral Development and Function," *British Medical Journal* 1.3145 (April 9, 1921): 529. Cited in Bourke, *Story of Pain*, 216.

23. William Preyer, *The Mind of the Child: The Development of the Intellect* (New York: Arno, 1889), 147.

24. Ibid., 105.

25. Ibid., 147.

26. Millicent Shinn, *The Biography of a Baby* (Boston: Houghton Mifflin, 1900), 47.

27. Claudia Castañeda, *Figurations: Child, Bodies, Worlds* (Durham, N.C.: Duke University Press, 2002), 13.

28. James Sully, *Studies of Childhood* (London: Longmans, Green, 1896), 10. Stephanie Olsen has written about James Sully in the context of emotional education and masculinity. See Olsen, *Juvenile Nation: Youth, Emotions and the Making of the Modern British Citizen, 1880–1914* (New York: Bloomsbury Academic, 2014), 159.

29. Michael Wertheimer, "The Evolution of the Concept of Development in the History of Psychology," in Eckardt, Bringmann, and Sprung, *International William T. Preyer Symposium*, 13–26.

30. George Romanes, *Mental Evolution in Man: Origin of Human Faculty* (London: Kegan Paul, 1888), 7.

31. Carolyn Steedman, *Strange Dislocations: Childhood and the Idea of Human Interiority, 1780–1930* (London: Virago, 1995), 83.

32. For Romanes's experiments with his child and the chimpanzee, see Rob Boddice, "Vivisecting Major: A Victorian Gentleman Scientist Defends Animal Experimentation, 1876–1885," *Isis* 102, no. 2 (2011): 215–37.

33. Romanes, *Mental Evolution in Man*, 324

34. Ibid., 324

35. Ibid., 324

36. For recent discussions on pain as a kind of practice, see Dolores Martín Moruno, "Pain as Practice in Paolo Mantegazza's Science of Emotions," *Osiris*, 31 no. 1 (2016): 137–68; In a similar line, historian Joanna Bourke has described pain as "a type of event": Bourke, *Story of Pain*, 5–9.

37. *The Lancet*, 1833–34, no. 1 (1824): 367.

38. On the history of paediatrics, see A. R. Colón and P. A. Colón, *Nurturing Children: A History of Pediatrics* (Westport, Conn.: Greenwood,1999); F. Garrison and A. Abt, *Abt-Garrison History of Paediatrics, with New Chapters on the History of Paediatrics in Recent Times* (Philadelphia: Saunders, 1965).

39. Charles West, *Lectures on the Diseases of Infancy and Childhood* (London: Longman, Brown, Green, and Longmans, 1852).

40. Ibid., 1–3.

41. Thomas Rotch, "Iconoclasm and Original Thought in the Study of Pediatrics," *Archives of Pediatrics* 7 (1891): 811.

42. M. J. Daunton, "Health and Housing in Victorian London," *Medical History* Supplement 11 (1991): 126.

43. Andrea Tanner, "Too Many Mothers? Female Roles in Metropolitan Victorian Children's Hospital," in John Henderson, Peregrine Horden, and Alessandro Pastore, eds., *The Impact of Hospitals* (Oxford: Peter Lang, 2007), 136. See also Andrea Tanner, "Choice and the Children's Hospital: Great Ormond Street Hospital Patients and Their Families, 1855–1900," in *Medicine, Charity and Mutual Aid: The Consumption of Health and Welfare in Britain, c. 1550–1950*, ed. Anne Borsay and Peter Shapely (Aldershot, U.K.: Ashgate, 2007), 141.

44. See Louise Hide, Joanna Bourke, and Carmen Mangion, "Perspectives on Pain: Introduction," *19: Interdisciplinary Studies in the Long Nineteenth Century* 15 (2012): 5; Lucy Bending, "Pain and Religion in the Victorian Era," in *Pain: Passion, Compassion, Sensibility*, ed. Javier Moscoso (London: Wellcome Trust, 2004), vi–5.

45. Richard Tonson Evanson, *A Practical Treatise on the Management and Diseases of Children* (London: Fannin / Dublin, Renshaw and Longman, 1842), 63.

46. Louis Starr, "The Clinical Investigation of Disease and the General Manage-

ment of Children," in *An American Text-Book of the Diseases of Children*, ed. Louis Starr and T. S. Westcott (Philadelphia: Saunders, 1895), 3.

47. Evanson, *Practical Treatise*, 108.

48. Starr, "Clinical Investigation," 6.

49. Luther Emmett Holt, *The Diseases of Infancy and Childhood: For the Use of Students and Practitioners of Medicine* (New York: Appleton, 1899), 1–45.

50. Ralph Vincent, *The Nutrition of the Infant*, 4th ed. (London: Bailliere, Tindall and Cox, 1913), 198.

51. Starr, "Clinical Investigation," 3–4.

52. Andrea Tanner and Sue Hawkins, "The Sentimental Hard Sell: The Role of Early Patient Photography at Great Ormond Street Hospital," Society for the Social History of Medicine Conference, Durham University, July 2010. Unpublished paper.

53. Great Ormond Street Hospital GOS/9/1/2; GOS/9/1/3, Hospital's General Admissions Registers, 1865–1872, 1872–1878.

54. Great Ormond Street Hospital GOS/9/1/2; GOS/9/1/3, Hospital's General Admissions Registers, 1865–1872, 1872–1878.

55. Great Ormond Street Hospital GOS/9/1/2; GOS/9/1/3, Hospital's General Admissions Registers, 1865–1872, 1872–1878.

56. For a discussion on representations of pain, see Bourke, "The Sensible and Insensible body: A Visual Essay" *19, Interdisciplinary Studies in the Long Nineteenth Century* 15 (2012): 15.

57. See Tanner, "Too Many Mothers?," 135, 64.

58. Gatty, Alfred, ed., "Report of the 'Aunt Judy's Magazine Cots' at the Great Ormond Street Children's Hospital," in *Aunt Judy's Christmas Volume for Young People* 8 (London: Bell and Daldy, 1870).

59. Katharina Boehm, *Charles Dickens and the Sciences of Childhood: Popular Medicine, Child Health, and Victorian Culture* (London: Palgrave Macmillan, 2013), 99.

60. "Lady Amateur," "How I Photograph My Little Ones," *British Journal of Photography*, March 28, 1872, 146–47.

61. See Mario Biagoli and Peter Galison, *The Disunity of Science: Boundaries, Contexts, and Power* (Stanford, Calif.: Stanford University Press, 1996), 1–37.

62. For example, see: Bernard Harris, *The Health of the Schoolchild: A History of the School Medical Service in England and Wales* (Buckingham: Open University Press, 1995); Deborah Dwork, *War Is Good for Babies and Other Young Children: A History of the Infant and Child Welfare Movement in England, 1898–1988* (London: Tavistock, 1987); Anna Davin, "Imperialism and Motherhood," *History Workshop Journal* 5 (1978): 9–65; and Harry Hendrick, "Child Labour, Medical Capital, and the School Medical Service, c. 1890–1918," in *In the Name of the Child*, ed. Roger Cooter (London: Routledge, 1992), 45–71.

5. Photographing the Emotional Body

Performing Expressions in the Theater and the Psychological Sciences

BEATRIZ PICHEL

Oh! que de beaux gestes perdus, évanouis!
Que reste-t-il d'un geste?
—Francisque Sarcey, "Le théâtre instantané," 1898

IN JANUARY 1898 the first issue of *Le Théâtre* came out. Like many other magazines, it covered some of the most important plays in national and international stages and published pieces on actors, clothing, and fashion.[1] But *Le Théâtre* aimed at being unique and thus accompanied all its articles with photographs of actors and scenes, including two full pages of color photographs, one of them always on the front cover. The overwhelming presence of photography in the magazine indicates that the images were not mere illustrations but were central to the communication of the information. The prominence of the visual over the textual was not only an aesthetic choice but also the result of what the articles were intended to convey: the actors' performances.

The French journalist Francisque Sarcey dedicated the editorial of the first issue of *Le Théâtre* to this topic. Sarcey defended that the actors' gestural skills were their most valuable patrimony. To illustrate this point, he put as an example the most renowned actress in France at the time, Sarah Bernhardt, who had been characterized by the poet Edmond Rostand as "the queen of the attitude, and the princess of gestures."[2] Sarcey regretted that her performances would not be properly remembered. Unlike the inflexion of the voice, gestures were of a fleeting nature, and therefore the audience was not able to keep good memories of them. Sarcey was not alone in voicing concerns about preserving and understanding the actors' gestures. Around the same time, authors such as Alfred Giraudet and Charles Aubert published acting treatises aimed at teaching actors how to express emotions onstage.[3] In the discussion around the nature of emotional expressions, Aubert referenced the works of Charles Bell and Darwin, who had published *The Expression of Emotions in Man and Animals* some years earlier.[4] In it, Darwin complained, just as Sarcey had, that the study of emotional expressions was difficult because these only lasted for a few instants. Both Sarcey and Darwin found in photography the best tool to capture those gestures and attitudes in "faithful plates."[5] Photography helped scientists such as Darwin to study expressions and helped spectators to remember what they had seen.

Sarcey continued his article suggesting that *Le Théâtre* would create a photographic archive that would allow future generations to learn the stock of conventional gestures common around 1900. According to him, the actors' acting style had changed over time, and comedy and tragedy had not always been expressed through the same means. In fact, Sarcey admitted that some gestures could be considered ridiculous by later generations, while they were perfectly adequate by the standards of the time. But photographs captured those gestures, which allowed keeping a record of changes in the performance's style.[6] Photographs thus enabled a history of gestures.

This chapter takes up this idea, asking which kind of history of gestures we can do by examining photographic sources. While expressions have often been examined in the history of emotions, less has been written about the photographic construction of gestures.[7] I argue that photography became a central device in the understanding of embodied expressions of emotions. Photographs served scientists and laypeople in grasping the gestures' *meaning*—that is, the emotions that they were supposed to communicate—as well as their *materiality*, the nervous and muscular processes that produced them. Both questions, as this chapter shows, permeated scientific and artistic life in France in the late nineteenth century.

To examine how photography constructed the meaning and materiality of gestures, I focus on the production of the photographer Albert Londe around 1890. Hired in 1882 as a chemist at the laboratory of the Parisian hospital La Salpêtrière, Londe became the chief of the photographic service two years later and served as one of the editors of the famous journal *Nouvelle iconographie de la Salpêtrière* in 1888.[8] As a result, Londe specialized in medical photography and published *La photographie médicale*, one of the first treatises on this matter, in 1893.[9] This book covered a broad range of aspects of photographic practices at the hospital, from the installation of the laboratory to the diversity of technologies available. *La photographie médicale* was richly illustrated with some of his most renowned photographs, such as the series taken in 1891 that recorded the expressions produced by the sensorial excitation of hysterical patients under hypnosis, and the chronophotographs he took for Paul Richer's studies on the physiology of movement in 1893.[10]

Londe's interests, however, went well beyond the medical realm. He was an active member of the Société Française de la Photographie, where he often presented his technological innovations, and president of the Société d'excursionistes amateurs de photographie.[11] Among his projects outside La Salpêtrière, his efforts in the development of artificial lighting and indoor photography stand out.[12] Particularly relevant for the purposes of this book are the series of stereoscopic photographs of the representations of the pantomimes *Jeanne d'Arc* and *Néron* he took at the Parisian Hippodrome de L'Alma in 1890 and 1891.[13]

A common thread in Londe's three projects (medical photography, chronophotography, and theatrical photography) is a shared concern regarding the reproduction and production of gestures. Hysterical patients, models of physiological studies, and theatrical actors had in common the performance of emotional gestures in front of the camera. Scholars such as Georges Didi-Huberman, Rae Beth Gordon, and others have already established parallels between hysterical and theatrical performances in the Parisian fin de-siècle, and, in this volume, Rob Boddice has examined the performativity of pain in hysterical attacks.[14] As a consequence, some have described hysteria as a performative disease.[15]

This chapter takes a different tack, discussing the performativity of photographic practices through the lens of new materialism, following Karen Barad's feminist approach. As the introduction to this volume has explained, Barad understands bodies as processes of materialization whose boundaries depend on the scales of observation.[16] What we call "emotional bodies" are, in this sense, the result of a particular configuration of matter in which emotions are a driving force. In this chapter I combine nineteenth-century understandings of emotions as bodily dispositions (and therefore, *material*) and, following Barad, emotions as *processes of materialization*. My case study will show that photography offers a privileged perspective to examine this issue. As previously mentioned, Londe's photographic sessions were intended to understand the meaning and nature of emotional expressions. The repetition of photographic images, as well as the repeated enactment of gestures in front of the camera, had, therefore, performative effects on the patients' and actors' bodies. In Londe's practice, photography was an act of intervention that had material effects on the photographed person. Photographic practices became, in this sense, performative practices that articulated emotional bodies.

Experimenting with Hypnosis at the Salpêtière

Photography had been a usual activity at the Salpêtrière since the 1870s, when Jean-Martin Charcot started to collaborate with *Revue photographique des hospitaux de Paris* (1896–1872), the first medical journal illustrated with photographs, and founded the renowned *Iconographie photographique de la Salpêtrière* (1875–1880). The Salpêtrière also hosted a museum of pathology and opened the first photographic service in 1879.[17] The fact that the successive photographic laboratories were always publicly funded indicates Charcot's power among French authorities as well as an increasing institutional—and governmental—interest in photography. Charcot's clinic, therefore, became not only the main place to study and treat hysteria; it was also, by virtue of the key role images and visual objects played in the making and dissemination of knowledge, turned into a role model for modern institutions at the end of the nineteenth century.[18]

Albert Londe became the most prolific photographer at the Salpêtrière, although he was neither the first nor the only one. Before him, Paul Regnard, Bourneville, and Loreau had been in charge of photographing the patients' attacks of *grande hystérie*.[19] Theirs are the famous images of Augustine's *attitudes passionnelles*, where she represents ecstasy, eroticism, or amorous supplication in her bed, only dressed in her white nightdress.[20] These photographs were later collected and reproduced by Paul Richer, who made a synoptic table of drawings that classified the different stages of the hysterical attack.[21]

By 1890 clinicians had lost interest in this classification. Gilles de la Tourette, Georges Guinon, and Richer himself had turned their attention to nervous disorders associated to hysteria or not, and the possibilities of hypnosis as a method of research and treatment. Photographic practices had also changed. Londe had systematized the photographic procedures, so patients were not photographed outdoors or in their rooms anymore but at the photographic studio instead.[22] All the elements of his studio, including its size, orientation, stage, color of background, cameras, and development techniques, were measured and calculated with precision. Londe's aim was to produce images that not only represented faithfully the condition of the patients but also allowed easy comparison among them.[23]

Figure 5.1 is an example of this photographic enterprise.[24] The four photographs of the series depict the experiments that Guinon and Sophie Woltke

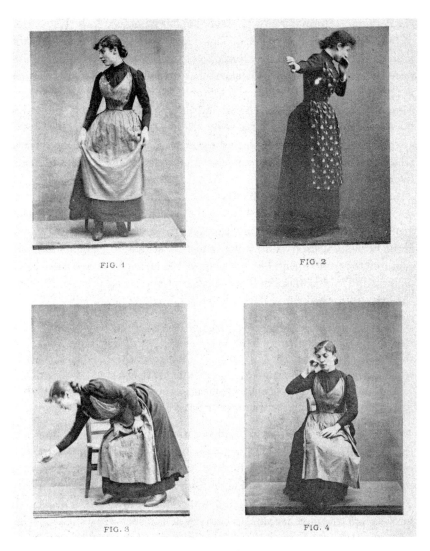

Figure 5.1: "Suggestions par le sens dans la période cataleptique du grand hypnotisme," pl. IX. *Nouvelle Iconographie de la Salpêtrière* 4 (1891). Photographs by Albert Londe. Wellcome Images.

(d'Odessa) carried out at the Salpêtrière in 1891. They aimed to test the excitability of hysterical patients during the cataleptic phase of the hypnotic sleep. With this aim, they stimulated the women's senses of vision, smell, touch, and hearing. One year later, Guinon and Woltke published their results in the article "On the Influence of Sensitive and Sensorial Excitations in the

Cataleptic and Somnambulist Phases of Major Hypnotism," which appeared in the *Nouvelle Iconographie de la Salpêtrière*.[25] In line with the spirit of the journal, the article included sixteen photographs of the experiments, reproduced in four separate plates, all taken by Albert Londe.[26] Although the article accounted three cases, all the photographs reproduced the same patient: Mme *Schey . . .*, a twenty-three-year-old woman who had been admitted at the Salpêtrière in 1886.[27] In these years, she had suffered from all the typical symptoms related to hysteria, such as paralyses, deliriums, and contractures, which made her the perfect patient to explore the characteristics of major hypnotism.

In the article, Guinon and Woltke described the reaction of the patient to stimulus such as a red glass. In this case, they explained, "the face immediately acquires the expression of [great] fear. Her arms go up and her eyes, looking at the horizon, seem to contemplate a terrible spectacle."[28] The photograph captured the woman with her arms raised and an apparent lost gaze. Later, Guinon and Woltke described the satisfaction the young woman felt when she was approached with a dark green glass. They reported:

> She smiles and does a gesture of satisfaction. She brings her hand close to her nose and smells a flower she holds in her fingers. She then puts it in a button of her corset. She gets out of the chair where she was sitting and looks down around her. Then she bends out, strips off with her right hand a flower within some distance from the floor, in an imaginary bush, and passes it to her left hand. . . . She will start this little scene again if we do not stop her.[29]

The article included two photographs of the woman, one scene of her collecting the imaginary flowers and another of her smelling them. In the first image, the hand appears a bit blurred, which served to indicate that the patient was actually moving and not posing for the photograph. For its part, the stimulation of the ear by making noises similar to a ringing bell "made her very sad. She puts her hand over the eyes, as if she were someone crying or praying. She obviously attends a funeral or a sad event at the church."[30]

However, not all the sensorial excitations led to meaningful reactions. For instance, the excitation of the skin by means of stings provoked a "banal movement that does not say anything about what happens in the brain."[31] In the picture, the reader could see the same woman with a different dress doing a side gesture with her arms and upper half body. Guinon and Woltke also explained that the three patients experienced different effects to the same stimulus. The blue glass provoked in *Schey . . .* such that "she raise[s] her eyes to the sky, join[s] her hands in the air, like in the attitude of the prayer, and ends up kneeling down," as evoked in the two photographs that illustrated this case.[32] However, the blue glass made the other two patients frown and provoked the physiognomy of sadness in *Witt . . .* and an expression of disgust in *Cless. . . .*[33] This discrepancy proved, according to the clinicians, that the responses to the stimulus depended on the memories, the "psychic substratum," and the personality of the patients.[34] Reactions were different, therefore, because each patient was different.

Londe, Guinon, and Woltke were not the only ones doing this kind of experiment. Since the 1880s scientists had been examining how the excitation of the senses and the muscles of hysterical patients produced emotional expressions. The aims and the instruments varied from one case to the other, but photography was often part of the experiment. In 1881, Charcot and Richer were the first to publish in *Archives de neurologie*, a series of articles on the hyperexcitability of the muscles of hysterical patients.[35] The piece included several photographs taken by Loreau, which showed Charcot and Richer pressing stings on the patient's face. This pressure produced muscular contractions that resembled emotional expressions. Three years later, in 1884, Richer reinterpreted these experiments in the light of Duchenne de Boulogne's experiences on the faradization of facial muscles.[36] He applied electricity to certain points of the face of the patient that provoked facial expression accompanied by bodily gestures, while Londe was taking the photographs.[37]

Outside the Salpêtrière, others replicated these experiments. In 1890 Jules Bernard Luys, a controversial doctor, published *Hypnotisme expérimental: Les émotions dans l'état d'hypnotisme.*[38] In this book, Luys tested the remote action of different scents and liquids, such as water and cognac, in the experimental induction of emotions in hypnotized patients. He also photographed some of the experiences, focusing on the face of the patient. In 1891 Albert Pitres, a Charcot's student working in Bordeaux, published his lessons on hysteria and hypnotism.[39] At the end of the second volume, Pitres included some case studies of particular individuals, such as Marie Louise. He examined the hypnotic suggestions that provoked the excitation of her facial muscles or the doctor moving her arms, for instance. Fernand Panajou, chief of the photographic service at the Faculty of Medicine, took a series of photographs that depicted two crystal batons pressing on particular points of the face, provoking expressions of laughter, sadness, and contempt.

This kind of research was not limited, however, to the field of hypnosis. As will be explained later, the Salpêtrière circle considered hysteria and hypnosis as two related phenomena. This is why, in 1891, Guinon and Woltke complemented their previous experiments with research on the sensory and sensitive excitability of patients during the phase of *attitudes passionnelles.*[40]

The aim was to demonstrate that the hallucinatory state in which the patients were plunged was independent from the doctors' will but could be modified through sensorial excitation—exactly as it happened during the cataleptic sleep. Inspired by the experiences of Dr. Motchoutkowsky (d'Odessa), Guinon and Woltke performed their own version of the experiment at the Salpêtrière. They again approached Mme. *Schey* . . . (one of the patients examined before, during the hysterical delirium) with colored glasses and scents.[41] Her reactions to ether, chloroform, a blue glass, and perfume provoked the same set of gestures, although in other cases the gestures changed.

All these experiments were intended to shed light on the nature of hysteria and hypnoses. Unlike the Nancy School, the Paris—Salpêtrière School argued that hypnotism could only be practiced on hysterical subjects.[42] Understanding hypnosis and hysteria under the same theoretical framework led doctors to consider hypnosis as a neurological disorder. They denied, therefore, that patients could act by mental suggestion. In their experiments, the transmission of the stimulus by approaching the patient with colored glasses or making noises proved that hypnosis worked through the manipulation of the body. Not only was the hypnosis achieved by pressing the muscles or approaching the hysterical women with colored glasses; all the reactions that happened during hypnosis were nervous responses.

These experiments contributed to understanding, therefore, the materiality of bodily expressions of emotions. At the core of the research on hypnosis and the hyperexcitability of the muscles, the fundamental question was the eventual correlation between *doing* gestures and *feeling* the corresponding emotions. These experiments asked whether the production of gestures provoked real emotions in the patients.

The Performativity of Medical Photographs and Experiments

These questions reflected contemporary concerns about the bodily roots of emotions. As Thomas Dixon and others have argued, a major shift happened during the second half of the nineteenth century.[43] The emergence of scientific psychology, based on the discoveries of physiology, promoted understanding emotions as bodily process rather than attributes of the soul. In France, Théodule Ribot, the main proponent of scientific psychology in France, also wrote in these years that feelings, passions, and emotions were the result of bodily changes in our needs and instincts, rather than the consequence of intellectual states.[44] According to Ribot, the essential elements of the affective life were desires, tendencies, needs, instincts, and inclinations, which manifested externally through gestures, attitudes, modifications of the voice, blush, paleness, trembling, and secretions.[45] This denial of the primacy of ideas in the emergence of feelings meant that psychologists started to consider bodily changes and movements not as mere reactions but as the essential component of emotions.

It is not surprising, therefore, that this debate permeated the experiments carried out at the Salpêtrière. Ribot was a regular attendant of Charcot's lessons (he was portrayed in the famous painting "Une leçon Clinique à la Salpêtrière" by André Bruillet—see figure 1.2 in chapter 1 of this book), they both founded the Société de Psychologie Physiologique in 1885 and were prominent figures at the first international conference of physiological psychology, held in Paris in 1889.[46] Although their work was different in many aspects, they shared concerns regarding the relationship between the body, the affective life, and mental states.

Charcot and Richer had argued in the mid-1880s that the production of gestures did not lead the subject to feel the related emotions. The results of the cardiograph and the pneumograph, they said, showed that there were no internal changes related to the stimulation of facial and bodily nerves.[47] This position coincided with the thesis defended by Duchenne de Boulogne, who denied in his *Méchanisme de la physiognomie humanie* (1862) that acting at the muscular level could have any effect on the passions of the subject.[48] But the 1890s brought about a change in this view. Pitres and Luys explicitly argued that the manipulation of the body of the patient led her/him to actually feel emotions. Pitres observed that "the contraction of the muscles has an immediate effect on the subject's intelligence, and provokes in his spirit ideas, *feelings* and other hallucinations according to expressions on his face."[49]

Guinon and Woltke never wrote such a categorical sentence, but their articles suggest a position closer to Pitres than to Charcot, Richer, and Duchenne. "The sensorial excitations," they noted, "are perceived by the subject and provoke her suggestions, which she communicates through perfectly appropriate mimicry and expressions."[50] They recognized that the patient was actually feeling what she was expressing. Following this interpretation, gestures had a twofold function: they were, at the same time, the effect of the sensorial manipulation and the external sign of the suggested hallucination. Therefore, in line with what Ribot defended, Guinon and Woltke's and Pitres's experiments proved that feelings were the result of a bodily change. These experiments were, in this regard, performative. The excitement of their senses provoked sensations in the patients, but it was the *doing* of the gesture what made the patient feel particular emotions, such as fear or sadness. As mentioned before, Guinon and Woltke deemed some bodily movements "banal" because they did not reveal what was happening in the brain. Doctors needed, therefore, recognizable gestures in order to access the internal life of the patients. Without these gestures there were no emotions, only muscular and physical reactions. The experiments, therefore, combined questions on the materiality and the meaning of emotional expressions.

In order to prove the theory of the bodily roots of emotions, doctors needed to demonstrate that the subject had reacted in particular ways to each stimulus and that these reactions corresponded with the memories she had of the hallucination. Photographs became the essential evidence in this process. Doctors took notes of the patients' recollections of their hallucinatory dreams, as well as photographs of the gestures they performed, so they could compare both accounts later. But photographs did not work exactly as written records did. In *La photographie médicale*, Londe explained that

> there is no doubt that some diseases modify the organism in the same way in different individuals. However, these characteristic modifications can escape even the most skilled eye if the observations are isolated from one another—although this does not happen if we collect a certain number of them. Thanks to photography, we can achieve this result by collecting similar prints. By doing this, we will come to recognize that these changes, which are not particularly prominent by themselves, have on the contrary a very high value from the point of view of the condition.[51]

While written descriptions of the patient depended on the subjective eye of the doctor, who decided what was relevant to record, the photographic plate recorded everything that was posing in front of the camera. For nineteenth-century photography critics, this property was an ambivalent feature. For some it was a cumbersome, as the lack of a selective focus meant that all details, relevant or not, would be included in the image. But for others like Londe, this was the real value of photography.[52] By recording everything and not only the intended details, one could discover things that might have escaped the informed eye. Images allowed the doctor to see different patients at the same time and fixed the position of the patient, so it could be carefully examined. Moreover, the photographic procedures Londe implemented meant that doctors could also compare these images among them, as all the photographs had been taken under the same conditions. This comparison was essential to determine that some attitudes were not part of the patient's idiosyncrasy but a symptom of the disease. Photographs constructed these attitudes as *symptoms*.

Londe used photographs like those in figure 5.1 precisely to capture the unnoticed symptoms of hysteria. All the images show the same space, recognizable by the chair, the background, and the stage. The clothes of the patient reveal that the photographic sessions had taken place in different days, but the perspective and the distance to the women was the same. The photographs printed in the journal were also of the same size. The standardization of these elements guaranteed that gestures could be easily compared. Photographic images, therefore, became an essential aid for the doctors to determine if the bodily movement revealed what was going on in the brain of the patients, in which case the gesture was classified as pathological. This is important because the gestures performed by the patient did not present anything special: they were not pathological in themselves. They became pathological because they appeared in medical photographs that identified them as such. Photographs functioned, therefore, as performative devices, as the repetitive comparison of these photographs created new entities: the gestures as symptoms of hysteria.

Photographing Actors

As mentioned before, Londe also engaged with nonmedical photographic projects outside La Salpêtrière during the 1890s. Together with other photographers who belonged to the Société Française de la Photographie, he endeavored to take photographs of onstage theatrical performances. The photography of actors had been a consolidated business at least since renowned photographers such as Nadar took the portraits of famous actresses like Sarah Bernhardt. In these photographs, actors would pose dressed as the character they were playing at the time, holding objects and doing gestures that were recognizable by the audience. These images were displayed on the windows of the photographic studios, printed as cartes-de-visite that people could buy at popular prices, and published in illustrated magazines such as the abovementioned *Le Théâtre*.[53]

By the end of the nineteenth century, theatrical photography had benefited from innovations such as color. However, capturing actors while they were performing onstage still presented a challenge. Recording this movement required very short exposure times, highly sensitive emulsions, and, more important, a good source of light. Photographing actors became a scientific and technical problem discussed in the pages of scientific journals such as *La Nature*, which included the special section on "Science in Theater." In 1888 G. Mareschal dedicated one of his articles to the photographs that M. Balagny had taken at the Théâtre du Châtelet in Paris during the representation of *Chatte Blanche*.[54] Thanks to the electric lighting of this theater, Balagny had managed to take six photographs of the main tableaux during the performance, with exposure times as short as a quarter of a second. Mareschal claimed that these were the first photographs to show actors without holding their poses. Like Sarcey at the beginning of this chapter, he recognized the potential value of these images as sources for the history of theater.[55]

Balagny's success depended on the artificial lighting of the theater and the use of a particularly sensitive paper he had developed. However, not all theaters in Paris had electric lighting. Photographers like Londe started then to experiment with different kinds of flash in an attempt to illuminate the stage only during the instant in which the photograph was taken. He specialized in the development of magnesium powder, which he applied to the photography of the pantomimes *Néron* and *Jeanne d'arc* in 1891, both performed at the Parisian Hippodrome de l'Alma.[56] The hippodrome's stage was circular, which was problematic from the point of view of the scenery, as it meant that the public completely surrounded the stage. Hippolyte Houcke, director of the venue, therefore invented a new system: a metallic web that, depending on the light, was invisible for the spectator or reflected the painted scenery.[57] Londe not only took a photograph of this system but also wrote a piece for *La Nature* on the subject.[58] Surprisingly, he did not mention his own photographic work in the article but only later in his book *La photographie à la lumière artificielle*, published in 1914.[59] Taking advantage of the ninety-meters length of the hippodrome, Londe placed white targets every ten meters. In the first one he put the magnesium powder, in the second the photographic camera, and, at the end, another camera that would record the magnesium lighting. He then made several tries with different magnesium loads to calculate the quantity he needed to capture the more distant targets and how far the system could reach. He concluded that the farthest targets the light could reach were at forty meters and that beyond sixteen grams of magnesium the improvement was negligible.[60]

The outcome of these experiments was a series of photographs of the main scenes and characters of the plays (figures 5.2 and 5.3). The images portrayed Britannicus, Agrippine, Neron, the Roman soldiers and the lions of Neron, as well as Joan of Arc being taken to torture, praying, brandishing a sword, or waving the French flag.[61] In line with the tradition of the pantomime, actors performed very expressive gestures to play their characters.[62] The portraits of Joan of Arc in scenes like figure 5.3 were emotionally loaded. Like the images published in *Le Théâtre* and *La Nature* just discussed, Londe's photographs were published in illustrated magazines such as *Photo-Journal* to accompany the critique of the play.[63] Although the text did not mention Londe's experiments in photographing at the hippodrome, the independent character of the photographs was affirmed. They were printed on a separate page, and preserved their stereoscopic form.

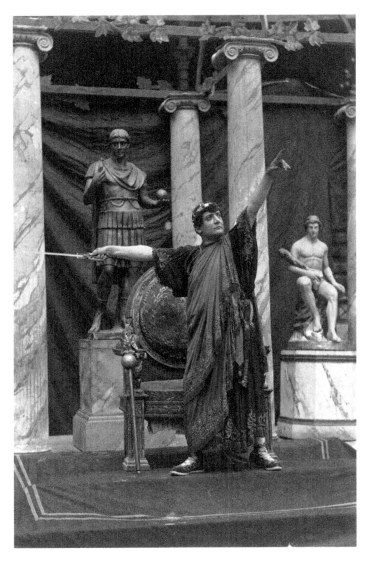

Figure 5.2: "Néron levant le bras au ciel" (Neron raises his arms towards the sky), RF MO PHO 2014 2 240, Hippodrome de l'Alma, Pantomime Néron, 1891. Photograph by Albert Londe. Album composé dans l'entourage d'Albert Londe. Musée d'Orsay/ RMN Grand Palais.

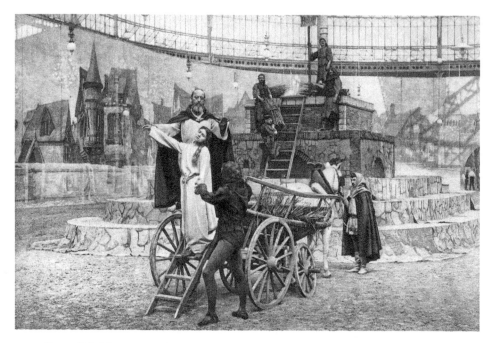

Figure 5.3: "Jeanne conduite au supplice" (Jean d'Arc being carried to torture), RF MO PHO 2014 2 34, Hippodrome de l'Alma, Pantomime Jeanne d'Arc, 1891. Photograph by Albert Londe. Album composé dans l'entourage d'Albert Londe. Musée d'Orsay/ RMN Grand Palais.

As in the case of Balagny's photographs, these portraits and scenes were Londe's attempts to take photographs of live performances. In spite of his progress, Londe complained as late as 1914 that the photographic technique was not developed enough, and he wished to see the day when "it will not be necessary to advise actors to hold a pose which will never be natural."[64] The Lumière brothers had insisted on the same point in front of the Société Française de la Photographie in 1891.[65] They stated that

> we have made a complete study of the question and, after taking more than 200 photographs both at the Theatre of Châtelet, l'Opéra and the Hippodrome, we have to recognize that . . . even under the best conditions, the pose has never been less than a quarter of a second. However, this exposure time is still too long to capture actors during their performance. . . . Unfortunately, the lighting is not fast enough, and actors have to be warned and being completely immobile.[66]

The photographs taken with the help of artificial lighting were not completely disconnected from his work at the Salpêtrière. From his experience at the

110   Photographing the Emotional Body

medical photography laboratory, Londe also experimented with the effects of the magnesium flash on the performance and physiology of actors. He recognized that "the magnesium lighting produces a brilliant, sudden light which dazzles our eye. It acts upon our nervous system to produce a range of phenomena of physiological nature."[67] Among the main effects were the occlusion of the eyes and the contraction of the facial features, giving an appearance of "fear and horror."[68] Londe also suggested using the magnesium flash in rooms with enough lighting, because when the room was too dark, the pupil dilated too much, producing another undesirable effect on the physiognomy.[69] His investigations concluded that photographers should use magnesium powder that could burn in 1/8 of a second in order to prevent making the model blink. Clearly, Londe had learned about these physiological reactions at the Salpêtrière. In *La photographie médicale* he explained the ways in which they had already incorporated artificial lighting into their practice at the clinic. He noted that the magnesium flash was helpful in capturing patients who could not be immobilized and were in rooms without enough light, "without having to alert them first."[70] His practice at the clinic had also revealed that using the flash could also induce the state of catalepsy in hysterical people.[71] While these effects should be avoided outside the hospital, Londe found them useful at the Salpêtrière, as photographing hysterical patients using quick artificial lighting allowed taking a portrait just before the catalepsy or at the moment of the transition.[72] This new technique revealed, therefore, very fast physiological processes that were invisible to the naked eye.

Cameras, Chronophotography, and the Physiology of Emotions

In addition to improving artificial lighting, Londe was also known for his contributions to the development of photographic cameras. In 1884, when he was photographing the previously mentioned experiments on faradization of hypnotized patients, he realized that the gestures obtained by faradization were stable, but they did not last very long.[73] Therefore, he needed a device fast enough to record the patients' unstable poses. He fabricated a stereoscopic device whose exposure time was less than a second and that recorded two almost identical images on the same plate. Seen through the stereoscope, the stereoscopic photographs provided three-dimensional images that helped doctors to fully appreciate the pathological gestures. In 1891 Londe faced a similar problem when he had to photograph actors onstage, as they could make quick moves or long poses, but gestures had to be recorded in both cases. Some of the photographs he took of Jeanne d'Arc were stereoscopic, and journals such as *Photo-Journal* published them.[74] As in the medical context, the stereoscopic images also helped to communicate the affective life of the character and the quality of the performance of the actor effectively.

The most famous camera Londe designed was, however, a chronophotographic device, which captured a succession of images at regular intervals in a short period. Following the work of Eadweard Muybridge and Étienne-Jules Marey, in 1893 Londe built a camera with twelve shutters that were arranged in three parallel lines, which provided twelve images organized in three rows of four.[75] The aim of this device was not to take the greatest number of images in a short period but to capture enough of them in order to "seize the attitudes that can escape direct observation" and to discover the "general march of the movement under analysis."[76] The aim of these images was to provide data to Paul Richer's research on the anatomy and the physiology of movement.[77] Among the physiological reactions Richer and Londe studied was the expressive gait, which examined how the muscles of the body expressed the emotions felt by the subject.[78]

The research on artificial lighting also benefited from his work on chronophotography. In *La photographie à la lumière artificielle*, Londe included a series of chronophotographic images of a man during a session using the magnesium flash.[79] The short time of each exposure revealed the changes in physiognomy at each stage of light exposure, helping photographers to calculate the exact dose of magnesium powder that should be used. Equally, this experiment demonstrated how human eyes blinked as reaction to a sudden, bright light.

The connection between the photographs of hysterical patients, chronophotography, and the images of actors did not lie, therefore, in the particular gestures performed but in the understanding of those gestures as physiological reactions to photography. These projects were conceived as experiments in which Londe integrated physiology through photography. Just as psychologists used physiology to explain bodily emotional movements, gestures such as blinking and expressions of emotions such as terror were presented as physiological reactions to the photographic act. Either at the Salpêtrière or at the hippodrome, taking a photograph became more than the mere documentation of an event. In Londe's practice, photography was an act of intervention that had material effects on the photographed person. The nature of the human physiological constitution made people react to the sudden, brilliant light of the magnesium in ways that doctors and photographs could anticipate.

Photographers and actors alike had to be aware of these effects and of the technical requirements of photography. Actors needed to know how and when to hold their poses for the photographer to capture. Their performance was, therefore, a compromise between the requirements of the character and the technological constraints of the photographic camera and the artificial lighting. This compromise was based on what historian of science Otto Sibum has described as "gestural knowledge."[80] These are the bodily performances that are required to properly use instruments and other objects in the laboratory but that are not explicitly stated because they belong to common sense. "Gestural knowledge" would refer in this example to the gestures and actions made by the photographer and the photographed model that were intended to control the performance of movement, on the one hand, and to coordinate and synchronize the acts of the photographer, the model, and the camera, on the other. These were series of tacit actions—the way in which the photographer had to manipulate the camera and other elements in the studio, and the way in which the photographed person reacted to it. A routine that embodied the codes of the photographic act.

The photographic intervention was, therefore, performative: it produced the body of the patient or the actor in a particular way. For instance, the expression of resignation played by the actress of Joan of Arc descending the cart was the result of the pantomime's conventions to express this emotion as well as the photographic requirements to portray it. The wide-open arms of Neron were part of the expressiveness of pantomimes, but the actor playing Neron needed to know how long he should keep his arms raised and opened.

Theater also became a performative practice when psychological theories of the bodily roots of emotions started to inform actors' performances. In the first decade of 1900, the dramaturge Constantin Stanislavski elaborated his own method of acting based in part on William James's psychology and Ribot's research on memory and emotions.[81] Stanislavski borrowed from James the concept of "second nature," which referred to the habits that are ingrained in the body. By training the performers' second nature through physical exercises, Stanislavski's system would "unburden the attention," as actors would "respond automatically to performance conditions."[82] This automatic response was corporeal, as the second nature would translate into gestures and the inflection of the voice, but it was also emotional. As Rose Whyman explains, in the Stanlislavski's system an actor must "*experience a feeling previously experienced.*"[83] Inspired by Ribot's work on emotions, Stanislavski appropriated the psychologist's concept of "affective memory" to refer to the physical work that actors had to do in order to experience and embody the emotion required by a role.[84] The emotions performed onstage were not, therefore, only expressed through external movements but were originated in the body and its emotional memory—not its intellect. The Stanislavski's system—so different from previous models that encouraged actors not to feel their roles but only mimic the external gestures—shows, therefore, the broad influence of the new conceptions of the bodily roots of emotions put forward by scientific psychology.

Performing the Emotional Body in Photography

This chapter has explored three different ways of understanding performativity. The first case study has shown that the experiments on the excitability of muscles and nerves of hysterical patients were performative, in the sense that doing the experiment produced the body of the hysteric. Second, I have examined the performativity of medical photographs, whose repetition and comparison sanctioned certain gestures as pathological, creating thereby medical categories and symptoms. Finally, I have analyzed the performativity of the very photographic act by means of investigating the effects of cameras and artificial lighting in the physiology of actors and patients. The common threads of these three cases are the photographic projects of Albert Londe and the emergent psychological theory of the bodily roots of emotions.

While these three uses of the concept of performativity might seem disparate, they all respond to the same approach. I have followed Karen Barad's performative understanding of material and discursive practices in an attempt to understand bodies' processes of materialization.[85] The examination of the emergent psychological theories of emotion based on the physiological reactions of the body has allowed me to discuss the "emotional body" as prominently material—a body that is created in the doing of emotions and gestures. This characterization is in line with Barad's idea that matter is not a thing but a *doing*. In this sense, the emotional body cannot be passive: it is always in the process of constituting itself—it is intrinsically performative. From this perspective, Barad defends an "account of the body's historicity in which its very materiality plays an active role."[86] This chapter has attempted to offer such an account, showing that emotions are material as well as processes of materialization of bodies. This materialization is intrinsically historical, as it depends on particular performances, instruments, and technologies. The example of photography has allowed me to discuss the performative process of materialization of the emotional body through different enactments: the experiment, the photographic image, and the act of photographing. I have considered photography as a material and discursive practice that constructs the body in a particular way in each iteration. The emotional body is, therefore, ephemeral: it is the result of a particular materialization (the actor's performance in front of the camera at the hippodrome, for instance), which is only part of an ongoing process.

The theoretical approach and the historical example examined here contribute to a better understanding of emotions as practices, one of the key themes of this book. By situating photography in the broader context of psychological and physiological theories of emotions, this chapter has demonstrated that a full understanding of the material effects of emotions needs to take into consideration how gestures have been historically embodied, performed, and understood.

Notes

This research was carried out during my Wellcome Trust Research Fellowship in Medical Humanities, reference 103101/Z/13/Z. Previous versions of this paper were presented in research seminars at the Centre for the History of Medicine, University of Warwick, and the Photographic History Research Centre, De Montfort University. Many thanks go to the anonymous reviewers for their insightful suggestions and my colleagues at the PHRC for their continuous support.

1. See Chossimo Chiarelli, "Images en Jeu. Théâtre, Photographie et Pratiques Visuelles Dans *L'Illustration* (1843–1913)," *Revue d'Histoire du Théâtre Numérique*, Special Issue "Scenes de Papier. Les Images Dans les Revues de Théâtre." 2 (no year).

2. "*reine de l'attitude et princesse des gestes*," Sarcey, "Le théâtre instantanée," *Le Théâtre* 1 (1898).

3. Alfred Giraudet, *Mimique: Physionomie et gestes d'après François Delsarte* (Paris: Ancienne Maison Quantin, 1895); Charles Aubert, *L'art mimique* (Paris: Meuriot, 1901).

4. Aubert, *L'art mimique*, 13–14. Charles Darwin, *The Expression of Emotions in Man and Animals* (London: Murray, 1872).

5. Sarcey, "Le théâtre instantané."

6. Ibid.

7. See Danny Rees, "Down in the Mouth: Faces of Pain," in *Pain and Emotion in Modern History*, ed. Rob Boddice (Houndmills: Palgrave Macmillan, 2014), 164–86. For a history of gestures, see Michael Braddick, "Introduction: The Politics of Gestures," *Past and Present* 203, no. 4 (special issue, "The Politics of Gestures") (2009): 9–35. For its relation with the history of emotions, see Colin Jones, *The Smile Revolution in Eighteenth-Century Paris* (Oxford: Oxford University Press, 2014).

8. See Denis Bernard and André Gunthert, *L'instant rêvé: Albert Londe* (Nimes: Chambon, 1993).

9. Albert Londe, *La photographie médicale: Applications aux sciences médicales et physiologies* (Paris: Gautiers Villars, 1893).

10. Albert Londe, "Attitudes obtenues dans la catalepsie sous l'influence de divers excitations," *La photogrpahie medicale* 7:95.

11. Bernard and Gunthert, *L'instant rêvé*.

12. Albert Londe, *La photographie à la lumière artificielle* (Paris: Octave Doin, 1914). See also Denis Bernard, "La lumière pesée: Albert Londe et la photographie à l'éclaire magnésique," *Études photographiques* 6 (1999).

13. The Musée d'Orsay acquired in 2014 an album with the most complete collection of photographs of theater and circus made by Albert Londe. See Thomas Galifot, "Londe, Albert," *Sept Ans de Reflexion: Dernières Acquisitions du Musée d'Orsay* (Paris: Musée d'Orsay / Skira Paris, 2014), 261–62.

14. Rob Boddice, "Hysteria or Tetanus? Ambivalent Embodiments and the Authenticity of Pain," chapter 1 herewith; Georges Didi-Huberman, *The Invention of Hysteria: Charcot and the Photographic Iconography of the Salpêtrière*, trans. Alisa Hartz (Cambridge: MIT Press, 2003); Rae Beth Gordon, "From Charcot to Charlot: Unconscious Imitation and Spectatorship in French Cabaret and Early Cinema," *Critical Inquiry* 27, no. 3 (2001): 515–49.

15. See Felicia McCarren, "The 'Symptomatic Act' circa 1900: Hysteria, Hypnosis, Electricity, Dance," *Critical Inquiry* 21, no. 4 (1995): 748–74; and Joanna Townsend, "Elizabeth Robins: Hysteria, Politics and Performance," in *Women, Theatre and Performance: New Histories, New Historiographies*, ed. Maggie B. Gale and Viv Gardner (Manchester: Manchester University Press, 2001), 102–20.

16. Karen Barad, "Posthumanist Performativity: Towards an Understanding of How Matter Comes to Matter," *Signs* 28, no. 3 (2003): 801–31.

17. See Natasha Ruiz Gomez, "The Scientific Artworks of Dr Paul Richer," *Medical Humanities* 39, no. 1 (2013): 4–10.

18. See Mark S. Micale, "The Salpêtrière in the Age of Charcot: An Institutional Perspective on Medical History in the Late Nineteenth Century," *Journal of Contemporary History*, 20 no. 4 (1985): 703–31.

19. Marie-Rose Faure, "La photographie scientifique de Bourneville," *Communication et langages* 135 (2003): 104–24.

20. Planche XXII, "Attitudes Passionnelles: Extase," *Iconographie Photographie de la Salpêtrière* (Paris: Delahaye, 1876).

21. See Mary Hunter, *The Face of Medicine: Visualising Medical Masculinities in Late Nineteenth-Century Paris* (Manchester: Manchester University Press, 2016), esp. chapter 3, "Hysterical Realisms at the Salpêtrière: Images, Objects and Performances chez Charcot," 166–241.

22. Londe recognized that photographing at the studio was the rule except in the cases of instantaneous photography of movement (*La photographie médicale*, 86).

23. I have examined this studio in more detail in Beatriz Pichel, "Cuerpos patológicos: Fotografía y medicina en el siglo diecinueve," *Alcores* 19 (2017): 35–55.

24. "Suggestions par le sens dans la période cataleptique du grand hypnotisme," vol. 9, *Nouvelle Iconographie de la Salpêtrière* 4 (1891).

25. Georges Guinon and Sophie Woltke (d'Odessa), "De l'influence des excitations sensitives et sensorielles dans les phases cataleptique et somnambulique du grand

hypnotism," *Nouvelle Iconographie de la Salpêtrière* 4 (1891): 77—88. Reprinted in Jean-Martin Charcot, *Leçons mémoires notes et observations parus pendant les années 1889—1890 et 1890—1891 et publiées sous la direction de G. Guinon* (Paris: Le Progrès Médical, 1893), 482.

26. The quality of both the photographic reproduction, made by Photocollographie Chene et Longuet, and the paper became one of the main characteristics of *Nouvelle iconographie*.

27. Guinon and Woltke, "De l'influence des excitations sensitives," 83. The clinicians at La Salpêtrière almost never included full names of the patients in the published case studies, only the beginning of the surname followed by ellipsis.

28. Ibid., 83.

29. Ibid., 83.

30. Ibid., 86.

31. Ibid., 83

32. Ibid., 83.

33. Ibid., 78, 81.

34. Guinon and Woltke, "De l'influence des excitations des organes des sens sur les hallucinations de la phase passionnelle de l'attaque hystérique," *Archives de neurologie* 63 (1891).

35. Jean Martin Charcot and Paul Richer "Contribution a l'étude de l'hypnotisme chez les hystériques: Du phenomène de l'hyperexcitabilité neuromusculaire," *Archives de neurologie* (1881): 32–75.

36. Paul Richer, *Etudes cliniques sur la grande hystérie, ou hystéro-épylepsie*, 2nd ed. (Paris: Delahaye et Lecrosnier, 1885.

37. I have further analyzed these two sets of photographs in Beatriz Pichel, "From Facial Expressions to Bodily Gestures," *History of the Human Sciences* 29, no. 1 (2016): 27–48.

38. Jules Bernard Luys, *Hypnotisme experimental: Les émotions dans l'etat d'hypnotisme* (Paris: Baillière, 1887).

39. Albert Pitres, *Leçons cliniques sur l'hystérie et hypnotisme faites à l'Hôpital Saint André de Bordeaux*, vol. 2 (Paris: O Doin, 1891).

40. Guinon and Woltke, "De l'influence des excitations des organes," 346–65. Reprinted in Jean-Martin Charcot, *Clinique des maladies du système nerveux: Leçons du professeur, mémoires, notes et observations parus pendant les années 1889-90 et 1890-91* (Paris: Babé, 1892-93), 26:336-55.

41. In this text, the name of the patient was fully disclosed, probably because *Archives de Neurologie* had a different policy from *Nouvelle Iconographie*.

42. See Jacqueline Carroy, Annick Ohayon, and Regine Plas, *Histoire de la Psychologie en France* (Paris: La Découverte, 2006); Jacqueline Carroy, *Hypnose, Suggestion et Psychologie: L'invention des Sujets* (Paris: Presses Universitaires de France, 1991).

43. Thomas Dixon, *From Passions to Emotions: The Creation of a Secular Psychological Category* (Cambridge: Cambridge University Press, 2003).

44. Serge Nicolas and Agnès Charvillat, "Introducing Psychology as an Academic Discipline in France: Théodule Ribot and the Collège de France (1888–1901)," *Journal of the History of Behavioural Sciences* 37, no. 2 (2001): 143–64.

45. Théodule Ribot, *La psychologie des sentiments* (Paris: Alcan, 1896).

46. Carroy, Ohayon, and Plas, *Histoire de la Psychologie*.

47. Richer, *Études Cliniques*, 680.

48. Duchenne de Boulogne, *Mécanisme de la physionomie humaine, ou analyse électro-physiologique de l'expression des passions* (Paris: Renouard, 1862).

49. Pitres, *Leçons cliniques*, 309. Emphasis added.

50. Guinon and Woltke, "De l'influence des excitations sensitives," 86.

51. Londe, *La photographie médicale*, 5.

52. For a discussion of scientific uses of photography in the nineteenth century, see Jennifer Tucker, *Nature Exposed: Photography as Eyewitness in Victorian Science* (Baltimore, Md.: Johns Hopkins University Press, 2005).

53. See Laurence Senelick, "Melodramatic Gestures in Cartes-de-visite Photographs," *Theater* 18, no. 2 (1987): 5–13; Laurence Senelick, "Eroticism in Early Theatrical Photography," *Theatre History Studies* 11 (1991): 1–49; Chiarelli, "Jeu des images."

54. Mareschal, "La photographie au théâtre," *La Nature* 16, no. 1 (1888): 757–82.

55. Ibid., 94

56. Galifot, "Londe"; Bernard, "La lumière pesée."

57. Albert Londe, "La science au théâtre: 'Jeanne d'arc' à l'hyppodrome de Paris," *La Nature* 895. 2, no. 26 (1890): 125–26.

58. Londe, "Jeanne d'arc." The photograph that illustrates the article is available online at the website of the Musée d'Orsay (H.0.132; L.0.193).

59. Londe, *La photographie à la lumière artificielle*, 266–67.

60. This system had been discussed some years before in M. H. Fourtier, *Les lumières artificielles en photographie* (Paris: Gauthier-Villars, 1895).

61. Some of these images are accessible online at the website of the Musée d'Orsay.

62. See John McCormick, "Pantomime," in *Popular Theatres of Nineteenth Century France* (London: Routledge, 2003), 134–47.

63. Alexander Georget, "À propos de Jeanne d'arc," *Photo-Journal* 1 (1891): 173–76.

64. Londe, *La photographie à la lumière artificielle*, 238.

65. Auguste et Louis Lumière, "Développateur au paramidophénol," *Bulletin de la Société Française de la Photographie* (1890): 195–202.

66. Ibid., 201.

67. Londe, *La photographie à la lumière artificielle*, 87.

68. Ibid., 87.

69. Ibid., 92

70. Londe, *La photographie médicale*, 132.

71. Londe, *La photographie à la lumière artificielle*, 87, 92.

72. Albert Londe, "Contribution à l'étude des lumières artificielles en photographie," *Bulletin de la Société Française de Photographie* (1892): 102–3.

73. Albert Londe, "Photographies médicales," *Bulletin de la Société française de la photographie* 10 (1884).

74. Georget, "À propos de Jeanne d'arc."

75. See Marta Braun, *Picturing Time: The Work of Etienne Jules Marey* (1830–1904) (Chicago: Chicago University Press, 1992), and Braun and Elizabeth Whitcombe, "Marey, Muybridge, and Londe: The Photography of Pathological Locomotion," *History of Photography* 23, no. 3 (1999): 218–24.

76. Londe, *La photographie médicale*, 370.

77. Paul Richer, *Physiologie artistique de l'homme en movement* (Paris: Octave Doin, 1895).

78. Richer, *Physiologie artistique*, 302. I have examined these photographs in Pichel, "From Facial Expressions."

79. "Fig. 25: Chronophotographie de l'occlusion des yeux," in Londe, *La photographie à la lumière artificielle*, 89.

80. Otto Sibum, "Reworking the Mechanical Value of Heat: Instruments of Precision and Gestures of Accuracy in Early Victorian England," *Studies on History and Philosophy of Science* 26, no.1 (1995): 73–106.

81. Rose Whyman, *The Stanislavski System of Acting: Legacy and Influence in Modern Performance* (Cambridge: Cambridge University Press, 2011), 52–54.

82. Whyman, "The Actor's Second Nature: Stanislavski and Willian James," *New Theatre Quarterly* 23, no. 2 (2007): 115–23.

83. Whyman, *Stanislavski System*, 49. Italics in the original.

84. Ibid.

85. Barad, "Posthumanist Performativity."

86. Ibid.," 809.

6. Yolanda

Youth, Heroin, and AIDS through the Lens of Photographic Practices

MARÍA ROSÓN

YOLANDA, BY PHOTOGRAPHER Ignacio Navas (Tudela, b. 1989), is an artwork whose most representative component is a fanzine self-published in 2014. The piece arises from the artist's own experience of self-inquiry and occupies the intimate sphere as its privileged site of enunciation. In 2011 Navas was rummaging through the photographs of his family archive when he found a snapshot of himself as an infant at his christening. In the image, an unknown woman affectionately held him. Next to her stood Navas's uncle, Gabriel (b. 1965), who in the photograph looked directly at the camera as he laughed. The woman must have been someone important within the family, he thought, if she was photographed holding him on such an important day. From that moment forward, Navas yearned to know more about the mysterious female figure who appeared in the image. He began an investigation, in which the photographer would "try to get to know her through old family photo albums and conversations with [his] uncle."[1] He would soon find out that the woman was Yolanda (b. 1970), Gabriel's partner during his early youth, when both were hooked on heroin in Tudela, a small agricultural and industrial city in Navarre in the northern part of the Iberian Peninsula. In 1995, at only twenty-five years of age, Yolanda died from AIDS. Navas's inquiry into the past is based on his uncle's testimony—that is, his oral history—and the artists' own engagement with the personal photographs of both Yolanda and Gabriel. These images, as I will argue, are a resistant legacy of their lives. Just as in Roland Barthes's *Camera Lucida*, where the absence of his mother's portrait detonates the author's analysis, the image that triggers

Navas's project of personal reflection is not included in the pages of the fanzine. Different scholars coincide in the attention they pay to the importance of and the meaning produced by seeing an album in the company of its creator, its owner, or a person within its close social circle, given the implicit narrative qualities and the strong oral component of these objects.[2] This correlation between the photographic album and orality is based on memory, or the capacity to remember, given the fact that one of the most important functions of this kind of compilation is its status as a device for activating memories of the past.

Yolanda's emotional body is a body that has been erased from collective memory and from history. Navas himself is unaware of his identity, and when he begins to stir up the past in Tudela, people are puzzled by his interest in examining "the things that are not talked about within the family."[3] These are things that have been kept silent in the familial sphere, as well as things that have not been addressed in public space despite the fact that they point to collective problems of enormous depth in our present lives. Yolanda's body, the visual and conceptual axis of the fanzine that bears her name, represents, together with that of Gabriel, a collective identity. With this piece, Navas lays out a type of engagement that seeks to uncover and make evident the tension between a body and an individual or personal identity—in this case, that of Yolanda and Gabriel, which embodies experiences and collective memories of a subaltern group. This shared subalternity belongs to Spanish youth, more specifically to those who came of age in the 1980s and 1990s. The life experiences of the members of this generation provide different accounts—different narratives—regarding the political transition from Franco's dictatorship (1939–1975) to democracy.[4] These experiences and their related narratives have not been heard by Spanish society or incorporated into the country's historical accounts of the recent past despite their significant presence during the decade of the 1980s and the first years of the 1990s, only later to be disappeared in the most silent of ways. Their legacy affects, configures, and interferes with our present reality.

The aim of this chapter is to create a dialogue with memory, the emotions, and the bodies of the latest generation of Spanish youth who directly lived and experienced the transition, often in situations affected by the consumption of drugs and the spread of HIV. In order to do this, I will analyze the fanzine *Yolanda* and the elements that this work unfurls, particularly friendship and romantic love, drug consumption, the performance of identity through portraiture and self-portraiture, illness, and disappearance. For Yolanda and Gabriel, the contradictions and emotions of their youth generation are constructed in front of the camera and through the photographic medium, thereby situating photography as an essential practice in their daily lives and as a mode of expression and personal remembrance. *Yolanda* is composed by and in dialogue with one of the most significant memory mediums of the twentieth century, the photographic compilation. Ignacio Navas's work departs from a simple and effective exercise, in which his uncle Gabriel "tells" or "narrates his album" of photographic images. These compilations, together with other forms of photographic collection, like the images that accumulate in boxes and envelopes, are as much as repository of memory as they are an instrument of social performance.[5]

Yolanda: Forms and Memories

The first thing that catches readers' attention about *Yolanda* is the publication's back and front covers made of paper that imitates a photographic print, matte on the outside, gloss on the inside. A watermark is located on the outside covers, where the name "Yolanda" repeats over and over, a mustard yellow spelling of the title inspired by a particular type of Kodak paper known as "Royal," an iconic mark introduced onto the backside of photographs printed on this type of paper during the 1980s and 1990s. With this gesture, Navas anticipates in a concise and eloquent manner the material he will use to build his visual essay: vernacular photographs and amateur snapshots linked to an earlier time when people took analog pictures that were printed on paper. Surely, most of the fanzines' readers will easily recognize the visual play proposed by fusing Yolanda's name with the aesthetics of the mark in both its form and color. This recognition is perhaps produced automatically, as when one returns to a well-known place after a time of distance. Vernacular photographs were common, "ordinary" objects that inhabited the life experiences of a large part of the Spanish population during the last twenty years of the twentieth century, thereby situating them as essential pieces—vital things—in our contemporary visual memory. The somewhat stereotyped character of these images has another powerful side related to "its extraordinary capacity to represent" since every image from the family archive "is a condensation, a crystallization of hundreds, of thousands of analogue images."[6] And yet there are particularities in the photographs that make up *Yolanda*, thereby breaking away from a hegemonic regime of visibility. First, these photographs are not family snapshots, and here it is interesting to refer to the arguments put forth by Langford when she says, "The family photo album does not exist. Only personal albums that occupy a specific model of family and community or that situate themselves in relation to that model exist."[7] It is with this in mind that I here will discuss personal

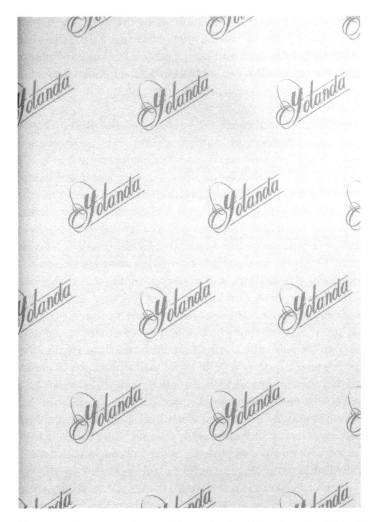

Figure 6.1: Front cover, Ignacio Navas, fanzine *Yolanda*, self-published in 2014.

or vernacular photography, rather than "family" photography. In this case, the community to which these photographs belong is not the family but rather the heterosexual couple immersed in a collectivity of young Spaniards.

There is another important aspect of the cover that allows one to understand the overall significance of the project: the importance of the name "Yolanda," which is repeated again and again in the playful fusion with the Kodak emblem. It is, therefore, this gesture—this expression—of her name that is made clear from the moment of seeing the work. The name creates identity; it is the name of exactly what is missing. Yolanda has her name while Gabriel has his voice and his memory, a kind of remembrance that structures the fanzine. Both individuals make their bodies present through the photographs, bodies made present during their youth through the consumption of heroin.

Yolanda takes form through the photographs that Ignacio Navas takes from his uncle Gabriel's family album and through the photographs that Gabriel took using a compact, second-rate camera so that he could share them with Yolanda. Both Yolanda and Gabriel were avid amateur photographers, and this kind of imaging practice intersected their everyday lives. In addition to these snapshots, the piece also includes a few images from the Municipal Archive of Tudela as well as a few taken by Navas himself. The fanzine is clearly structured and carefully elaborated.[8] Navas recounts that in the beginning he wanted to construct a story via a lineal narrative. However, he soon realized that this strategy did not work, which then pushed him to devise a more elliptical historical sketch, which would be defined by points of extreme tension. The work has three levels or layers of signification, the first and most central of which is configured through the photographs printed onto the page. These images establish an elliptic rhythm that rises, only then to recede little by little. In addition, the photographs are arranged and ordered from an inverse logic that allows a clear dialogue between the first and last images. In between the photographs, Gabriel's oral history is incorporated through the appearance of textual annexes that take the form of narrower pages that alternate throughout the publication. Finally, in between these capsules of meaning are the things that are caught in between, the ellipses, the things never said and never caught in image form. Navas makes these gaps and silences evident through the utilization of blank spaces on the printed page and through the inclusion of texts, where the artist selects parts of his uncle's memory—the places where he demonstrates doubt with phrases like, "I don't remember very well"—which, in turn, also make visible the very contradictions of one's own memory discourse.

The first photograph is a portrait of Yolanda taken at night. Her body, with her arms open and resting on a white banister, is trimmed against the black background of the night. The final photograph of the series is also an individual portrait of Yolanda, which is conceived as an inverse of the first. In this last luminous image, she stands next to the sea. It is a tribute, a homage, a visual obituary. For it is, according to Navas, Gabriel's favorite photograph, the one with which he wants to remember Yolanda. However, the power of the individuality that begins and ends the fanzine is placed in tension with

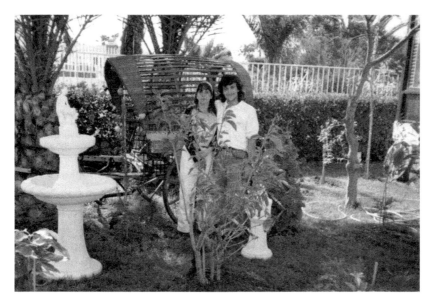

Figure 6.2: Yolanda at night. Untitled photograph published in the fanzine *Yolanda*, self-published by Ignacio Navas in 2014.

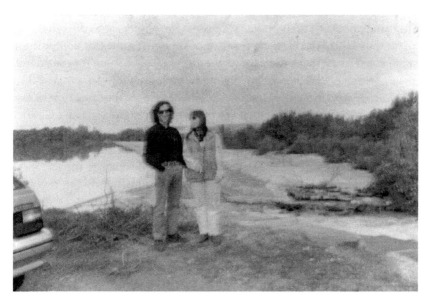

Figure 6.3: Photograph of the couple. Untitled photograph published in the fanzine *Yolanda*, self-published by Ignacio Navas in 2014.

the photograph of the couple that immediately follows. The image, printed to fill the bleed on the double page, situates the two subjects at the center of the composition, in a florid garden, thereby establishing a pattern that will repeat itself throughout the piece. As carefully noted by Isabel Cadenas, these "assembly marks"—that is, the traces left by the process of laying out the photographs—make it appear as if the couple is separated in the material plane of the publication.[9] The second-to-last photograph is again a portrait of the couple, where the mark left by the binding produces another separation. In this second case Yolanda and Gabriel are placed in positions that are inverted in comparison to those that appear in the first. It is a blurry image with a bluish patina, giving this second-to-last photograph in the sequence a spectral character.

The physical and mental separation of Yolanda and Gabriel is achieved through distinct strategies. For example, the couple is centered on the double page in a way that allows the bookbinding mark to cross down between the two subjects. It is a technique used in the examples previously analyzed as well as in other instances. There are also strategies of concealment and exposition, where textual interventions cover up parts of the pages or where the act of "uncovering," or turning the page, reveals something else. Finally, on various occasions, Yolanda and Gabriel can be found posing almost in the same positions, their bodies swapped. One photographs the other and, then, the reverse in the same scene, in a similar if not exact composition and pose. Navas places the photographs in parallel position on continuous pages, which establishes an interesting interplay among pairs that seeks a tension between individual identity and the couple. At the same time, it also acts as a prelude to the eventual separation between Yolanda and Gabriel, thereby transmitting a sense of solitude and disappearance. Some of the photographs, like the pair of positive parallel images printed on the double page that corresponds to the first trip that the couple made to the sea, spark a mix of sadness and affection.[10] They pose individually between two cars, having recently descended from their own in a dirty parking lot located in front of a dented, humidity-marked fence. The horizon is blurry, which causes the line of the sea to get mixed up with that of the sky in a weak mix of blue. These photographs of Gabriel and Yolanda, as well as all of the other photographs of the couple in their different trips and vacations, show us two persons who, despite being together, appear to be encapsulated in completely separate and different moments due to the effects that heroin had exercised on their bodies. They were snapshots of individuals who had never in their lives enjoyed a vacation: as Gabriel confirms in his narrative, these trips were often seen as an opportunity to wean oneself from drug addiction.

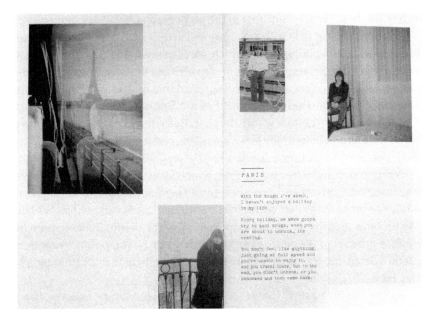

Figure 6.4: Untitled photograph published in the fanzine *Yolanda*, self-published by Ignacio Navas in 2014.

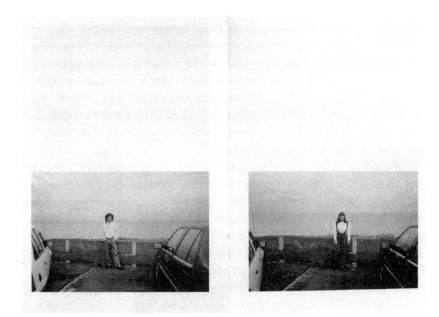

Figure 6.5: Yolanda, Gabriel, and cars. Untitled photograph published in the fanzine *Yolanda*, self-published by Ignacio Navas in 2014.

It is also important to note that in the photographs, Yolanda rarely smiles. This produces a rupture with the most widely repeated conventions of domestic and family photography, which are displayed after a double process of selection—the photographs that are "made" and the later the ones that are chosen or kept—where supposedly happy moments are conserved. In this case and especially within the context of the feminine portrait, the smile is the codification of a gesture within the pose. Referring to this first photograph of Yolanda and Gabriel in the garden, Cadenas refers to the cut produced by the binding, which in turn achieves a kind of separation: "This simple gesture forces us to stop and pause on the gaze, which up until this moment, we have not observed. Consequently, we realize that Gabriel is smiling as he hugs her, while she looks at the camera seriously with her hands gathered in her lap. We become attentive to the ominous quality of the photo: the ever-present mark, a product of the editing work completed by Navas, points to another mark, a detail that was already there is the very moment that the photograph was taken."[11]

As one begins to turn the pages of the fanzine, a knot of signification becomes apparent within the portraits of Yolanda. In this sense, the initial sequence is paradigmatic: a black-and-white portrait of Yolanda as a child wherein she sits on a chaise with a toy horse. Subsequently, another image appears. This time, it is a drawing, by Yolanda, of a woman whose head is cradled by a flowery crown and surrounded by serpentine forms, which easily relates to the subsequent photographic portrait of Yolanda, where she is surrounded on a bed by stuffed animals as a black shawl hanging from the wall seeps together with her dark hair. It is an encryption that makes patent the tension that moved Navas to reveal and answer the question, "Who is she?" What activates the artistic work of *Yolanda* is precisely his need to understand his identity in a context where his memory of something had been erased. As in other traumatic contexts that arise throughout the recent history of Spain, like the violence and repression suffered during the civil war (1936–39) and the first period of Franco's dictatorship ("franquismo," 1940s), these memories, in this case the artist's own photographs and Gabriel's own narrative, were not completely lost. Instead, it is simply that no one has asked about them, and few have wanted to hear the answers because there are many things that are still difficult to remember. They provoke pain. This is perhaps also because they disrupt hegemonic historical narratives, in this case those related to the transition from dictatorship to democracy, which will be analyzed in the second part of this chapter. In this respect, there is an important turn in the fifth double spread that provokes, in part, the reader's own understanding.

Yolanda and Gabriel are sitting on a sofa, petting their dog. The inexperience of the amateur photographer who took the snapshot or the insolent indifference of the group provokes a revelation. In the foreground of the image, a table is full of domestic and everyday objects typical to the period: magazines, a calculator, some glass bottles of orange soda, an ashtray brimming with cigarette butts and foil with the remains of heroin that surely served to "fumar un chino," a phrase used to describe a form of inhaling the powerful substance. With this image, the conventions of photographic compilation, in which a series of "implicit norms"[12] determine what is shown and what is kept from view in the album, are radically broken. After all, the consumption of drugs, like illness and death, generally pertains to the category of the "not visible." Navas will also be sure to emphasize this point by including successive close-ups of portions of photographs where the remains of drug consumption are apparent or by treating the narrative excerpts plastically so that these elements fulfill the role of covering or showing different traces of drug use. Here it is important to consider the reflections of Jorge Fernández Puebla, the publication's graphic designer, when he refers to the function of these narrative excerpts: "On one hand, they cover, occupying half of the page, those elements that we want [to show], in a way that allows one to turn the page and, in some cases, observe the before and after of some of the images." Navas and Fernández Puebla decided to cover up the drugs so that later they could be discovered as one flipped through the supplement, thereby also hiding from view the protagonist "in relation to her progressive disappearance."[13]

It is interesting to compare the principal compositional strategy, which is grounded in both concealment and visibility. One of the other key functions of the narrative segments is to emphasize an aspect through the inclusion of a small photograph with a selected framing in the upper part of the page. The images refer to iconic fragments of the material and visual culture of those years. For example, a typical pendent in the form of a Map of Navarre or the advertising balloons of Campsa, the state-owned petroleum products company, that plowed through the Spanish sky. In order to piece together his story, Navas employs a strategy that fluctuates between showing and hiding, between revealing and keeping from view. This strategy is exactly what vernacular photography and its related modes of compilation, especially those related to the creation of photographic albums, also bring into play. Critiques that have emerged from feminist reflections on the album have put into evidence the limited and desensitized content of its iconography, which full of absences and silences reifies idealized narratives regarding the individual and the collective.[14] As Teresa Vilarós has noted, the strategy of hiding and

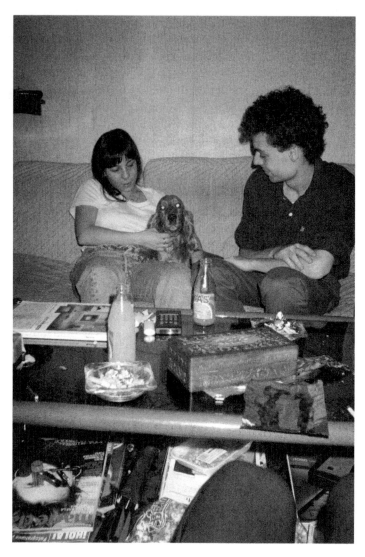

Figure 6.6: Yolanda, Gabriel, and their dog. Untitled photograph published in the fanzine *Yolanda*, self-published by Ignacio Navas in 2014.

revealing, or the "aesthetic of disappearance," is key to understanding other works that address HIV/AIDS.[15] This issue becomes more perceptible in the last pages of the fanzine, where Navas accentuates the "assembly marks" in order to evidence "noise"—that is, something that "destabilizes in sudden, unexpected, and very real ways."[16] He achieves this by materially breaking from the continuity between the photographs enlarged to fit the double page and interspersing them with other photographs, thereby dislocating the narrative direction. Finally, just before the end of the publication, the blank spaces begin to become more evident. The ellipses—what had appeared before, but now stands out—begin to occupy the complete space of the double spread that coincides with Yolanda's death announcement, which appears in the textual excerpts.

Yolanda can be understood as a postphotographic piece. This concept, developed by Joan Fontcuberta, refers to those creative practices that are interrelated with digital techniques conceived in a context like the present one, which is characterized by the massive production of images and their subsequent circulation. It is a new artistic paradigm that focuses on a "visual ecology" that "will penalize saturation and celebrate reuse." In this paradigm, forms of making, as occurs specifically in Navas's artistic practice, will have more to do with "the curator, the docent, the historian, and the theoretician."[17] One of the privileged poetics of the postphotographic creative currents is that of the "found photograph," or the *photo-trouvée*, which tends to contain a particular secret and, as we see in *Yolanda*, provides an encounter that "can catapult us toward a search for a lost truth, as well as toward the discovery of a sleeping one."[18] Navas creates a piece that is grounded in the formal strategy of showing/hiding by using found materials that emerge from the intimate sphere. His interest in the photographs taken by his aunt and uncle between 1985 and 1995 transcends his inquiry into his family genealogy in that the piece draws to the surface and makes clear the emotional experiences of his aunt and uncle, which are gathered against the grain of photographic practices that are collective. Yolanda and Gabriel's album is a repository, a legacy that is resistant to time and the cultural logics dominant in the "*fiesta*" that was the transition. Through their photographs a way of being young is put into action, which allows us not only to acquire a unique narrative regarding the lives of young, working-class Spaniards who experienced firsthand unemployment, the spread of heroin, and the expansion of speculative urban development, but also to see how these elements are performed. The images included in this piece are indicative of performative practices: the repetition of poses and gestures, rituals of young evolution. They are also remnants of a genuine material and visual culture that appears (and disappears) through its constant interest in photographing and capturing the objects and emotional landscapes of that time. Within this performative language, which produces and reproduces concrete effects in the lives and memory of individuals, photography and emotions are indistinguishable. The poses, the compositions, and the photographed objects allude not only to visual and material culture or to photographic techniques used in this context but also to the textures and emotional practices of those young Spaniards who used photography as a privileged medium for the expression of their affections.

Youth, Heroin, and Disenchantment

Yolanda is grounded in the recovery of memories belonging to a subaltern collectivity—Spanish youth from the 1980s and 1990s—through the collection of oral histories and the compilation of photographs. As the fanzine's author confirms, it is a publication that focuses on "being young" by exploring the central theme of "the emotions and contradictions of youth." Here, the author refers to a specific kind of Spanish youth, those who lived and grew up in the Lourdes neighborhood of Tudela, belonging to the popular and working classes of this particular small city located in the Province of Navarre. The piece is also about friendship and heterosexual love. In this sense, it addresses a series of affective and life practices that are related to being young in Spain during the end of the 1980s and the beginning of the 1990s—specifically, going to the "mili" or completing obligatory military service; "having a shit job" or having no job at all; consuming heroin and scheming to get it; and finally, taking photographs and making albums.

Yolanda and Gabriel only barely experienced the dictatorship, which began to decline when dictator Francisco Franco died in 1975. Nevertheless, they absorbed, confronted and were familiar with the dictatorship's social and cultural ecosystem through the regime's deep and abundant cultural residues. These traces included, on one hand, an education that was profoundly authoritarian and sexist, as well as fundamentally Catholic, and, on the other, a nationalist society that pivoted around the patriarchal family as the privileged social structure. Yolanda, born in 1970, and Gabriel, born in 1969, belong to a generational cohort that emerged following the close of the baby boom, which included Spaniards born until 1965. And while both were children rather than young adults during the second half of the 1970s and the first half of the 1980s, their lifestyles are closely connected with some of the collective habits belonging to those youth generations who experienced firsthand the death of Franco in 1975 and the subsequent political changes that led to the establishment of democracy. This specific "transition" generation included individuals born in between 1950 and 1955, which means they would have been between fifteen and twenty years old in 1975. Pablo Sánchez Léon argues that this transition generation "has established a pattern of collective habits and customs that have left and continue to leave a profound trace on those Spaniards who came of age and who entered into civic life [at this time of political change]."[19] This pattern has to do with this generation's direct experience with structural unemployment, the rise in delinquency, the eruption of drug consumption as a mode of socialization, and the rise in mortality rates. As Sánchez Léon notes, the data regarding this last issue are noteworthy: members of the generation born around 1955 experienced birth rates much higher than those born around 1940. However, data also show that by the end of the 1990s there were more living Spaniards from the generation born in the 1940s than the generation born in the 1950s.[20] Finally, there is another opening characteristic that marks the experiences of the youth generation of 1975 as well as the generations of Spaniards that would follow: the institutionalization of a stigma related to apathetic attitudes and stances, described in local argot as being "pasota." As Sánchez León notes, to describe someone as *pasota* "was a way to summarize a set of traits and attitudes condemned as antisocial and hedonist, whose common denominator would be a reprehensible apathy and a lack of commitment with the new democratic institutions."[21]

The adult world understood youth as a kind of identity in terms of otherness, where the stereotypes represented by the images associated with "pasotas," and later with "quinquis" and "yonkis," embodied the fears associated with political change and new, complex ways of life. According to Germán Labrador, Spanish youth in the 1970s emerged (from the intergenerational conflict that characterized the transition) as a new historical subject linked to ideas of change. In this way, youth generations were capable of transforming the most fundamental social and cultural values of Franco's regime and did so by successfully implanting four metamorphoses within Spanish culture: a turn toward secularization, the embrace of the sexual revolution, the celebration of pacifism, and the identification of a crisis regarding forms of state nationalism.[22] These shifts were structural and continue to act as points of political debate in Spain. However, other radical aspects of the political imagination that first appeared in the 1970s developed around an idea of the political that, by the 1980s, was increasingly related to ways of framing and carrying out institutional and representative democracy. The modernization of Spain and the beginning of economic normalization was based on neoliberal policies that also prevailed in other latitudes with the rise of conservative governments to power. In Spain, the process coincided with the PSOE's (Spanish Socialist Workers Party) incorporation into governing bodies in 1982 and the party's responsibility to carry out economic reforms based on industrial reconversion, thereby giving way to processes of decentralization and the outsourcing of production.

The transformation of Spain from a national-Catholic dictatorship to a social-democratic democracy reached a visible milestone within the cultural arena in 1992 with the inauguration of the Olympics in Barcelona and the celebration of the Universal Exposition in Seville. These cultural phenomena, rooted in Spain's embrace of the tourism industry, were fundamental in producing and shaping an idea of democratic Spain within an international imaginary. The end of the transition embraced these international cultural events as a way of apparently demonstrating its ability to shake off Francoist scurf and to open the country toward an acceptance of global capitalism. Within this context, one could observe a profound urban remodeling of the postindustrial city in which public space was deregulated and privatized. Factories were dismantled and, with that, a large part of the working class's claim to power was also undone. Unemployment emerged as an increasingly urgent problem, especially for Spanish youth. From the mid-1980s onward, when countercultural synergies that had developed in the previous decade had been devoured by the market, a new order of representation based on a separation between politics and culture gained force.[23] It is from within this cultural field that Spanish counterculture became inextricably associated and socially embedded with a way of being young that was rooted in the experience of nightlife as an engine of leisure and drug use.

According to Labrador, Spain's young baby boom generation and their early access to transitional freedoms conditioned their behavior in relation to heroin, making it possible to "complete the whole cycle more quickly," meaning that many would begin consuming the drug during their adolescence.[24] By understanding heroin use as "a way of being young," members of this generation created their identity in relation to forms of addiction and social exclusion. Taking up the argument developed by psychiatrist González Duro, Labrador focuses on the idea that drug use was related to a feeling of disaffection experienced by Spanish youth in relation to the values that prevailed during the Franco dictatorship, which they also identified as principles that their parents held in high regard. For González Duro, this is indicative of a clinical expression of a social fracture. While adults feared the bodies and lifestyles of the transition's youth, this very generation also reacted drastically to the imaginaries, values, and experiences that their parents represented and that were closely associated with the Franco regime.

Labrador develops an analysis of a unique testimony, the written memoirs of two heroin addicts, Jancho and Javi, titled "Notes for a History of *Yonqui* Zaragoza."[25] In the memoirs, three periods——or three ways of understanding and consuming heroin———each following generational differences, are established. During the first stage, at the beginning of the 1970s, heroin consumption is linked to a smaller number of individuals coming from hippie environments, who link the drug with psychedelic culture. Here, heroin consumers are members of the middle class who are introduced to the powdery substance through the consumption of prescribed drugs, like opiates, obtained in pharmacies and later, after 1974, through the use of morphine.[26] The second period, spanning from 1978 and 1982, corresponds with the brutal expansion of heroin within Spain.[27] It is during this period that Jancho and Javi, the narrators of the text Labrador analyzed, "get hooked." Both narrators belong to the generation that was young in 1975, before "getting high" was linked to leftist political militancy and/or Spanish countercultures. When Jancho and Javi write their story, they describe the large number of "junkies" who belonged to this generation who died as a result of their addiction. Many say that there was a preconceived government-backed plan to promote the rapid spread of heroin and, by extension, the onset of the HIV/AIDS crisis, as a strategy for calming the creative, radical dynamics that were used to imagine alternative political and cultural strategies during the transition. However, there is no evidence that proves this. Although not a power conspiracy, the truth was that the increase in drug use certainly played an undeniably important role within the political field.

Finally, the third stage began in 1983. In many ways "Notes for a History of *Yonqui* Zaragoza" was written to those who got hooked on heroin during this period. As the text states, "The immense majority of people from Zaragoza who were initiated into heroin use did so after the decriminalization of the drug consumption in 1983. The decriminalization of drug consumption radically transformed the entire 'smack' map."[28] With the drug's falling prices and its decreasing quality, a massive number of young people got quickly addicted to the substance. Its subsequent expansion through working-class neighborhoods brought many to the brink of marginality. The problem, then, radically relapsed into the performativity of being a "*yonqui*" (junkie), which Labrador reiterates when he describes this third generation as "being *yonqui* before even being *yonqui*."[29] In other words, there is a generational discourse that establishes itself in relation to this very identity. Jancho and Javi explain with clarity the performative effects of the yonqui identity for Yolanda and Gabriel's generation when they write,

> Now there are kids, and not so kids, that think it's cute to want to shoot up, even though they don't have the smallest of symptoms that come with abstinence. They think they are "hooked" (with the terrible consequences that this bears), just because they have injected four times with a product that is only four percent heroin. The most serious issue is that these people think they are hooked, and psychologically they become hooked, and so if they hear that an addict steals, kills, and has AIDS, it becomes a serious problem for society (something that is monotonously repeated everywhere), because this means

that they are just one step away from stealing, killing, getting AIDS, and thinking of themselves as being really important.[30]

This text allows us to face the heart of the problem: How can we understand the embodiment of an identity that passes through rapid self-destruction and marginality and that in many cases ends in physical disappearance? Through the photographs of Gabriel and Yolanda that appear in the fanzine, one can begin to understand how this process affects the third generation of heroin addicts. It also provides performative keys, embedded in the publication itself, by emphasizing the constant effort exerted to make and configure physical and symbolic bodies through photographic practice and its ability to record and compile.

Completing military service—or "hacer la mili"—was one of the most significant milestones in the life of young male Spaniards until 2001, when the practice was declared no longer obligatory. Gabriel keeps a portrait of himself dressed in a military uniform with his hair shaved short that is recovered in *Yolanda*. For many Spanish youth who came of age during the transition, the ritual of shaving one's head was a castrating experience. Once forced to remove their long locks in order to complete military service, many young men saw hair as an important sign of physical identity that could potentially challenge the established order. In the photographic portrait, Gabriel exhibits a pouting, harsh face, perhaps an effect of having "gone cold turkey" after being forced to abstain from drug consumption.[31] His facial expression is reiterated in his own testimony transcribed onto one of the fanzine's textual fragments: "Military service. A waste of time. They took a year of your life and didn't teach you anything. You just learned to be lazy, to be a bastard and to pass the buck." Like Gabriel, young Spaniards, many of whom strongly identified with pacifism and antimilitarism, felt that military service limited their freedoms and their life agency. "La mili," without a doubt, was replete with characteristics that could be linked with *franquismo*, the dictatorial regime that celebrated fascism and militarism. After all, the coup d'état in July 1936 that provoked the civil war was, in fact, a military uprising against the democratic Popular Front government. It is, therefore, important to note that the youth of the extended Spanish transition developed an identity that was radically opposed to that of their "francoist" parents, as well as the conservative powers and forces of the status quo that were clearly inherited from the dictatorship and its legacy.

This conflict between parents and children is powerfully addressed in the film *El Pico*, directed by Eloy de la Iglesia and released in 1983. The feature examines a friendship, marked by heroin consumption, between two young

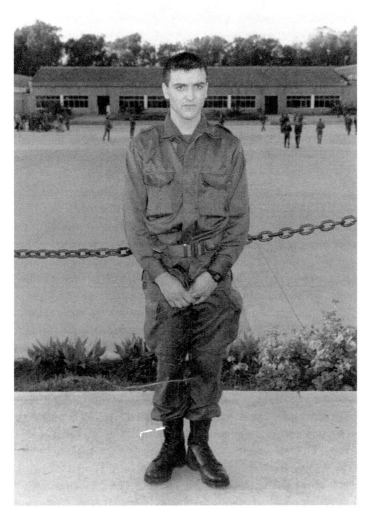

Figure 6.7: Gabriel. Untitled photograph published in the fanzine *Yolanda*, self-published by Ignacio Navas in 2014.

boys who live in the grey, industrial city of Bilbao. Urko, played by Javier García, is the son of Basque left nationalist parliament representative; Paco, played by José Luis Manzano, is the son of a Civil Guard major. In the film, generational conflict is fundamental to the narrative, especially within the relationship described between Paco and his father, Major Torrecuadrada, played by José Manuel Cervino, who wants his son to follow in his footsteps by immediately entering into the military academy. Again and again, Paco rejects the idea, suggesting repeatedly that he does not want to be like his father. In a key sequence, during Paco's eighteenth birthday, the audience observes the family celebration. Clearly uncomfortable, Paco can only think about leaving his family home in order to shoot up with heroin. His father, hopeful and excited, takes Paco aside and suggests that he dress in the Civil Guard uniform as a surprise for his mother and sisters. Paco agrees. It is here that a true exercise in what Judith Butler calls performativity begins. By "dressing up," Paco becomes a "true man"—that is, a violent civil guard, a father of a family, who is sexist, homophobic, and conservative. The father draws a moustache on his son's upper lip before taming his unruly, curly hair with gel. He then dresses Paco in the stiff uniform and places the "tricornio," the special three-cornered Civil Guard hat, on his head. Finally, he secretly tells his son that they will celebrate his coming of age by visiting prostitutes. Paco is unaware and unaccustomed to the dynamics imposed by his father and eventually chooses to become a man quite different from the model proposed by the family patriarch. The final sequence of the film artfully reveals this choice. Father and son stand together on a cliff overlooking the sea. The father places a large bag of heroin that his son had recently stolen from a dealer inside his three-cornered hat. Before throwing the goods into the water below, Paco's father says, "This garbage can destroy a life." His son responds ironically, "Are you talking about the powder or the hat?" thereby, emphasizing the complexity of the lives and identities of Spain's transitional youth.

    One of the photographs that appears in Yolanda shows a cake, a birthday cake, with the words "Life is disgusting" written on the top in whipped cream. The image is not from Gabriel's personal album but instead was found and recuperated by Navas, thanks to a Facebook publication that he dedicated to Parrys, the bar frequented by Tudela's youth and known for being full of "junkies and fags." The owner of the image is not important. It is instead the phrase that deserves attention, a set of words that violently refers to a sense of disenchantment, or *desencanto*, made material through an object used to celebrate life. *Desencanto* is the emotion or affective condition that young Spaniards began to experience at the end of the 1970s and that subsequent generations continued to experience with some variations. It was a disenchantment that, in conjunction with the expansion of the drug-induced narcosis, served as a reaction to attitudes of suspicion and rejection that young generations had toward the future. It was a kind of postrevolutionary melancholy that followed the euphoria of the first months of the transition.[32] At the beginning of the transition, this initial disenchantment was most likely related to highly conflictive reactions toward franquismo, as well as the unconscious addiction to such contention.[33] However, by the mid-1980s it had transformed into a kind of boredom, fatigue, and even desperation. In contrast, Sánchez León offers an alternative interpretation of "desencanto" and suggests that the phenomenon was the result of a "clash between utopian and mesocratic utopias, a clash inevitably produced among the founding pillars of representative democracy: elections, parties, and constitution."[34] Spanish youth reacted in radical ways against the middle-class values that had been installed during the period of *desarrollismo*, the name given to Francoist-era, neoliberal economic development policies. And they did so by fostering transgressive attitudes toward social class, in which they emotionally self-projected and identified with the *lumpen* rather than with the disappearing imaginaries of the working class. Following the ideas put forth by Sánchez León, it could be said that as a result, these imaginaries found themselves in a state of retraction.[35]

This youthful disenchantment also possessed a creative potential that was translated, particularly in the international context, into a particular music culture based on radical rock, particularly punk. During the 1980s, many young people lived their lives from the nonsense that characterized the lack of opportunities brought on by the economic crisis and its related wave of structural unemployment, both of which fomented the idea that the future was uncertain. This experience with a "no future" defined the new global privatization that was analogous to the rise of neoliberalism. In this sense, the emergence of punk in Spain, developed first in Catalonia and the Basque Country, had much to do with the synergies of the genre's international development: "There are no major differences between European and Basque punk; they arise from similar events: crisis and anomie, being uprooted and facing a lack of opportunities, social schizophrenia and youthful rebellion."[36]

Returning to the photographs of Gabriel and Yolanda, one finds an apparent conglomeration of gestures, objects, memories, scenes, and practices—like heroin trafficking, a passion for race cars, and their inverse, car accidents—that are seamlessly related to working-class imaginaries, as well as those related to the quinqui subculture. At the same time, the protagonists who appear in the images demonstrate a resistance to loss and decadence in their ability to reflect through the photographic image the kind of precision and impulse, often exhibited by chroniclers and historians needed in order to capture the sentimental textures of the everyday life that surrounds them: images of the David Bowie poster and the samurai sword that decorate the bedroom; a ticket stub from a concert by The Cure; a snapshot of a dog; the landscapes with snow used as a metaphor for heroin; the picture of a

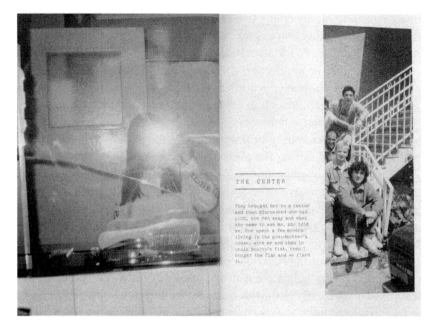

Figure 6.8: Flash. Untitled photograph published in the fanzine *Yolanda*, self-published by Ignacio Navas in 2014.

leather bomber jacket next to the television; and even the self-portrait of Yolanda wearing dark glasses in front of the bathroom mirror, taken before her entrance into a detoxification center when her hair had been cut short only moments before. The flash that covers her face reflected on the surface of the mirror foretells the erasure that her memory will undergo.

It is interesting to consider that in the face of her own erasure, Yolanda sought memory. She projected her identity and her emotions through personal photography, a medium especially adept for subaltern or marginal groups who seek to express or construct a memory that is distanced from hegemonic narratives. This genre provides a kind of visual agency that always exists in tension with the cultural norms that, as we have seen, determine the regime of what is photographable.[37] The visual repertoire of emotional bodies that are collected in *Yolanda* most certainly have to do with the creation of new modes of social belonging. The photographs are without a doubt an attempt, although small and perhaps mundane, to create a narrative faithful to Yolanda and her surroundings. This generation has failed to assume its own identity as a collective political group, perhaps because this narrative, as well as those cobbled together by many of the young Spaniards who experienced the transition, lack sufficient force and essence.[38] As Labrador confirms, "We do not have a civic, citizen-based memory of one of the most terrible chapters of our recent history, a chapter that tells the story of the tragic consequences of the exponential expansion and circulation of heroin."[39] And yet when we speak of Yolanda, we are not recounting her history, her memory, but rather writing ours. As Navas concludes, the final objective of his piece, that which moves us, is definitely the capacity to understand ourselves and our present.

Coda

Studying heroin consumption in transitional Spain is a way to confront my own ghosts. At the same time, it is an attempt to understand how my own genealogy activates emotions and processes of collective memory similar to that experienced by Navas. It is the memory of the orphans, of those who lost our fathers, our uncles, and our parents' friends during the 1990s. It is the memory of those who still do not understand what happened. It is also the memory of the mothers, like my grandmother, who buried their yonqui children. There are few spaces where one can talk across generations regarding the erasure of those young Spaniards who experienced firsthand the arrival of democracy. It is surely because of this that our sorrow—our ability to mourn—is still pending, both on collective and individual levels. We are not sure how to understand the young people who, between 1978 and 1985, became rapidly hooked on heroin. As we have seen, there are few frameworks—memory frameworks—that can help us understand ourselves, because there are few texts that conserve their ideas, because few people have expressed an interest in their lives. This is why it is difficult to confront these ghosts. It is more productive, more useful, to direct our gaze forward in that Spain that during the 1990s was launched into modernity through urban change while also burying, without sorrow or glory, the damaged, leftover, and monstrous bodies of addicts.

It was with a photograph that I was finally able to talk to my mother about the death of my father. A high school teacher asked us to complete autobiographic narratives that would recount the micro-histories of our families. We had to collect documents regarding our lives as well as the lives of our family members and friends: birth certificates, childhood drawings, and snapshots from our photo albums. As I shuffled through envelopes stuffed with photographs and kept together in a box, I found a portrait of my father with my brother in a small boat. Behind them, the blue sea. The photograph was taken in Cadiz, where we spent our summers. My father wore a cloth hat and a white t-shirt with a logo advertising the photographic brand Fuji. His arm was extended as he rested it on the edge of the boat. In the image, I could see perfectly the marks on his arm, the typical prick wounds or "*picos*" produced by heroin injected with a hypodermic needle. By looking at the photograph, I confirmed what I had always known, even though no one had told me, that my parents had consumed heroin and that he had died as a result of a related illness, most likely AIDS.

I showed the photograph to my mother, and we were able to talk about everything. That is where the most significant emotional, performative, and memory-related effects of personal photography dwell. Surely because of this, I labor to recover the history of common folk, the history of those whose stories are never told, by examining and analyzing vernacular photography. I know that now. And, surely because of this, *Yolanda* made such a profound impact on me. I never thought I would tell this story in a book written in English and published in a place as distant as Illinois. Perhaps because of this, I decided to do it. I realize now that there are few casualties. You may ask yourself what I did with that photograph. I cut the fragment of the image where my father's arm was so alarmingly visible, and I pasted the rest of it onto my school project. Individuals, like the societies they inhabit, exert agency over the ways we remember.

Notes

The research described in this chapter was completed in conjunction with the project "Género, emociones y subjetividad en la relaciones de pacientes/profesionales sanitarios" (HAR2016-78223-C2-2-P), financed by the Spanish Ministry of Economics and Competitiveness (MINECO) and made possible through the support of the State Research Agency (SRA) and the European Regional Development Fund (ERDF). The essay was also written with the support of a "Juan de la Cierva Formación" postdoctoral fellowship (MINECO), University of Valencia.

1. These are Ignacio Navas's own words, as published in http://www.yorokobu.es/yolanda.

2. See Andrew L. Walter and Rosalind Kimball Moulton, "Photo Albums: Images of Time and Reflections of Self," *Qualitative Sociology* 12, no 2 (1989): 155–82; Carmen Ortiz, "Fotos de familia: Los álbumes y las narrativas domésticas como forma de arte popular," in *Maneras de mirar: Lecturas antropológicas de la fotografía*, ed. Antonio Cea Gutiérrez; Carmen Ortiz García and Cristina Sánchez-Carretero (Madrid: CSIC, 2005), 189–210; Martha Langford, *Suspended Conversations: The Afterlife of Memory in Photographic Albums* (Montreal: McGill-Queen's University Press, 2001).

3. These are, again, Navas's own words, as cited in http://www.yorokobu.es/yolanda.

4. Here "transition" is understood as the political passage from the militaristic and dictatorial regime of Francisco Franco to an established democracy. I use the expanded chronological arc proposed by Teresa Vilarós that begins in 1973 with the attack against General Carrero Blanco perpetrated by the terrorist organization ETA and ends in 1993, when Spain definitively becomes a member of the European Union with the signing of the Maastricht Treaty. See Teresa Vilarós, *El mono del desencanto: Una crítica cultural a la transición española (1973–1993)* (Madrid: Siglo 21, 1998) 1–2.

5. Martha Langford, "Speaking the Album: An Application of the Oral-Photographic Framework," in *Locating Memory: Photographic Acts*, ed. Annette Kuhn and Kirsten Emiko McAllister (New York: Berghahn, 2008), 223–46.

6. Roger Odin, "El film familiar como documento: Enfoque semiopragmático," *Archivos de la filmoteca* 57–58, no. 2 (2007): 203–4, cited in Isabel Cadenas Cañón, "Poética de la ausencia: Formas subversivas de la memoria en la fotografía y el cine de la España contemporánea" (PhD diss., New York University, 2016), 209.

7. Martha Langford, "Contar el álbum: Una aplicación del marco oral-fotográfico," in *Álbum de familia: [Re]presentación, [re]creación e [in]materialidad de las fotografías familiares*, ed. Pedro Vicente (Madrid: Diputación Provincial de Huesca, 2013), 79.

8. I had the opportunity to speak with Ignacio Navas about *Yolanda* on May 13, 2017. I am thankful to the photographer for his kindness and for all of the ideas he shared with me.

9. Cadenas, "Poética de la ausencia," 51–53.

10. In Spain at the time of the transition, traveling to the sea for the first time was often a milestone in the lives of Spanish working-class youth who did not live on the coast. This kind of practice is depicted in a key film from the time, *Deprisa, Deprisa* (Carlos Saura, 1981), where heroin, youth in marginal environments, and, in this case, delinquency take center stage. The film follows a group of friends who make a living by robbing banks. *Deprisa, Deprisa* is one of the best cinematographic examples of what is often referred to as cinema "quinqui." The word is a derivative of *quincallero* or *merchero*, meaning traveling merchant, which was a derogatory nickname used during the first years of Spanish democracy, in order to refer to adolescents or young adults from poor, suburban neighborhoods who often consumed drugs and participated in criminal or delinquent activities. Ángela, one of the film's protagonists, can be compared to Yolanda, given that the quinqui subculture predominantly focused on the socialization of men, which means that the presence of women—be it in fiction or in real life—was both powerful and complex. For a description of the quinqui subculture, see Joaquín Florido Berrocal et al., eds. *Fuera de la ley: Asedios al fenómeno quinqui en la Transición española* (Granada: Comares, 2015).

11. Cadenas, "Poética de la ausencia," 52.

12. Pierre Bourdieu, *Photography: A Middle-Brow Art* (Stanford, Calif.: Stanford University Press, 1990).

13. See the website http://graffica.info/jorge-fernandez-puebla-yolanda-fanzine-fotolibro.

14. The book *Beyond the Family Album* (1978-1979) by Jo Spence is a paradigmatic example of a feminist analysis of the photographic album.

15. Vilarós, *El mono del desencanto*, 246. Vilarós draws on this concept developed by Smith in order to refer to the subject represented through his or her absence, a kind of praxis in which remains and traces refer to illness and death; see Paul Julian Smith, *Vision Machines: Cinema, Literature and Sexuality in Spain and Cuba, 1983-1993* (London: Verso, 1996), 2.

16. These are the exact words used by the author.

17. Joan Fontcuberta, *La furia de las imágenes: Notas sobre la postfotografía* (Barcelona: Galaxia Gutenberg, 2016), 39.

18. Fontcuberta, *La furia de las imágenes*, 142. *Recopilar imágenes sin memoria* (2012-2015) by Lúa Cordech is a piece that is closely related to Navas's creative impulses. In the piece, Cordech examines his family albums in order to select those photographs for which no surviving kin can identify the circumstances wherein the images were taken or the persons who appear in it. Other important works that use found photographs include *Mujeres, amor, mentiras* (2003) by Carmela García; *Los Modlin* (2013) by Paco Gómez; and *Orphan Photo* (2004) by David Trullo.

19. Pablo Sánchez León, "Estigma y memoria de los jóvenes de la Transición," in *La memoria de los olvidados: Un debate sobre el silencio de la represión franquista*, ed. Emilio Silva et al. (Valladolid: Ámbito Ediciones y Asociación para la Recuperación de la Memoria Histórica, 2004), 168-69.

20. Ibid., 167.

21. Ibid., 169.

22. German Labrador Méndez, *Culpables por la literatura: Imaginación política y contracultura en la Transición española (1968-1986)* (Madrid: Akal, 2017), 65.

23. Ibid., 575.

24. Ibid., 561. There are few works that seek to understand youth generations belonging to the extended transition (1973-1993). Fortunately, the few analyses that exist are eloquent in their treatment of this subject. Germán Labrador dedicates a chapter of his recent book *Culpables por la literature: Imaginación política y contracultura en la transición española (1968-1986)* to an analysis of those Spaniards born from 1960 onward, who are often identified as members of the *movida madrileña* and connected to the decade of the 1980s. Yolanda and Gabriel would have been a bit younger than the generation Labrador analyzes. However, as we have seen through the reflections made by Sánchez León, they are generations that indeed adhere to similar patterns.

25. This text can be found in Gonzalo García Prado, *Los años de la aguja: Del compromiso político a la heroína* (Zaragoza: Mira, 2002), where it is located between Jancho's memoirs, taken from a series of interviews of more than twenty-four hours in length, conducted by García Pardo in between 1997 and 1999, Javi's diary, and transcriptions of some of his letters.

26. García Prado, *Los años de la aguja*, 65-69. The film director Iván Zulueta develops his relationship with heroin during this period. His film *Arrebato* (1979) is

paradigmatic of the radically underground film created in relationship with heroin addiction.

27. The year 1978 was a moment of inflection within the expansion of heroin addiction in Spain. This was not a product of the increase in the drug's consumption but rather a reflection of the growing public attention paid to the drug. The mass media transformed heroin addiction into a "problem" before it was actually an issue. As if in a self-fulfilled prophecy, this epidemic state was massively promoted before addiction took hold of Spanish youth; see Juan Carlos Usó, *Drogas y cultura de masas: España (1855–1995)* (Madrid: Taurus, 1996), 325. On the other hand, 1978 also marks a moment of inflection in the political field since it coincided with the moment in which the open institutional dynamics, like the Moncloa Pacts—two agreements that were signed between the government, the Congress of Deputies, employers' associations, and the Workers' Committee Union and that regulated fundamental political and economic matters pertaining to the transition, such as free-labor dismissals and freedom of the press—were established via the passage of the democratic Constitution. As Labrador affirms, "The institutionalization of the political and its definition as consensual made the forms of protest, public opinion, and dissidence that remained outside of parliamentary margins invisible." Labrador, *Culpables por la literatura*, 539.

28. García Prado, *Los años de la aguja*, 87–88. In the original text, the authors use the word *caballo* to refer to heroin. This word is commonly used in Spanish argot to refer to the drug. Here the word is translated to a similar form of English slang, "smack," which is also used to refer to this particular narcotic. To clarify, drug consumption was decriminalized, while drug possession and drug trafficking were not.

29. Labrador, *Culpables por la literatura*, 564.

30. García Prado, *Los años de la aguja*, 89.

31. Military service was a place for drug withdrawal, or "going cold turkey," but also a space in which Spanish youth continued or reaffirmed their consumption of narcotics. This kind of experience is narrated in Javi's diary (García Prado, *Los años de la aguja*, 77).

32. German Labrador Méndez, *Letras arrebatadas: Poesía y química en la Transición española* (Madrid: Devenir Ensayo, 2009), 107.

33. Vilarós, *El mono del desencanto*, 18.

34. Pablo Sánchez León, "Desclasamiento y desencanto: La representación de las clases medias como eje de una relectura generacional de la transición española," *Kamchatka* 4 (2014): 89.

35. Sánchez León, "Desclasamiento y desencanto," 88.

36. Jakue Pascual, "El Punk: De England a Euskadi bailando un pogo," *Inguruak: Asociación Vasca de Sociólogos* (1987): 47, quoted in Jakue Pascual, *Movimiento de resistencia: Años 80 en Euskalherria. Contexto, crisis y punk* (Tafalla: Txalaparta, 2015), 93. For more on Basque punk, see also the documentary *Bilbao, Aste Nagusia de 1986*, directed by Mikel Arce y Gisella Keller. For more on the Barcelona punk scene,

see Jordi Llansamà, *Harto de todo: Historia oral del punk en la ciudad de Barcelona 1979–1987* (Barcelona: Jordi Llasamà@BCore Disc., 2011).

Sánchez León, "Desclasamiento y desencanto," 89.

37. Catherine Zuromskis, *Snapshot Photography: The Lives of Images* (Cambridge, Mass.: MIT Press, 2013), 33–34.

38. Sánchez León, "Estigma y memoria," 165.

39. Labrador, *Letras arrebatadas*, 19.

PART III

Making Social Bodies

This section shifts the focus away from individual actors—hysterical women, patients suffering from either cancer or AIDS, children in pain, criminals of passion, and even photographic cameras—in order to examine the capacity of emotions in building collectives. Historians of emotions have, from the beginning, advocated for analyzing the affective life of the past within the contours of societies. Moving beyond psychology, the initial impetus of this historical enterprise was to shed light on the ways through which institutions had reinforced emotional behavior through the prescription of laws and codes.

This was Lucien Febvre's very premise when he claimed the urgency of writing a history of sensibilities in order to forbid the eruption of a wave of violence similar to the rise of Hitler's Nazism in Europe.[1] Febvre went so far as to say that if historians did not engage with the study of hate, fear, and cruelty, humanity would finish looking like "a stinking pit of corpses."[2] More than sixty years after, Jan Pampler would note a renewed interest in emotions among historians, which he identified with the terrorist attacks perpetrated on 9/11 because of the highly emotional nature of this event, provoked by media communication.[3] Even though theses linking the emergence of—both the old and new—history of emotions to past and present atrocities have not attained historians' unanimity, what seems clear is that emotions cannot be correctly approached without situating them at the heart of social and political debates.[4]

In the 1980s, Peter and Carol Stearns also called for studying the attitudes or the standards of groups of people toward basic emotions and their expression, what they understood under the term of "emotionology," a conceptual tool they introduced in order to frame the history of emotions as a development of social history.[5] We have learned over time that there are emotions we have lost and whose absence reveals major structural changes in our present societies, as Ute Frevert has shown.[6] Scholars like William Reddy have, moreover, opted for demonstrating that emotions make history—a history that can help us to integrate social interactions within major political transformations, such as the French Revolution.[7] Beyond the modern nation-state, emotions have also become for other historians like Barbara Rosenwein the lenses with which to venture in more distant epochs, such as the medieval age, and examine how people organized their life around institutions like families, schools, or churches.

Taking Rosenwein's work on "emotional communities" as starting point, this section precisely investigates how emotions like joy or fear have prompted to the emergence of social bodies. The two chapters in this section contribute to rethinking the creation of religious communities or revolutionary crowds thanks to the work of emotions.[8] Most specifically, the case studies proposed here contribute to showing that emotional practices are at the roots of the process through which social groups constituted themselves as having a common identity and not inversely, by previously supposing them before their formation. The focus on the performativity of emotions thus allows a reexamination of Rosenwein's emotional communities both real and fictional in the light of practices, such as religious adoration and political abjection.

Piroska Nagy's chapter recreates the first celebration of Christmas in Greccio by Saint Francis of Assisi as a multisensorial experience: visual, auditory, even gustative. Nagy's attention to the sensory elements allows her to reinterpret this religious ceremony as an event that created an emotional body through the collective experience of an emotion lived in the early-twelfth-century Franciscan hermitage based in the mountains. As ephemeral as this body was, it is important to highlight this moment as a performative practice, as doing emotions together created a new evangelic community. Nagy argues, therefore, that observing the emotional embodiment can account, in this case, for social and religious change.

Dolores Martín-Moruno completes this section by examining the emergence of a fictional collective, the incendiary women of the Paris Commune, as a result of the performative nature of fear. Like Nagy, Martín-Moruno interprets the formation of this female terrorist body in the light of a politics of emotion, which consciously erased what happened in late-nineteenth-century France: the hope for social revolution. By looking at Louise Michel's judgement, she analyzes abjection as a common practice among conservative military officials, journalists, and even evolutionary scientists that led to the transformation of working-class women into the *pétroleuses*: an organized criminal group threatening the Third Republic. As she argues, women revolutionaries also contributed to the making of this terrorist body when they recognized themselves as abject. By comparing past and present fears, the performative effects of this emotion led the author to problematize terrorist bodies as an expression of state terrorism.

Notes

1. Lucien Febvre, "Sensibility and History: How to Reconstitute the Emotional Life of the Past," in *A New Kind of History: From the Writings of Febvre*, ed. Peter Burke, trans. K. Folca (London: Routledge and Keagan Paul, 1973), 12–26. For other contemporary influential work for the history of emotions, see Norbert Elias, *The Civilizing Process* (1939), trans. Edmund F. N. Jephcott (Oxford: Blackwell, 2000).

2. Febvre, "Sensibility and History," 26. On the importance of Fevbre for the history of emotions, see also Rob Boddice, *The History of Emotions* (Manchester: Manchester University Press, 2018).

3. Jan Pampler, *The History of Emotions: An Introduction*, trans. Keith Tribe (Oxford: Oxford University Press, 2015), 60–66.

4. On the political origins of the history of emotions, see Thomas Brudholm, ed., *Emotions and War Atrocities. Philosophical and Theoretical Explanations* (Cambridge: Cambridge University Press, 2018), 1.

5. Peter N. Stearns and Carol Z. Stearns, "Emotionology: Clarifying the History of Emotions and Emotional Standards," *American Historical Review* 90, no. 4, (1985): 813–36.

6. Ute Frevert, *Emotions in History: Lost and Found* (Budapest: Central European University Press, 2011).

7. William Reddy, *The Navigation of Feeling: A Framework for the History of Emotions* (Cambridge: Cambridge University Press, 2001).

8. Barbara Rosenwein, *Emotional Communities in the Early Middle Ages* (Ithaca, N.Y.: Cornell University Press), 2.

7. Making a Collective Emotional Body

Francis of Assisi Celebrating Christmas in Greccio (1223)

PIROSKA NAGY

IN 1223, THREE YEARS before his death, Saint Francis of Assisi was spending the month of December in the little hermitage of Greccio, situated upon the hills that overhang the valley of Rieti, in the Latium (central Italy). Greccio was one of several hermitages in these mountains,[1] established by Franciscans as a quiet place to stay, an alternative to the already great collective houses that the order, which numbered then three thousand members, occupied in the swarming towns of flourishing Italy. Two weeks before Christmas, Francis called to him a man named Giovanni, whom he knew and liked, a man "of good reputation and even better life,"[2] living in the little town of Greccio. This man was most probably Giovanni Vellita, a friend of Francis and the lord of Greccio. Francis explained his project to him: he wanted to celebrate the Nativity of Jesus in Greccio with great solemnity and fidelity and asked Giovanni for his help. I quote here from the first biography of Francis of Assisi, by Thomas of Celano:

> For I *wish to do something that will recall to memory* the little Child who was born in Bethlehem and *set before our bodily eyes* in some way the inconveniences of his infant needs, how he lay in a manger, how, with an ox and an ass standing by, he lay upon the hay where he had been placed.[3]

According to Celano, Christmas came, and an event was prepared; laypeople, friars, and Francis himself arrived from the surrounding area. The celebration, as we shall see, was a success: the guests shared a beautiful feast, a strong sensory and emotional experience with the holy man. Proving the mystic realization of the event, a miracle occurred. A person of virtue (*a quodam viro virtutis* [I Mach. 5: 50]) from the audience—perhaps Giovanni Vellita, according to later sources, and first to the *Legenda maior* of Bonaventure—received a vision of the baby Christ sleeping, or inanimate, in the crib and then woken up by Saint Francis. At the end of the celebration, all the guests, deeply moved by what they lived and saw, went home filled with "holy joy," the most appropriate feeling for the birth of the Savior and its commemoration.

This is the story, as told by Thomas of Celano, who wrote this first biography (generally called *Vita prima*) in 1228–29, on a pontifical command just after the canonization of the saint who died two years earlier.[4] The scene is well known, conveyed in the "general culture" of the West as the moment of the invention of the scene of Christmas crèche (in all likelihood, the French word "crèche" comes from the name of the town, "Greccio"). Later written sources mentioning the event quote and rewrite it after Thomas's account.[5] His narration is also the source of the iconography of the scene. The episode describing in detail how Francis acted the memory of the birth of Jesus occupies chapter 30 (84–87) of the *Vita prima*, which ends the first part (opus) of the *vita* before turning to his death and the last two years that preceded it, in a second *opus*. The four paragraphs of the chapter are divided as follows: Francis explains his project (84), the feast is prepared (85), it is related in detail until the miracle occurring at the end of the celebration reveals the meaning of it (86); a last paragraph discusses the posterity of the place (87).

Noted as an important episode in the life of Francis, the scene enters quickly in the iconographic cycles of the life of the saint. The first representation (fig. 1) is that of the dossal of the Maestro of the Bardi chapel, in the Franciscan convent of Santa Croce of Florence, a hotspot for spiritual Franciscans in the late thirteenth and early fourteenth centuries. Dated 1254–57,[6] it was placed in the chapel of the Bardi family in Santa Croce at the end of the sixteenth century.[7] This hagiographic dossal,[8] based on the *Vita prima* of Celano, stands out from the other surviving dossals of its kind by virtue of the large number of narrative scenes of the life of Francis that it contains as opposed to posthumous miracles. The dossal contains twenty scenes (life and miracles) around a huge standing figure of saint Francis: the scene of Greccio (fig. 2) concludes the first six biographic scenes, in the bottom and on the left of the saint. Next come two scenes in the predella and a second series of scenes on the right, which need to be read from the bottom to the top.[9]

In what follows, I shall discuss this famous, frequently commentated event,[10] mainly on the basis of these first two sources, the *vita prima* of Celano and the Bardi dossal.[11] Focusing on this unique sensorial and emotional moment, I shall argue that the event created a collective emotional body, in the sense the editors of this volume understand it, where all the people present could participate. In what follows, we shall focus on the role of emotions in this celebration, which constitutes an event, a ritual, and a performance at the same time. An event is first something that interrupts the course of things, producing a break that frequently confers a new meaning or that changes the direction of current happening.[12] In any case, this change produces emotions, just like emotion produces this change.[13] The event we are concerned with is a ritual and a performance, specifically orchestrated toward the production of an event taking shape in the form of a shared affective experience. Identifying the transformative power of the shared experience occurring during the event, we can question, in broad terms, the importance of emotional happenings in the production of what becomes considered a historical event and, more specifically, the relationship between the *action of emotions* shared and, as a result, the birth of collective emotional bodies capable of registering and commemorating the event of which they are the result. In so doing, this study opts for a vision of emotions as *emotives*, to use a concept coined by William Reddy,[14] who considers that emotions, as they are expressed, change the world around them in the manner the performative statements of John Austin do.[15] In this sense, this paper tries to contribute to the ongoing reflection on the relationship of emotions and change in society by offering a case study on how emotions, either springing up or performed around an event, participate actively to the creation of collective emotional bodies, united by the experience of an emotion lived. This approach, which confers *social agency* to the performance of emotions akin to the proposition of Monique Scheer,[16] may help us understand what Francis of Assisi really meant by creating, staging, and conducting the event.

Before going further in the reflection on the sources, let us take a little tour of historiography. What does emotion change in history—and how does emotion affect change in history? Almost twenty years ago, Barbara Rosenwein elaborated the notion of emotional communities as a way of explaining the affective dimension of social and cultural groups linked by common aims and values.[17] She argued that when there is change in power, values, and relationships in a society, emotional communities—based on the sharing of emotional values, standards, and aims—also change.[18] In this sense, emotional change is subordinated to political, social, and cultural change, as well as to the change of theories encompassing affective life.[19] For Rosenwein, emotional community is an analytical tool, helpful for understanding and dissecting affective "standards" as well as their uses, transformations, and limits, but it does not serve to report and analyze change—among others, the change that gives birth to emotional communities themselves. It is in this perspective that observing emotional embodiment, the creation of ephemeral emotional bodies that can be stabilized (or not) in emotional communities, may be particularly useful.

Indeed, there is a strong interrelation between cultural, political, religious, and emotional change, which can follow different scenarios or trails.[20] The question of the relationship between emotions and change turned out to be an important concern for another pioneering historian of emotion, William Reddy. Reddy—who works as an anthropologist methodologically speaking, rather than as a historian—is extremely sensitive to what constitutes a major topic of history: social change. While Rosenwein criticized the Eliasian grand narrative of a simplistic relationship between emotion and (Western) historical change, Reddy was the first historian who tried to formalize the tools for thinking of emotion and change together in history. His notions of "navigation of feeling" and "emotives" both draw attention to the fact that emotional expressions *are movements*, and even processes: their performance can provoke movement and change.

Yet before emotion initiates a process, and before it becomes part of a set of accepted social norms, an emotion is a sudden movement. From a historian's point of view, the emotion is something that "pops up" in a document: it comes to the foreground of narration with immediacy, and sometimes even unexpectedly, and creates an event.[21] It *is* an event, as it forms a breach in the way reality is structured, at least for the person who feels, expresses, or describes it. An event, a breach: both designate a movement creating discontinuity, one felt as such by the people who witness or share it, something that requires a reflection to produce new meaning. An emotion may suddenly reveal a current transformation, or it can induce change, transmitting the produced breach in waves to other persons, provoking emotional, bodily, and intellectual reactions and processes, which may produce new emotional bodies. It is this aspect of emotion in history I shall investigate here, this aspect that melds "emotion" and "event" and is necessary when considering emotion in relation to any kind of social or historical change.

Greccio: The Stage

In 1223, Greccio was a very little town. According to Thomas of Celano, Francis likely stayed at an old hermitage, "a place of the friars near to Greccio where the saint liked to stop, because he saw it *rich of poverty*" and, as he says, because in the cell constructed on the rock he could easily dedicate himself

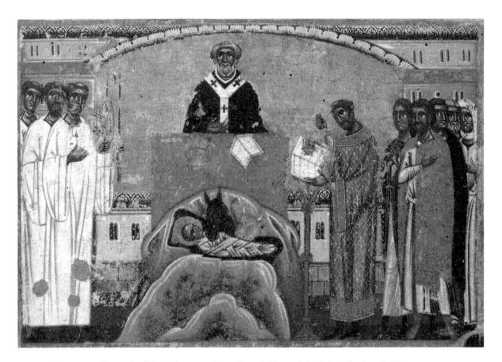

Figure 7.1: Dossal of the Master of the Bardi Chapel (1254–57), detail: The Invention of Greccio. Florence, convent of Santa Croce, capella Bardi. Scala/ Art Resources, New York.

to contemplation.[22] Fiercely opposed to any stable installation, for the sake of the humility and minority of his *religio*, Francis did not construct, in any case, convents or houses; he used only existing places, mostly humble ones. At the end of chapter 30, Celano suggests that any construction of a chapel (*templum*) in Greccio was consecutive to this celebration and the subsequent miracle. Some historians working on the topography of the place even believe the crib was constructed outdoors in a natural cave.[23] In the *vita prima* we learn only that the mass was celebrated *over* or *on the crib* (*celebrantur missarum solemnia supra praesepe*), which was used for the occasion as an altar. This symbolic unification of the birth and death of Christ, Incarnation and Passion, beginning and end, joined in the thought and devotion of Francis,[24] makes the crib an Incarnational and Eucharistic one at the same time;[25] the faithful could thus reflect about its meaning as a crib for the second birth, or Resurrection, after Christ's sacrificial death. The author of the Bardi dossal chose to juxtapose, visually, two spaces and elements of the scene. In the center top, the altar is depicted with a priest celebrating; just below, the rocks refer to the cave, with the baby Jesus and the head of the ox and ass near to him. On the two sides of the image, between laypeople and clerics, Francis is figured alone in front of the lay group; an arch linking the two sides indicates an urban setting.[26]

The question one cannot avoid at this point concerns the very place of the celebration. Can we imagine that Francis wanted to celebrate Christmas outdoors, outside of a church, as Celano suggests—in nature, even if it would appear somewhat subversive? Chiara Frugoni and Louis Gougaud note that, contrary to popular opinion, the very idea of constructing a crib was not a novelty in itself, and it could take place outside or inside a church. Liturgical "theater"—we had better say *performances*—celebrated around Western Europe included plays on the Nativity, involving clerical or lay actors. These plays were given the days after Christmas and used a crib on their stage from at least the eleventh century on.[27] Staged by priests, deacons, and subdeacons, some of these plays became satiric and were explicitly forbidden by the Pope Innocent III in a *decretale* of 1207.[28]

At this moment, the crib of the Nativity had been an object of veneration for several centuries. The church of Santa Maria Maggiore in Rome, constructed in the fourth century, when the date of Christmas had been stabilized, slowly became a *Betlemme di Roma*, especially after Bethlehem was occupied by the Muslims in 638. It was here that the relics of the real crib were then transferred[29]—a fact that involved, in turn, the construction of an *oratorium presepii*, an oratory of the crib, and of a specific altar, *altare presepii*.[30] Last but not least, it was here that the pope would celebrate Christmas, most probably from the eleventh century on, though there was also a permanent crib in Santa Maria di Trastevere.[31] Just before the episode of Greccio, in the final years of his pontificate (1213–1216), Innocent III renewed the *ordines* of the papal court. According to the new ordinal, the pope celebrated the mass of midnight at Santa Maria Maggiore at the altar of the crib, "ad presepem."[32]

Deciding to create a living representation of the Nativity a few years after his unvictorious return from the Holy Land in 1219, where he might have encountered the scenery of the crib in Bethlehem, Francis was conscious of this complex background. He took the inspiration of the celebration most probably in the ceremony practiced in Rome and well described in the recent papal ordinal.[33] In terms of spirituality, his vision of Christmas and of the baby Jesus was not far from that of Bernard of Clairvaux, according to the sermons for Nativity the great Cistercian abbot had written.[34] So, when preparing to celebrate Christmas in Greccio by constructing the first "living" representation of Nativity of Christian history,[35] he drew on a lively tradi-

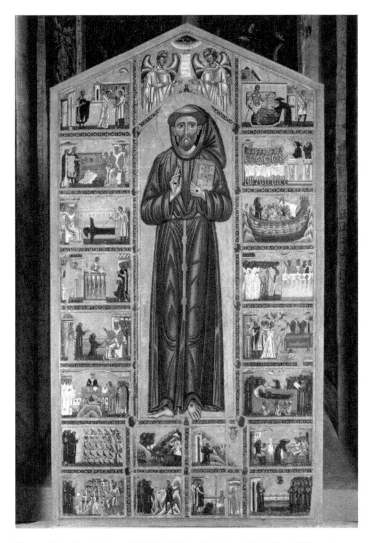

Figure 7.2: *Bardi dossal* (1254–57), by Master of the Bardi Chapel; Florence, convent of Santa Croce, capella Bardi. Scala/ Art Resources, New York.

tion and simultaneously transgressed part of it, abandoning the great urban churches for a place that symbolized, in his words, the richness of poverty,[36] and by imagining a series of details.

Francis of Assisi was a man who preferred to preach by his actions, so the scene was staged for a multisensorial experience: visual, auditory, even gustative. On his request, a *grandeur-nature* crib was constructed, with hay in it, and an ass and an ox were brought. In the staging, Francis omitted and added elements, compared to those usually characterizing medieval Christmas crèches, as far as they are known.[37] On the one hand, he added living animals. The event of Greccio, likely staged outdoors, underlines the natural environment and the animals, as well as the hay in the manger, the presence of which was important to Francis. This is not surprising: besides his intent of faithfulness to Bethlehem, Francis had a special affinity for nature and animals, a sensory relationship to all the elements and creatures belonging to the Creation and celebrating it, known from his own writings as well as from the written and iconographic sources concerning him.[38] On the Bardi dossal, the famous scene of his preaching to birds follows immediately that of Greccio (and is figured under it).[39]

On the other hand, Francis omitted key figures of the scene in his staging. Instead of actors who would play the Virgin, Joseph, and Jesus, Francis elided the persons of the scene, creating a void. Offering emptiness for contemplation, metaphorically figuring Jesus Christ who became invisible after his death, was a frequent procedure in the medieval Church.[40] Chiara Frugoni interprets this absence as an invitation for spectators to use, as customary in the monastic tradition, imagination and meditation for visualizing the baby Christ.[41] The efficacy of this procedure is the miracle offered to a virtuous man, at the end of the scene, the miraculous "incarnation" of the Child. In accordance with a method used since the eleventh and twelfth centuries in monastic spiritual texts,[42] Francis proposed his participants put themselves in the place of the Holy Family and experiment mentally the scene, as it is both staged and recalled verbally.

Sharing a Sensory and Emotional Event

When shaping the event, Francis specifies to Giovanni that the experience is intended to involve both inner and outer senses (*intus* and *foris*), referring to the inner (spiritual) and outer (bodily) man:

> For I *wish to do something that will recall to memory* the little Child who was born in Bethlehem and *set before our bodily eyes* in some way the inconveniences of his infant needs, how he lay in a manger, how, with an ox and an ass standing by, he lay upon the hay where he had been placed.[43]

In this way, the mental act of commemoration ("volo enim illius pueri *memoriam agere*," says Francis) became an act of bodily re-presentation, or presentification—in the same way the Eucharist, with Transubstantiation, came to make present, and not only represent, the body of Christ. Francis invites the public to complete with their inner eyes the scene they perceive with their outer, bodily eyes. The emptiness of the crib—the absence of Jesus—then foments a powerful symbolic meaning, at the end of the celebration, when miraculously, vision is granted to a faithful, allowing him to see the baby Jesus in the crib-altar, in an Incarnational and Eucharistic miracle.

The scene is prepared; laypeople from the surrounding areas and friars arrive with joy; Francis himself comes by. Perhaps because the event is taking place outdoors, Celano is careful to underline all the sensorial effects involved in any liturgical celebration:[44] here they participate to mobilize emotions that coalesce, as we shall see, in the creation of a new emotional body. The first experience is both visual and emotional. It is the night. Candles and torches are brought by the laypeople, arriving with "joy and exultation"; literal illumination brings the light of God, and its pleasant and joyful effects are extended to the surrounding nature as well:

> The night was lighted up like the day, and it delighted men and beasts. . . . The woods rang with the voices of the crowd and the rocks made answer to their jubilation.[45]

The liturgical celebration begins, passing from light and vision to voices, the auditory experience produced collectively. The friars chant; Francis, standing in front of the crib, is deeply moved: "uttering sighs, overcome with love, and filled with a wonderful happiness."[46] The priest, about whom no source speaks, seems to celebrate the mass over the crib, as the pope does it according to the ordinal of Innocent III. Francis himself, dressed "as a levite," a deacon, which he actually is, sings and preaches. The chant of Francis has a series of qualities in the text of Celano: strong, sweet, clear, sonorous; his preaching is qualified *mellifluous*, tasting honey, a term coming mostly from spiritual literature—the *epitheton ornans* of Bernard of Clairvaux, *doctor mellifluus*, and Gregory the Great, who were both great preachers.

Besides the quality of his voice and words, the very fact of Francis's predication is extraordinary, as he is not a priest. The other well-known occasions of his preaching—to the sultan in Egypt (1219) and to the birds—can be qualified as *exhortations*, according to the nomenclature of the thirteenth-century Church, opposed to formal predication to the faithful. But in Greccio, Francis preaches in the midst of a liturgical celebration to a Christian community. A simple deacon, Francis has not the right to preach to Christians, according to canon law; rather, it is his special, charismatic authority, testified by the qualities and effects of his sermon and a specific authorization of the pope, which allows him to do so.[47] After the chanting, Francis himself preaches on the Nativity, speaking of Christ as *Jesus*, in an intimate way:

> And speaking the word *Bethlehem*, his voice was more like the bleating of a sheep. His mouth was filled more with sweet affection than with words. Besides, when he spoke the name *Child of Bethlehem* or *Jesus*, his tongue licked his lips, as it were, relishing and savoring with pleased palate the sweetness of the words.[48]

Francis, who almost identifies himself to the sheep, signifying thereby the continuity of Creation and the equality of its humble creatures, tastes, almost eats the loving words he pronounces, savoring and relishing their meaning and sweetness in his heart and mind. This sweetness is also sensorial—he can lick it on his lips—and witnesses thereby the extension of love and joy to sensory feelings too.

The term *mellifluus*, quoted above, helps here to qualify the delight Francis feels and shares when pronouncing the name of Jesus with love.[49] The sweet words Francis savors and pronounces become, by his *mellifluous voice*, sensorial, affective, and spiritual nourishment, just like the host of the Eucharist, when given to the faithful audience. Francis shares what he tastes himself, and this is the case with emotions too. He shares the sweet experience of his words and feelings about the meaning of the Nativity and of Incarnation with all those present, whether ecclesiastic or lay.

As we can see, the whole performance and sensory experience prepares, through the shared embodiment of an emotional event, the creation of a new, collective emotional body. We can consider it "embodied" as the sensory experience brings up emotions that will, in turn, be shared. Here, emotions are anything but "*motus animae*": they are inseparable from the sensory experience as described above. This embodiment of emotions is a well-known feature of thirteenth-century Western Christian anthropology, specifically (but not only) developed by Francis.[50] Bodily signs and expressions of the moving soul are frequently emphasized in all kinds of sources, written or iconographic, and express an important turn. Emotions appear, all of a sudden, "incarnate," embodied—and belong, as they do here, to the embodiment, or incarnation, of spirituality. In our case, this *embodiment* is threefold. It concerns the nature and the manifestations of the sacred as it is lived by sensory and emotional experience; the composition of a collective emotional body, moved by the shared experience, by those who are living them; and the Eucharistic miracle, to which we shall return, when the little Jesus is visualized, suddenly "embodied," incarnate, in the Incarnational and Eucharistic crib: an event that reinforces the emotional unification of all those present who are witnessing the miracle.

Observing the emotions involved in the scene, it is important to underline that the celebration in Greccio is introduced, at the beginning of Celano's chapter, with a reminder that Francis wanted to live strictly according to the Gospel:[51]

> Francis's highest intention, his chief desire, his uppermost purpose was to observe the holy Gospel in all things and through all things and, with perfect vigilance, with all weal, with all the longing of his mind and all the fervor of his heart, "to follow the teaching and the footsteps of our Lord Jesus Christ." [Regula 1, c.1]

In the light of this paragraph, we can read the whole scene as organized in order to introduce a new start for Christianity, an emotional recreation of the primitive Church. During the celebration, only two traditional Christian emotions are evoked, both of which express, or refer to, *inner conversion*: Francis sighs alone in contrition, and the priest is touched, alone again, by a "new consolation" while listening to him. Aside from these two, the remaining feelings and emotions are shared by all the people. The joyful event of a healthy but also miraculous and divine birth is certainly even greater in the thirteenth century than in our world, where low infant mortality has become the norm. The shared emotions are all pleasant and positive: joy, exultation, happiness are the dominant ones, from the beginning of the scene:

- Joy: *gaudium, laetitia* and their verbal forms
- Exultation, entranced by joy, satisfaction or enthusiasm: *exultatio,*
- Jubilation, the shared expression of joy: *jubilatio*
- Sweetness: *dulcedo, melliflua*
- Expressions of love: *amor, cordis fervor, dulcis affectio*

Certainly joy, love, and exultation, emotions linked to the miracle, can be perceived as the most suitable feelings and expressions mobilized for celebrating Christmas, a major Christian feast, which honors the birth of Christ, the mystery of Incarnation, and the promise of Salvation. Still, these have not always been the feelings evoked at the feast of Nativity: if we find comparable feelings expressed in the preaching of Cistercian monks in the twelfth century, we would look for them in vain in Carolingian times.[52] On the other hand, these emotions of joy and jubilation belong to the universe and vocabulary of mysticism, of *raptus*, in Christian texts, where they describe other-worldly meeting with God. Yet they are also the specific emotions characterizing Francis of Assisi's path in this world. Francis was a holy man frequently performing emotions, particularly joyful all the time, since his conversion—inverting thereby the traditional Christic image, that of a suffering saint (that Francis eventually became in the last years of his life). In this sense, these joyful emotions belong to what Francis brought to Western Christianity:

he lived the joy of being with God in his earthly life, an experience that gave him a taste of the joy of Salvation. Sharing positive emotions, the specific flavor of the "religio" of Francis, during Christmas celebration thus prepared and undergirded the creation of a new emotional body in Greccio, enriched with a mystical, miraculous taste. We can speak of a new emotional body as an emotional melting that is happening during the feast, especially around the miracle—and this, in spite of the difference and hierarchy of *status*, of life states, always recalled, as it can be seen in the image of the Bardi altarpiece. The sharing of emotions suggests the erasure of social order and borders, occurring at the moment of the miracle: emotional and mystical union happens then, in what we, after Victor Turner, can call a liminal community.[53] Instead of a traditional liturgical spectacle, which involves clear spatial boundaries between clerics and lay folk, the accent, put-on sensory, emotional, and mystical experience transforms the celebration in a participative performance. This can be read as a manifesto for the unification of the whole Creation, the abolition of social distinctions in a new conception of the Church—at a moment when, after the council of Lateran IV, clerical control on the access of the brethren to the sacred is stronger than ever before. The main object of this shared happiness is the "Incarnation"—embodiment—of *simplicity, poverty, and humility* in this little, simple hermitage. The real meaning and "novelty" of Greccio, according to Celano, is this: "almost a new Bethlehem is made of Greccio," says the text, *quasi nova Bethlehem de Graecio facta est*. We can read here a return to the origins of Christianity: through the shared and living experience of this special and mystic event, on a symbolic level Francis re-founds the Church. This "new Bethlehem," founded in communion of pleasure and joy, peace and spiritual love, has to be read in the light of the opposition of Francis to any kind of war, among which first to the Crusades, as well as in the light of his own failure in the Holy Land.[54] Celano emphasizes this "novelty" several times—a novelty that recalls, and even replicates, the "good news" of the Gospel:

> There simplicity was honored, poverty was exalted, humility was commended, and Greccio was made, as it were, a *new Bethlehem*. The night was lighted up like the day, and it delighted men and beasts. The people came and were filled with *new joy over the new mystery*. [. . .] The solemnities of the Mass were celebrated over the manger and the priest experienced a *new consolation*. [. . .] At length the solemn night celebration was brought to a close, and each one returned to his home with *holy joy*.[55]

Unified by the shared joy and sensations of the event, reinforced by the miracle of the vision of the baby Christ, the micro-society assembled for

Christmas in Greccio appears as united by the exceptional, holy feelings, making a new emotional and social body—one that not only suppressed social borders but even transcended the frontiers of humanity, according to Celano, since for Francis, animals could understand and participate in the Revelation.[56]

Feast or Foundation?

On these bases, let's observe what we can say about the meaning of this event and chronology. Christmas 1223 is located near to the end of Francis's life, as he would die three years later, in October 1226. Also, the celebration in Greccio took place a month after the Franciscan order received its consecration from Pope Honorius III: the papal recognition of its rule, the *Regula bullata*. Considering this larger context, do we exaggerate by saying that Greccio was not only a feast, a commemoration of the birth of Christ, in the special style of saint Francis, reactivating the identity of Franciscan "religio"? Replacing the moment in its immediate context in the life and the *vita prima* of Francis, we realize that this emotional event was most probably intended to be, or due to become, more than a feast: the celebration gave birth to an emotional body, a new community, that Francis, a recognized and venerated saint, intended to found here of new. Let's reread Thomas of Celano's description of the miracle at end of the scene:

> The gifts of the Almighty were multiplied there, and a wonderful vision was seen by a certain virtuous man. For he saw a little child lying in the manger lifeless, and he saw the holy man of God go up to it and rouse the child as from a deep sleep. The vision was not unfitting, for the Child Jesus *had been forgotten in the hearts of many*; but, by the working of his grace, he was brought to life again through his servant St. Francis and stamped upon their fervent memory.[57]

Here, the biographer makes a parallel between Francis (not yet considered *alter christus*) and Jesus Christ. Francis resurrects (*suscitare*), as from a long sleep, the inanimate child (*videbat puerulum exanimem*): by an interesting inversion, Francis takes the role of Christ, who could perform resurrections, thereby resurrecting Jesus in the heart. By this immense miracle—which can also be read in parallel with the divine insufflation of the soul to the embryo[58] or by analogy with the animation of Adam by God—Francis gives birth to a new humanity. Actually, while the text says that "a certain virtuous man" saw the baby Christ being reawakened by Francis "as from a deep sleep," the event was "stamped upon *their* fervent memory," the memory of the whole group being present. The grace of God was diffused to the whole

Piroska Nagy 163

assistance, of which "each one returned to his home with *holy joy*."[59] In this perspective, the new emotional and social body created by the celebration takes a symbolic significance.

Actually, Christmas in Greccio occurred at the end of 1223, at the end of three years during which, putting forward his poor health, Francis had been moving away from the Franciscan order. As the friars chose the path of institutionalization and integration in the Church, against the narrow path of the early Franciscan poverty and minority, he took his leave of the management of the order in 1220. In the last years of his life, while he suffered from various ailments, Francis spent more and more time alone as a hermit, taking a path of reorientation and of mystic rebirth. Turning away from the order, Francis turned directly to Christ and to those who were "minor," precarious and poor, like the beasts.

This turn was well illustrated by his choice to stay in Greccio for a long time—either the whole month of December 1223 or the period of Lent in 1224, perhaps both.[60] As to show this, the episode of Greccio concludes, in the *vita prima* of Celano, the first part of the text, devoted to the earthly path of Francis; the second part concerns the last two years leading to his death. In the economy of the *vita*, the next moment recalled in the life of Francis after Greccio is his stigmatization, in September 1224. During the very special feast celebrated in Greccio, the Eucharistic miracle of the mass is doubled by the miracle of the Incarnation—just like "the humility of incarnation" was joined to "the charity of the passion" in the devotion of Francis and in his life. The social reformer traded his role for that of the charismatic *alter Christus*, acting in the footsteps of Christ: when "the solemn night celebration was brought to a close, [. . .] each one returned to his home with *holy joy*."[61]

The particular celebration of Christmas appears, then, as a new way to recreate what Francis believed the Church should be: a new community composed of humble laity and of a few friars, all unified by simplicity, humility, love, and joy. This foundational event happens in a context when the Church, a strongly hierarchized institution, was at the zenith of its medieval power and wealth; it controlled lay religious practice and everyday life more than ever after Lateran IV. Recreating Bethlehem *in absentia* in the West, at a moment when the failure of the Crusades was more than evident, meant a symbolic act of recreation of the first evangelic community as a peaceful, loving, nonhierarchic group. The miracle seen by the faithful, the effect of which was a collective holy joy, appears then as the divine validation for the celebration, in all its mystical sense. Within this context, the celebration of Greccio was much more than a commemoration: the new emotional body created there was intended to incarnate and materialize a new evangelic community, in some way a new Church.[62]

Conclusion

Let's return for a while to the question of methodological tools. What does the analysis of this well-known scene in terms of senses, emotions, and experience teach us of new? What do we learn about the way emotions act in history—and about the process by which a new emotional body, ephemeral or long lasting, may be born?

The experience of shared emotions takes action at three levels: in social interaction; in discursive formations; and in the "co-creation" of the miracle as an event and a breach in continuity, in the flow of time as it was lived. This case study may illustrate, first, how emotional experience works in society. It is Francis, a holy man living emotionally, who diffuses his emotional state and intention to others: sensory and emotional action is his *modus operandi*, his charismatic tool, as the celebration of Greccio shows it well. Let us note that frequently, this way of being and acting is assigned to holy women, not men, both by medieval (mostly male) authors and modern historiography; however, the case of Francis, though unique for other reasons, is not the only male case in this regard.[63] Second, the analysis shows that emotions can be used by a *discourse* (written or iconographic) in order to manifest, create, or prove—or even hide, erase, or negate—that *something is happening*, that there *is* an ongoing change. This is what we can call the "politics of emotion" in different Franciscan sources, a notion to which we shall return. Third, going beyond a simple celebration, the emotional event of Greccio produced a threefold "embodiment." The sacred or spiritual was embodied as sensed; the miraculous vision revealed an "embodiment" of the infant Christ; and, last but not least, the emotions experienced by all those who witnessed it created, as if "embodied," a collective emotional body.

Now the question arises whether we can speak about a new community—or, in other terms, if the emotional body created survived the event shared. On the very local level, the crèche was maintained in its place and became the place of a new devotion.[64] Since the crib produced miracles, first for animals and then for women in difficulty of delivery, Greccio was destined to grow into a pilgrimage site. Still, it remained for almost the whole century a hermitage, where the most faithful followers of Francis liked to come and even sojourn. On the general level of the history of Francis and his order, the vivid battles dividing the order all along the century are well known between, on one side, those who were faithful to the radical idea of poverty and minority of Francis and, on the other, the "conventuals," supporters of institutionalization and monachization. The story of this well-documented battle shows that the emotional community created and recreated by Francis was difficult to stifle. Though the emotional embodiment of Greccio was ephemeral, this event became an important common reference for at least one more century in the circle of those friars who tried to revive and reinvigorate the ideals Francis cherished.

Later Franciscan sources frequently treat the scene of Greccio: all of them receive and reinterpret the scene according to their agenda, presenting a different politics of emotion *à l'oeuvre*.[65] Among the written sources, the relation of the *vita prima* of Thomas of Celano remains the longest and the most detailed. Later sources all depend on him for their account of this scene, mostly mentioning the event and the miracle. Bonaventure, at the head of the order in 1263, wrote his *Legenda major* to replace earlier circulating documents and set out an order to destroy them all. Many were lost forever; the *vita prima* of Celano reemerged only in the eighteenth century. The bonaventurian legend, which became the official *vita* of the Order of Saint Francis for several long centuries, still used Thomas of Celano as his main source. Yet, insisting on the virtues of Francis as a holy man, as well as on the miracle instead of the collective experience, it discusses Greccio with much less details.

A cumbersome memory for the order as it became increasingly institutionalized, Greccio remained an important *memorial* for some of its members.[66] Accordingly, the emotional body unified by the miraculous vision of the baby Christ is different in size and nature; also, the position of Francis varies. The Bardi dossal (see fig. 7.2)—one of the earliest iconographic cycles on Francis, dated probably from the 1250s—proves the survival of the radical ideal of the saint. Not only does the whole cycle show a peaceful and charismatic Francis, related to nature and to simple laypeople, but the image of Greccio itself is also one that figures Francis as a deacon, standing and celebrating; on the side of the laymen, equal to the friars in the image; and as occurring both "in and out" of a church.

In contrast, the dossal of the Siennese anonyme (fig. 7.3), now in the Pinacoteca of Siena,[67] dated around 1270, gives a representation of Greccio inside a little church, with Francis wearing Franciscan habit, kneeling before the crib where the child is laying; there are no animals or laypeople in the scene, and there are only three clerics behind, among whom is the priest, celebrating at the altar behind the crib. The scene of the crib is situated on the right side of the dossal and precedes the last scene, that of the death of Francis. Separated from its context, the meaning of the whole scene changes,

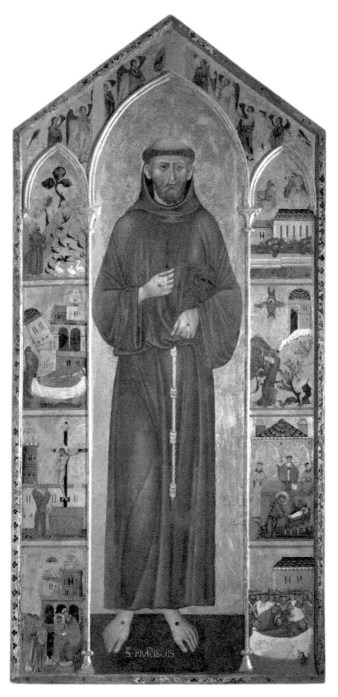

Figure 7.3: Anonymous Siena master, Dossal 1270. Siena, Pinacoteca.

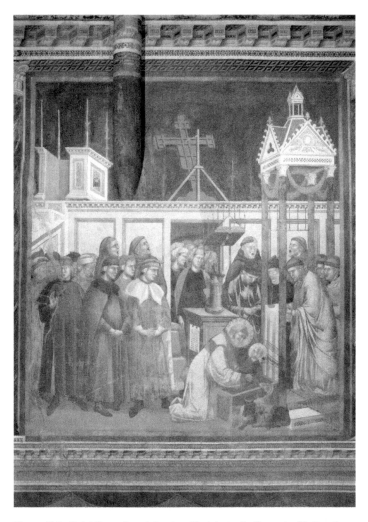

Figure 7.4: *Saint Francis celebrates Christmas in Greccio*. Giotto di Bondone, 1290–1300, fresco, Assisi, Superior basilica, *in situ*. Scala/Art Resources, New York.

indeed; it loses a part of its symbolic as well as its public character. A further transformation, in the most well-known representation of Greccio, in the Assisi upper church (fig. 7.4), most likely by Giotto and dating from 1290 to 1300, shows a crèche inside a huge urban church. Francis, kneeling humbly in front of the crib, is surrounded by friars—chanting or enchanted—on the right, a crowd of laymen standing behind him on the left, and laywomen looking at the scene from the doorway.[68] Francis holds the baby Christ in his hands. There are two small animals, a cow and a sheep of the same size, hardly larger than the baby Christ himself, on the side of the crib—they seem to be placed there in order to *represent* animals. The architecture of the scene is dominated by the institutional context: the huge church, the jube separating lay folk and clerics, men and women, structuring a hierarchically ordered scene to liturgical action, where a vertical line links, from heaven to earth, the reversed, red cross regarding the nave and up, as a memory of the death of Christ; the open Scriptures, ready to be proclaimed by the celebrant; and the kneeling Francis with the infant Jesus in his hands. On the horizontal line, all the postures and gestures, the gazes and facial expressions of the participants demonstrate their attention and curiosity, turned toward Francis and the miraculous child, as if it was to teach how far lay participants take their part in the building of an emotional body—and the communal meaning of the scene.[69] While this figuration of Francis at Greccio with the infant Jesus in his hands becomes, in the subsequent decades and centuries, one of the most widespread presentations,[70] the liturgical celebration itself is represented most frequently as clerical or strictly Franciscan; laypeople disappear from later iconography of the event of Greccio.

Notes

I am happy to express my gratitude to those with whom I could discuss this research: besides the editors and anonymous readers of this volume, Damien Boquet, Giulia Puma, as well as diverse colleagues of the Centre of Excellence for the History of Emotions in Australia during my stay with them as a partner investigator, and primarily Charles Zika and Constant Mews. A special thanks to Lauren Mancia for her revision of my English and to Chiara Frugoni for her generous iconographic help.

1. François Delmas-Goyon, *Saint François d'Assise. Le frère de toute créature* (Paris: Edition Parole et Silence, 2008), 166–67.

2. "bonae famae sed melioris vitae," Thomas of Celano, *Vita prima*, 30, 84, *Legendae s. Francisci Assisiensis, saeculis XIII et XIV conscriptae* (Firenze: Collegio San Buonaventura di Grottaferrata, 1926–1941), AFH X, I-IV, Fasciculus I: Thomas of Celano, *Vita prima s. Francisci Assisiensis*, trans. Placid Hermann (Chicago: Franciscan Herald, 1963), 63. *Saint Francis of Assisi* (Chicago: Franciscan Herald, 1963), 75–78. I use mainly the translation from John Raymond Shinners, ed., *Medieval Popular Religion, 1000–1500: A Reader* (Peterborough: Broadview, 2008), 73–75.

3. "Volo enim illius pueri memoriam agere, qui in Bethlehem natus est [Mt 2:1–2], et infantilium necessitatum eius incommoda, quomodo in praesepio reclinatus [Lc 2:7] et quomodo, adstante bove atque asino, supra foenum positus exstitit, utcumque corporeils oculis pervidere." Celano, *Vita prima*, 30 and 84 in Shinners, *Medieval Popular Religion*, 88.

4. See the introduction of Jacques Dalarun to the last French translation of the *Vita prima*, in *François d'Assise. Écrits, Vies témoignages* (Paris: Le Cerf—Editions franciscanes, 2010), 429–56, especially 444–48.

5. This mention especially concerns the *Officium rythmicum* attributed to Julian of Spire (ca. 1232-35) and of course the *Legenda maior* of Bonaventure (1262–63), which were the texts most used by the Franciscan order for many centuries, during and outside of liturgy. In his *Vita brevior*, written between 1232 and 1239, Thomas of Celano conserves a slightly abbreviated version of the event, which shows its importance in his eyes. See Thome Celanensis, *Vita Patris nostri Francisci (Vita brevior)*; Jacques Dalarun, ed., "Présentation et édition critique," *Analecta Bollandiana* 133, no. 1 (2015): 57–58. As this contribution is intended for a volume on the notion of "emotional body," destined for a public of historians who most probably are not medievalists, my choice here is to limit the discussion to very few sources, putting aside the erudite questions of the transmission of texts and ideas, which would have produced a much more complicated text and required a huge *apparatus criticus*.

6. This dating, quite large, results from Judith E. Stein, "Dating the Bardi Saint Francis Master Dossal—Text and Image," *Franciscan Studies* 36 (1976): 271–96, for whom the date is 1254–57; and Chiara Frugoni, *Francesco: Un'altra storia, con le immagini della tavola della cappella Bardi* (Genova-Milano: Marietti, 2005 [1988]), 9, who dates the *pala* from around 1240. See also Michel Feuillet, *Les visages de François d'Assise: L'iconographie franciscaine des origines 1226-1282* (Paris: Desclée de Brower, 1997), 95; and Giulia Puma, "La Nativité italienne: Une histoire d'adoration (1250–1450)" (PhD diss., Université Paris III, 2012), who both adopt this later dating.

7. Feuillet, *Les visages de François d'Assise*, 95.

8. "retable hagiographique." Expression of André Chastel, *La pala ou le retable italien des origines à 1500* (Paris: Lévi,1993), 72.

9. Puma, *La Nativité italienne*, 88.

10. This prominent episode of the life of Saint Francis has engendered countless commentaries. Among the last and most lavish ones, see two excellent studies: Chiara Frugoni, "Sui vari significati del Natale di Greccio, nei testi e nelle immagini," *Frate Francesco: Rivista di cultura francescana* 70, no. 1 (2004): 35–148; and Puma, *La Nativité italienne*, 87–89.

11. Giulia Puma, primarily in, *La Nativité italienne*, and in "Présence des animaux et place de la louange dans les textes et les images du Noël à Greccio (XIIIe—XVe siècles)," in *Des animaux dans la nature: Images antiques et médiévales*, ed. N. Kei and S. Wyler (forthcoming). It discusses all the relevant sources, both written and iconographic, of the thirteenth century.

12. On the question of event in history, see first two major works: François Dosse, *Renaissance de l'événement: Un défi pour l'historien; Entre sphynx et phénix* (Paris: Gallimard, 2010); and Paul Ricoeur, *Temps et Récit* (Paris: Seuil,1983–85), 3 vols., and a short article summing up much of his ideas for historians: Paul Ricoeur, "Événement et sens," in *L'espace et le temps* (Paris-Dijon: Actes du XXIIe Congrès de l'Association des Sociétés de Langue Française, 1991), 9–21. For a short approach, see Michel Ber-

trand, "'Penser l'événement': En histoire; mise en perspective d'un retour en grâce," in *Les sciences sociales face aux ruptures et à l'événement*, ed., Michel Grossetti, Marc Bessin, and Claire Bidart (Paris: La découverte, 2010), 36–50. This article reuses, going further, many of the reflections of Jacques Revel, "Retour sur l'événement: Un itinéraire historiographique," in *Le Goût de l'enquête: Pour Jean-Claude Passeron*, ed. Jean-Louis Fabiani (Paris: Harmattan, 2001), 95–118; and Arlette Farge, "Penser et définir l'événement en histoire: Approches des situations et des acteurs sociaux," *Qu'est-ce qu'un événement? Terrain* 38 (2002): 67–78.

13. The importance of the link between emotion and event has been already noted by Farge, "Penser et définir l'événement en histoire," 73–74, and underlined by Dosse, *Renaissance de l'événement*, 135.

14. William M. Reddy, *The Navigation of Feeling: A Framework for the History of Emotions* (Cambridge: Cambridge University Press, 2001).

15. John L. Austin, *How to Do Things with Words* (Oxford: Oxford University Press, 1962).

16. Monique Scheer, "Are Emotions a Kind of Practice (And Is That What Makes Them Have a History?): A Bourdieuian Approach to Understanding Emotion," *History and Theory* 51, no. 2 (2012): 193–220.

17. Barbara H. Rosenwein, "Worrying about Emotions in History," *American Historical Review* 107 (2002): 821–45.

18. Barbara H. Rosenwein, *Emotional Communities in the Early Middle Ages* (Ithaca, N.Y.: Cornell University Press, 2006); Barbara H. Rosenwein "Theories of Change in the History of Emotions," in *A History of Emotions, 1200–1800*, ed. Jonas Liliequist (London: Pickering and Chatto, 2012), 7–20; Damien Boquet, "Le concept de communauté émotionnelle selon B. H. Rosenwein," *BUCEMA*, Hors-série no. 5, 2013.

19. See also Rosenwein, "Theories of Change," 7–20.

20. On this question, see a few contributions in Damien Boquet and Piroska Nagy, eds., "Histoire intellectuelle des émotions de l'Antiquité à nos jours," *Ateliers du Centre de Recherches Historiques* 16 (2016): David Konstan, "Their Emotions and Ours: a Single History?," in *Histoire intellectuelle des émotions*, https://journals.openedition.org/acrh/6756; and Angelika Messner, "Knowing and Doing Emotions in Times of Crisis and Radical Change," in *Histoire intellectuelle des émotions*, https://acrh.revues.org/6736.

21. Farge, "Penser et définir l'événement," 67–78.

22. "In loco fratrum de Graecio sanctus placito morabatur, tum quia paupertate divitem esse cernebat, tum quia in remotiore saxo prominente constructa, vacabat liberius caelestibus disciplinis." See also François Delmas-Goyon, "Compilation d'Assise," in *François d'Assise: Écrits, Vies et témoignages*, ed. Jacques Dalarun (Paris: Editions Franciscaines, 2010) 1:1301.

23. Massimo de Angelis, "Analisi storico-architettonica dell'eremo di Greccio," *Frate Francesco* 70, no. 1 (2004): 149–88.

24. "Summa eius intentio, praecipuum desiderium, supremumque propositum eius erat sanctum Evangelium in omnibus et per omnia observare ac perfecte omni

vigilantia, omni studio, toto desiderio mentis, toto cordis fervore, 'Domini nostri Iesu Christi doctrinam sequi et vestigia' [Regula 1, c. 1] imitari. Recordabatur assidua meditatione verborum eius et sagacissima consideratione ipsius opera recolebat. Praecipue incarnationis humilitas et charitas passionis ita eius memoriam occupabant, ut vix vellet alius cogitare." Thomas of Celano, *Vita prima*, 30, 84, Shinners, *Medieval Popular Religion*, 73.

25. Partly from Frugoni, "Sui vari significati," 44.

26. Puma suggests the arch is part of the church. Puma, *La Nativité italienne*, 88.

27. Frugoni, "Sui vari significati," 39–40; Louis Gougaud, "La crèche de Noël avant saint François d'Assise," *Revue des Sciences Religieuses* 2 (1922): 26–31.

28. Gougaud, "La crèche de Noël," esp. 27–32. Gougaud argues that this can explain why, in the *Legenda major* of Bonaventure, Francis asks for the authorization of the pope to celebrate Christmas in Greccio. See also Frugoni, "Sui vari significati," 73 and n121.

29. Probably under Pope Theodore 1, 642–649, who was of Palestinian origin, illustrating by his career the ongoing transfer of legitimacy.

30. See Charles M. de la Roncière, "La Nativité dans la dévotion de saint François d'Assise," in *La Nativité et le temps de Noël. Antiquité et Moyen Age*, ed. Gilles Dorival and Jean-Paul Boyer (Aix-en-Provence: Presses universitaires de Provence, 2003), 236; Henri Leclercq, "Crèche," in *Dictionnaire d'Archéologie chrétienne et liturgie*, 3/2 (1914): 3021–29.

31. See Puma, *La Nativité italienne*, 16–17.

32. Roncière, "La Nativité," 237; Stephen J-P. Van Dijk OFM, *The Ordinal of the Papal Court from Innocent III to Boniface VIII and Related Documents*, comp. Joan Hazelden Walker, (Fribourg: The University Press Fribourg, 1971), 121.

33. See Roncière, "La Nativité," 238–40.

34. Jean-Hervé Foulon, "La Nativité dans la prédication de saint Bernard, abbé de Clairvaux," in *La Nativité et le temps de Noël*, 213–29.

35. Puma, *La Nativité italienne*, 69.

36. See the text at n. 19 above. Rosenwein, "Theories of Change," 7–20.

37. Details on what we are used to understanding as theater, a field in historiographical renewal, are essentially known for the later Middle Ages. On the time of Greccio, besides a few hints in Gougaud and Frugoni, see Marie Bouhaïk-Gironès, ed., *Le théâtre de l'Église (XIIe-XVIe siècles)* (Paris: LAMPO, 2011).

38. See Jacques Dalarun, *Le Cantique du Frère Soleil: François d'Assise reconcilié* (Paris: Alma, 2014).

39. This scene is always mentioned, just like some others that involve Francis with the animals, in the abbreviated versions of his life.

40. See on this point the interesting article of Didier Méhu, "L'évidement de l'image ou la figuration de l'invisible corps du Christ (IXe—XIe siècle)," *Images Re-vues* 11 (2013), http://imagesrevues.revues.org/3105.

41. Frugoni, "Sui vari significati," 39.

42. See for instance the spiritual texts and letters of John of Fécamp and Aelred

of Rievaulx in Damien Boquet and Piroska Nagy, *Sensible Moyen Âge: Une histoire des émotions dans l'Occident médiéval* (Paris: Seuil, 2015). For an English translation established by Robert Shaw, see *Medieval Sensibilities: A History of Emotions in the Middle Ages* (London: Polity, 2018).

43. "Volo enim illius pueri memoriam agere, qui in Bethlehem natus est [Mt 2:1–2], et infantilium necessitatum eius incommoda, quomodo in praesepio reclinatus [Lc2:7] et quomodo, adstante bove atque asino, supra foenum positus exstitit, utcumque corporeils oculis pervidere." Celano, *Vita prima*, 30, 84. Shinners, *Medieval Popular Religion*, 73

44. On the sensorial dimension of liturgy, see Eric Palazzo, *L'Invention chrétienne des cinq sens dans la liturgie et l'art au Moyen Âge* (Paris: Cerf, 2014).

45. Celano, *Vita prima*, 30 and 85; and Shinners, *Medieval Popular Religion*, 74.

46. Celano, *Vita prima*, 30 and 85; and Shinners, *Medieval Popular Religion*, 74.

47. "Ne vero hoc novitati posset adscribi, a Summo Pontifice petita et obtenta licentia, fecit praeparari praesepium, apportari foenum, bovem et asinum ad locum adduci." Doctoris seraphici s. Bonaventurae, *Legenda Maior s. Francisci* in *Legendae s. Francisci assisiensis, saeculis XIII et XIV conscriptae*, ed. Collegio San Buonaventura di Grottaferrata (Firenze, 1926–1941), Fasciculus V, 604.

48. Celano, *Vita prima*, 30, 86; and Shinners, *Medieval Popular Religion*, 74.

49. See Puma, "Présence des animaux," (forthcoming).

50. On this question, see Boquet and Nagy, *Sensible Moyen Âge*, 267–97.

51. Celano, *Vita prima*, 30 and 84; and Shinners, *Medieval Popular Religion*, 73.

52. Foulon, "La Nativité," 219–20.

53. See Victor Turner, "Liminality and Communitas," in *The Ritual Process: Structure and Anti-Structure*, ed. Victor Turner (Chicago: University of Chicago Press, 1969), 94–113; and 125–30.

54. On Francis and war, see Frugoni, "Sui vari significati," 51–57 and 58; on the message of peace of Greccio, see John Tolan, *Le Saint chez le sultan: La rencontre de François d'Assise et de l'Islam, huit siècles d'interprétation* (Paris: Seuil, 2007).

55. Celano, *Vita prima*, 30, 85–86, Shinners, *Medieval Popular Religion*, 74.

56. Giulia Puma, "D'Assise à Santa Croce: L'empreinte franciscaine sur la nativité du Christ (fin duecento—premier tiers du trecento)," *Chroniques italiennes* 26, nos. 3–4 (2013): 3–4. See also the writings of Francis himself.

57. Celano, *Vita prima*, 30 and 86; and Shinners, *Medieval Popular Religion*, 74.

58. Maaike Van der Lugt, "L'animation d el'embryon humain et le statut de l'enfant à naître dans la pensée médiévale," in *Formation et animation de l'embryon dans l'Antiquité et au Moyen Âge*, ed. L. Brisson, M.-H. Congourdeau, and J. L. Solère (Paris: Vrin, 2008), 233–54.

59. Celano, *Vita prima*, 30 and 86; and Shinners, *Medieval Popular Religion*, 74.

60. Delmas-Goyon, *Saint François d'Assise*, 150–59 (on the turn in the life of Francis and its reasons, between 1220–23), 166–67 (for the month of December in Greccio). See also Frugoni, "Sui vari significati," 51–57 and 58.

61. Celano, *Vita prima*, 30 and 85–86; and Shinners, *Medieval Popular Religion*, 74.

62. See also Caroline Walker Bynum, *Christian Materiality: An Essay on Religion in Late Medieval Europe* (New York: Zone, 2011); Dominique Iogna Prat, *La Maison Dieu: Une histoire monumentale de l'Église au Moyen Âge (v.800–v.1200)* (Paris: Seuil, 2006).

63. On this question, see Boquet and Nagy, *Sensible Moyen Age*, 267–97.

64. Frugoni, "Sui vari significati," 38.

65. See Damien Boquet and Piroska Nagy, eds., *Politiques des émotions au Moyen Âge* (Florence: SISMEL, Edizioni del Galluzo, 2011).

66. Frugoni, "Sui vari significati," 73.

67. Its original place was of the dossal was on the high altar of the church dedicated to San Francesco, in Colle Val d'Elsa (Tuscany).

68. Richard Read, "Boosting the Emotional Power of New Liturgy: The Hidden Sides of Things in Giotto's Crib at Greccio," in *Performing Emotions in Early Europe*, ed., Philippa Maddern, Joan McEwan and Anne M. Scott (Turnhout: Brepols, 2018), 201–20.

69. See Read, "Boosting the Emotional Power of New Liturgy," 201–3.

70. On the long-term transformations of the iconography of the theme, see the blog of Giulia Puma, "La Nativité italienne," https://nativita.hypotheses.org.

8. Fearful Female Bodies

The *Pétroleuses* of the Paris Commune

DOLORES MARTÍN-MORUNO

Fear of Terrorism

It could seem that writing about fear is more than ever a timeless issue in our twenty-first-century globalized world. Not that long ago, a Jihadist attack took place in Barcelona, when the driver of a van killed sixteen people and wounded dozen more on the intersection between Las Ramblas' Boulevard and Catalonia Square.[1] A week before, white North American supremacists manifested proudly in Charlottesville, leading to a counterdemonstration, which also ended with a car attack, costing the life of a thirty-two-year-old civil right activist, Heather Heyer.[2] Both of these stories reveal a common pattern: they are what we call today "terrorist actions" perpetrated by collectives, which are fueled by a careful cultivation of hatred against an imagined *other* who is considered, in their ideological worldview, as an essential threat against their own existence.[3] If these stories have the power of horrifying us, this is because we may feel their violent repetition as a kind of emotional bomb, as a stressful experience that not only reminds us the uncertainty of our future but also of those situations that represent our past suffering because they lay bare our vulnerability.[4] Barcelona's attack reminds us of those of Manchester, Nice, Paris, London, Madrid, and New York. When we feel fear in the Global North, we also tend to forget the fear that people feel in other parts of the world.

Current discourses establishing *dangerous liaisons* between refugees and terrorists are tragic consequences of the workings of fear in international politics and how they have led us to the creation of fictional enemies from whom we need to protect ourselves, putting them outside our frontiers.[5] As Judith Butler explains, "this is the mode by which Others become shit": through the expulsion and repulsion of their bodies, which are felt as abject, because they incarnate all those attributes that we cannot assume as our own.[6] Sara Ahmed has also written extensively about how "the performativity of disgust" allows us to marginalize the racial others according to an "affective politics of fear," which she particularly links with George W. Bush's war on terror.[7]

Following these feminist interpretations, my aim here is to show that fear of terrorism is not just an affective economy that encompasses our present society but is, rather, an old one whose history goes back much further in time. More specifically, this chapter retraces terrorism's past within the French revolutionary tradition, when the word "terror" and "terrorist" appeared for the first time.[8] This is the period that has usually been designated as the Reign of Terror (1793–1794) because of the guillotine executions carried out under the Jacobin's rule. After their creation, those two terms would become recurrent in allusion to further nineteenth-century revolutionary upheavals, such as the revolutions of 1830 and the 1848, as well as the Paris Commune (March 18–May 29, 1871). As this study argues, the Commune provides a rich example with which to study how the performativity of emotions led to the shaping of fearful bodies, such as the *pétroleuses*, a group of organized working-class women who were accused of having burnt the Court of Accounts, the Council of the State, the Ministry of France, the Palais Royal, the Louvre library, the Hôtel de Ville, and the Tulleries Palace by throwing bottles of petrol and kerosene during the last days of the Commune's existence.

In spite of the persistent news spread in the French capital, the historian Edith Thomas concluded in the 1960s that there was not enough evidence to claim that those revolutionary women had deliberately provoked those fires.[9] For her, the pétroleuses were more likely fictional creatures resulting from a manifestation of "collective fear" or a "mass hysteria," in which "delusions took over the population through the dissemination of rumours and terror."[10] Little matters if revolutionary women really burned the main buildings of the capital, as they merged in public opinion as the evilest enemy of French society. In other words, what matters here is to analyze the affective mechanisms through which they came to be a criminal body living at the margins of the late-nineteenth-century Western civilization.[11]

With this aim in mind, I will delve into Thomas's hypothesis by combining emotion and gender histories in order to understand the production of the pétroleuses as a consequence of what Piroska Nagy has termed in the previous chapter a "politics of emotion," which was exerted during the Commune and its aftermath in order to consciously negate something that had happened: social revolution.[12] This politics of emotion is intimately related to what has come to be known as the "dark legend of the Commune," according to which this episode simply constituted "the parodic end of the French revolutionary tradition."[13] Within the context of the French civil war, conservatives' fear revealed a powerful capacity by defining the female revolutionary body as a danger, whose very existence became a threat to the whole existence of the Third Republic.[14] Revolutionary women were considered to be more fearsome than men, because they were imagined as having participated in the Commune just like their male comrades, raising barricades and fighting, which means breaking with late-nineteenth-century gender ideologies about femininity.[15]

By naming them pétroleuses, judges, literary men, journalists, and even evolutionary scientists mobilized fear as a social practice, which led to the emergence of an "emotional body," a social group whose identity was identified by repetition with the execution of a terrorist action.[16] While writing, drawing, and theorizing about the dark legend of the women incendiaries, those conservative agents were, furthermore, symbolically inscribing working-class women's bodies within past stories of fearsome female bodies, such as the Amazons, the furies, the witches, and, namely, the *tricoteuses*, those who were remembered for knitting during the public executions perpetrated in the French Revolution.[17] What "doing fear" is here—paraphrasing Joanna Bourke's word—is negotiating "the boundaries between one community and another" by distributing power within the social space. Fear is, therefore, not simply an inner state but rather "a social enaction," which involves a variety of actors navigating through complex power relations in order to put this emotion into action.[18]

Taking Louise Michel's testimonies during her war trial as starting point, I will show that fear was also a matter concerning revolutionary women, because they contributed to establishing an emotional economy that led them to feel others' fear as their own such that "it is felt as an impossible or inhabitable body."[19] When internalizing this painful experience, which I will interpret in the light of the notion of abjection, revolutionary women came to feel enclosed within the contours of their fearful female bodies, once the Commune was crushed and many of them were incarcerated in the prison camp of Satory close to Versailles.[20] This conclusion will lead me finally to establish a broader comparison between past and present fear in order to think about the importance of the performativity of emotions for the creation of fearful bodies, such as those of the terrorists whose limits still today remain blurred halfway between fiction and reality.

Who's Afraid of Louise Michel?

On December 16, 1871, Louise Michel (1830–1905),[21] the famous anarchist schoolteacher, writer, and activist, was judged before the 6th Court-Martial Board for having participated in the revolutionary self-government ruling in the French capital during the springtime of the same year.[22] Coming into being just a month after the end of the Franco-Prussian War (1870–1871), the Commune was the result of working class's growing discontent toward the politics implemented during Napoleon III's empire and, later on, by the provisional government established during the war against Prussia.

After having dramatically struggled against famine, disease, the extreme cold winter temperatures, and constant shell bombardments during the four-month Prussian siege, Parisians felt outraged by the humiliating terms under which the armistice had been signed by Jules Favre, the minister of foreign affairs, and the Prussian general Otto von Bismarck.[23] Once the war was over, the new elected president of the recently created Third French Republic, Adolphe Thiers (1797–1877), would not hesitate to push policy measures contributing to an increasing feeling of resentment among the most radical sectors of the population.[24]

The ruling that ended the moratorium on mortgages and rents during wartime, the detention of charismatic leaders, such as Louis Auguste Blanqui (1805–1881) and Gustave Flourens (1838–1871), the censorship of left-wing journals, as well as the suppression of the daily wage of National Guardsmen, made Thiers an especially hatred figure among Parisian workers.[25] Although they were overcrowded in the outskirts of the city, they were extremely well-organized within a network of revolutionary clubs that had provided them with an intensive training on social contestation, as shown by their political agenda throughout the long nineteenth century.[26]

Thiers's order to seize the cannons, for which Parisians had paid with their own money to defend the city during the Prussian siege and which were still held by the National Guard at Montmartre, was the catalyst for the March 1871 uprising. The French army failed in their attempt to retrieve them, and soldiers ended up fraternizing with the people living in Montmartre's neighborhood, as well as with members of the National Guard, who proclaimed the self-rule of the city of Paris. The sole casualties related to the initial insurgent movement were Generals Claude Lecomte (1817–1871) and Jacques-Léonard Clément Thomas (1809–1871); both were executed.[27] In an atmosphere of hope, the population was called on to participate in new elections at the Hôtel de Ville; a wide range of left-wing representatives would win: Jacobins, Blanquists, Internationalists, as well as radical socialists.[28] As

Louise Michel enthusiastically reported, "The revolution was already done."[29] This state of affairs forced Thiers to flee to Versailles, where he provisionally established the French government during the two and a half months that the Commune would last.

Those two and a half months were also marked by a civil war confronting the French regular army against the Communards, in which fear was used by each side as a weapon in order "to break the opponent's will."[30] Its dramatic end took place during the last week of May, when Marshal Patrice MacMahon's troops entered the city and killed around ten thousand people and arrested 43,500, who were sent to a prisoner camp at Satory and, later on, judged by summary war tribunals.[31] This episode, also known as the bloody week, was one of the most frightening massacres perpetrated in the nineteenth century. Still today, it is remembered in a pilgrimage site, which left-wing activists visit each May: the Communards' Wall at the Cemetery of Père Lachaise, where around 150 combatants were executed and thrown into a mass grave.[32]

Among those who were captured, fiercely repressed, and imprisoned, there were a great number of women. Like Louise Michel, those women were suspected of having burned the main governmental buildings during the last week of existence of the Paris Commune. In her trial, Michel proudly recognized her involvement in those fires that had devastated the French capital. She also defied the president of the court, Colonel Delaporte, when she suggested that she should be sentenced to death for the charges held against her.

> I wished to oppose the invader from Versailles with a barrier of flames. I had no accomplices in this action. I acted on my own. [. . .] Moreover, I am honored to be singled out as one of the promoters of the Commune. It had absolutely nothing to do with assassinations or burning. I attended all the sessions at the Hôtel de Ville, and I affirm that there never was any talk of assassinations or burning [. . .] If you are not cowards, kill me![33]

As reported in the *Gazette des Tribunaux*, Michel's testimony caused a great commotion in the courtroom. Her words were subversive because she recognized with conviction the perpetration of a violent action whose central motivation was political passion; a behavior that was culturally associated with male patterns.[34] Nevertheless, the utterance of Michel's words—namely, when saying that she had no fear of dying for the ideals represented by the social revolution—would not have the implications that she originally expected. The judges interpreted her declaration as lacking accuracy because she could not be imagined as the only pétroleuse having acted during the bloody week.

Indeed, Michel was never condemned to death but rather to lifetime deportation in New Caledonia, even though she would remain in the French colony for only seven years until the armistice granted to the Communards in 1880. She would also become the heroine of the European left, known as "the Red Virgin of Montmartre."[35] Acclaimed as a kind of martyr of the revolution, she represented the sacrifices carried out by all those people who had fought for a better world in the streets of Paris and, particularly, those women who had been summarily killed, or persecuted, arrested, and forced into exile when not condemned to death, because of their commitment to the Commune.

But who were those women who were suspected of having put Paris to the flame? Victorine Brocher (1838–1921), Anna Jaclard (1843–1887), André Léo (1824–1900), Victoire Léodile Vera's literary pseudonym, and Julia Béatrix Euvrie (1849–unknown), also called Béatrix Excoffons, were some of them.[36] Like Louise Michel, they provided emergency relief assistance to the wounded soldiers in provisional hospitals that were scattered around the city.[37] With rare exceptions, such as in the case of the *Légion des Fédérées*, women were not officially allowed to use weapons, a prohibition that revealed male's communards anxieties toward women's increasing agency in the public. This is why Michel altogether with Excoffons decided to channel their activism into organizing ambulance work and other social healthcare activities, such as the distribution of food in canteens or the protection of orphaned children.[38]

Although ambulance women belonged to the National Guard's army, their recruitment was managed by women's committees and female revolutionary clubs, such as *L'Union des femmes pour la défense de Paris et les soins aux blessés* (The Women's Union for the Defense of Paris and Aid to the Wounded) or the Women's Vigilance Committee of Montmartre.[39] Those revolutionary clubs had been created during the Commune, because working-class women did not feel that their specific needs were recognized within the general objectives identified by the ongoing revolution.[40] Indeed, to achieve gender equality seemed to be a more distant utopia than to establish a self-government in Paris.

Working-class women were the powerless in late-nineteenth-century French society. Most of them worked in the industrial sector for between twelve and fifteenth hours in exchange for a salary that could range from 50 centimes to 2.5 francs per day—half that earned by men. As many working-class women lived in concubinage, they were charged with the major part of family responsibilities. This situation often obliged them to resort to prostitution in order to feed their children. The French expression "faire le cinquième quart de la journée" reflects to what extent prostitution was a common practice among those women who did not have sufficient economic resources.[41]

Louise Michel tried to help prostitutes by training them to be nurses, who—she hoped—would one day replace Catholic nuns in French hospitals. Her initiative would be, however, not well accepted by the Commune's leaders who considered prostitutes a potential danger for the achievement of the social revolution.[42] Whether they were imagined as libidinous prostitutes or compassionate nurses, women were not warmly welcomed by their male comrades, as André Léo explained it in an article published in early May at *La Sociale*.

> We are well aware that in every district of Paris, groups of devoted and courageous female citizens have been formed in order to assist in the defense of Paris. Some are engaged in the preparation of our fighters, generally very undernourished, with warm and healthy food, others go onto the battlefield to bring first aid to the injured and dying. [. . .] We are also aware, however, that in Paris there are a large number of [. . .] Republicans who find this love shown by women for the Republic unworthy and distressing.[43]

Léo's words expressed lucidly the constraints women faced during the Commune when acting beyond the borders of the private realm, even if it was as the subalterns. Working-class men were scared of losing their hegemonic position and, therefore, reinforced a patriarchal vision of the social revolution, which was still chained down in gender-role expectations according to Pierre-Joseph Proudhon's misogynistic ideas about the physical and intellectual inferiority of the female sex.[44] Thus, male communards' fear worked toward impeding women's movement within the social space in order to assure a distance between their bodies and those of their female counterparts, which became a threat when occupying what men considered their own natural place: politics.[45] As I will explain in the following section, working-class leaders were not the only agents afraid of women like Louise Michel. There were also many serious military officials, judges, journalists, and scientists who animated a feeling of abjection in order to instigate terror among the population toward the most dangerous criminal body scowling at the society of the fin de siècle: the pétroleuses of the Paris Commune.

The Making of the Women Incendiaries

On December 16, 1871, while attending Louise Michel's trial, the *Gazette des Tribunaux* portrayed her in the following terms:

> Louise Michel is thirty-six years old, petite, brunette, with a very developed forehead which recedes abruptly. Her nose, her mouth and chin are very prominent, and her features reveal an extreme severity. She dresses entirely in black. Her temperament was excitable as it was during the first days of her captivity. When she was first brought in front of the court-martial, she suddenly raised her veil and stared at her judges fixedly.[46]

Michel's detailed description reveals the importance that physiognomy played in late-nineteenth-century culture to scrutinize criminal's personality through physical traits—namely, by regarding facial features.[47] As stated by contemporary physicians such as Cesare Lombroso (1835–1909), a leading representative of the Italian Positivists, somebody does not become criminal; he is, rather, born as one.[48] Irregular facial traits, prominent lips, ears or noses, and receding foreheads were, thus, physical stigmata that reveal one's criminal nature.

By applying Herbert Spencer's Social Darwinism to anthropology, Lombroso studied criminal types as a scientific proof of atavism, a throwback in the evolutionary process "living amidst the very flower of European civilisation."[49] In so doing, Lombroso was integrating abjection as a scientific practice of observation in order to demonstrate that criminals' features were the definitive proof announcing mankind's degeneration into a primitive state.[50] "Criminals," wrote Lombroso, "speak differently because they feel differently; they speak like savages because they are savages."[51] As a liminal force that refused signification, criminals came to embody all those emotional traits that should be removed from humanity—notably, their inability to feel remorse.[52] In fact, one of Lombroso's Italian colleagues, the physician Angelo Mosso (1846–1910), noted in his work *Fear* (1884) that a criminal always "remains impassive before the traces of his crime," just as Louise Michel did during her trial.[53]

In Criminal Man (1876), Lombroso explicitly referred to the participants of "the Paris Commune that had employed petroleum" as a regression moving backward the bloodshed of the 1789 revolution.[54] He particularly examined Louise Michel as a rare case of what he termed as "mattoidism,"[55] a form of insanity, which he associated with criminals moved by political passion who revealed an "excessive altruism," as well as intellectual abilities such as "a particular mania for writing."[56] As Lombroso argued:

> Mattoids can be crafty and capable in daily life, succeeding as doctors, politicians, soldiers, professors and counsellors of state. [...] They are distinguished by a morbidly exaggerated energy for work. This energy resembles to that of the genius, but does not produce the same results.[57]

Michel's singularity stemmed from the fact that there were few female mattoids. Indeed, Lombroso pointed out that "only one female mattoid, Madame Michel, has been found in France."[58] This explained why she had a disgusting virile aspect. In a similar vein, on December 16, 1871, the judges asked Michel about her male physical appearance during the revolutionary upheaval.

> QUESTION: It seems that you wore various uniforms during the Commune.
> ANSWER: I was dressed as usual. I only added a red sash over my clothes.
> QUESTION: Did you not wear a man's uniform several times?
> ANSWER: Once. On March 18. I dressed as a National Guardsman so I would not attract attention.[59]

What seemed scandalous for the judges was that Michel had worn a military uniform, as this was perceived as a transgression against social expectations about her biological destiny, which was nurturing her tender feelings in the private sphere. By performing a disturbing female-male personality before the audience, Michel appeared as frightening because she was breaking with gender binary identity illusions. Her "ontologically unstable character" was, therefore, situating her revolutionary body in what late-nineteenth-century conservatives described as a "powerful and ravaged ugliness."[60]

However, the judges interpreted that her "gender trouble" could more likely be viewed as an "emotional trouble" throughout the statement of the court-martial.[61] In particular, they mentioned that "even if she was an illegitimate child reared by charity," she had "surrendered to her heated imagination and excitable character," which contributed to "exalt the passions of the crowd."[62] For that matter, the revolutionary crowd would be largely pictured as a group of working-class women looking like Michel, who would become the visible face of degeneration: those female arsonists who were supposed to put Paris to the flame during the bloody week.

As Lombroso clarified in other of his works, *Criminal Woman, the Prostitute and the Normal Woman* (1893), criminality during the Commune was an obvious case of epidemic cruelty having affected, overall, the female sex because of their weak brains and exalted passions.

> Women participated in the Paris Commune . . . with the greatest of violence. They were the most bloodthirsty heroes in the assassination of priests . . . and in the executions of hostages, surpassing in cruelty men themselves. . . . In the intense heat of passion, all the moral restraints that evolution has built up slowly over time dissolve in a flash. . . . Women, in these extraordinary, transient, atavistic reversions, become the cruelest of the cruel.[63]

Lombroso's explanation of women's cruelty as a result of their intense heat of passion was making reference to affections such as hysteria, which had linked ungovernable female emotional excess throughout the medical tradition with the fact of having a uterus.[64] As a variant form of moral insanity, hysteria was common in violent contexts, such as rebellions, because they had a direct repercussion on female oversensitivity.[65] For Lombroso, women's passion for arson was physiologically rooted in their voracious sexual desire.[66] The incontinence of their sexual fire, which was also fueled by their alcohol intake may probably be the reason that led them to ignite the fires during the bloody week. "A tendency to arson," Lombroso wrote, has been observed in women "during puberty, amenorrhea, and pregnancy," revealing the close connections between their criminal behavior and the critical moments of their sexual life.[67]

The pétroleuses thus came into being imagined not only as alcoholics but also as hysterics bringing into light to what point working-class's female sexuality epitomized late-nineteenth-century anxieties about potential attacks against the institution of marriage, notably after the legalization of free unions, which were regulated during the Commune.[68] Lombroso definitively turned those anxieties into a collective "fear of crime," while defining revolutionary women's sexual desire outside the limits of what it could be symbolically tolerated: promiscuity,[69] a promiscuity that became the object of Lombroso's abjection, even though it solicited, disturbed, and fascinated his monstrous male desire.[70]

Lombroso also referred to early conservative accounts of the Commune, such as Maxime Du Camp's *Les convulsions de Paris*, in order to complete the cultural assimilation by which the crowd would come to resemble a female hysterical body displaying a violent tendency to cruelty.[71] As Du Camp wrote, women "had but one ambition: to best men by exaggerating their vices. They were cruel when sent in pursuit of defaulters, they were implacable; when serving as nurses, they gave liquor to the wounded to kill them."[72]

Lombroso's criminology would have a wide reception in France in the aftermath of the Commune. Not only did Adolphe Thiers usually adopt the language of degeneration in order to describe the personalities that had been involved in the revolutionary upheaval, but also did those intellectuals who would become the Third Republic's ideologues: the historian Hippolyte Taine (1828–1893), the physician Gustave Le Bon (1841–1931), and the social psychologist Gabriel Tarde (1843–1904). Deeply inspired by Lombroso, Tarde portrayed the crowd "by its routine caprice . . . its credulity, its excitability, its rapid leaps from fury to tenderness, from exasperation to burst of laughter." "The crowd is a woman," Tarde insisted once again, "even if it is composed, as almost always happens, of masculine elements."[73] Like Louise Michel, the crowd appeared through Tarde's words as having committed crime because of an excessive passion whose expression was frighteningly relative to late-nineteenth-century France's normative gender ideologies. The powers of horror thus enabled conservatives to provoke an endless feeling of disgust toward revolutionary women, up to giving birth to a sort of "slim alien": a fearful female body materializing all those attributes that should be expelled from civilization, as if they were a kind of "excrement."[74]

Following the logic of abjection, Michel's prosecutor, Captain Daily, asked to the court on the December 16 "to excise the accused from society," as she "was a continuous danger to it." What seems most interesting is that Michel also demanded to be "cut off from society." "You have been told that, and the persecutor is right," she continued to explain. "If you let me live, I will not stop crying for vengeance."[75] In so saying, Michel's intervention during her war trial definitively proved the involvement of revolutionary women in the making of the pétroleuses. As I will conclude later in this chapter, abjection gave a meaning to revolutionary women's experiences in the Satory camp, where the people from Versailles walked along "to see the vanquished as if they were going to look at animals in the *Jardin des Plantes*."[76] Finally, they would come to feel themselves as abject bodies as the result of the Third French Republic's politics of fear, which appeared as Adolphe Thiers's particular contribution on what we call today "the war on terror."[77]

State Terrorism

On March 11, 2004, ten bombs exploded in four different trains killing 192 people in Madrid. Three days before general elections, José María Aznar, the former Spanish president, "blamed the Basque separatist group ETA" for having perpetrated the terrorist attack.[78] Even if Aznar did not have enough evidence, "he went so far as to phone newspaper editors" in order to communicate that it had been planned by the Basque organization.[79] People believed him, because ETA had repeatedly spread terror through bombing, assassinations, and kidnapping, even before what has been called the "Spanish Democratic Transition."[80]

After a massive demonstration that ended in Atocha train station, an Arabic tape with Koranic quotes was found in a van at Alcalá de Henares (Madrid). Throughout the night of March 12, doubts about the official version began to circulate, linking the attack to al-Qaeda. A photograph taken in March 2003 in the Azores, where George W. Bush, Tony Blair, and Aznar met to orchestrate the Iraq war, started to embody the dark nightmare that

Spanish people were assisting in a new type of global war. What we learned from the March 11 attacks, as well as those in New York, is that terrorism is the work not only of radical Islamists but also of democratic states when they consciously use people's fear in order to achieve their political goals.[81]

When Thiers's government accused working-class women of having put Paris to the flame, the French Third Republic set in motion a similar affective strategy, at the heart of which was fear toward a supposed enemy inhabiting its frontiers. As several historians have pointed out, the ignition point of horror was on the night of March 22, when Versailles's shells burned the Ministry of Finances.[82] By the March 23, the Palais Royal, the Louvre library, and the Palace of the Tulleiries were destroyed, probably by the communards to stop the advance of Thiers's army. In the following days, the Hôtel de Ville, the quartiers of La Villette, and Père Lachaise were also seen in flames.[83] The press widely reported that the fires had been provoked by a female petrol-bomber militia, even though, surprisingly, French conservatives had no correspondent in the capital. French journals such as *Le Galois*, *Le Monde Illustré*, *Le Figaro*, as well as the international press, repeated endlessly that there were pétroleuses everywhere, flinging "their little vials of petrol, their devil's matches, their burning rags into cellars."[84] By reproducing the horrible vision of this Paris in flames, journalists succeeded in focusing the French population's attention on fires while forgetting to mention what was really happening in the streets of the capital: the systematic murder of men, women, and children, whose corpses were buried in mass graves.

"Down in the catacombs under Paris," wrote Michel in her memoirs, "where the government chased the Communards with torches and dogs as if they were animals, there must be many modern skeletons among the ancient bones. Betrayals so numerous, they were nauseating, stupid fear, disgust, the horror—all this was the aftermath of the Commune."[85] Those who were not killed were arrested, having no idea what their final destination would be. "We were marching between the lines of a cavalry escort.... People said they were going to shoot us.... Thrilled by my perceptions... I only looked and now I remember," noted Michel.[86] Many prisoners died on their way to Satory, as the soldiers provided them with neither food nor water. Others were executed on their arrival at the camp after having previously dug their own graves. A group of women, including Louise Michel, were transferred to another prison in the rue de Chandeliers, where they slept on the floor. There were "so many lice that you believed you could hear the noise of their swarming."[87] Some of those women went mad. Others, like Michel, survived by paying the price of feeling their bodies as abject when they could not even change their underwear while being "constantly guarded by soldiers."[88]

Thiers took special care of making them feel their vulnerability in a radical way. They were dirty "in the mud, where they had lain down."[89] French conservatives' disgust and abjection worked here by showing no compassion for those who believed in the social revolution. In fact, they had never considered the communards as really human, as shown by the humanitarian intervention carried out by the French Red Cross during the Commune, assisting "only those who fought against insurgents."[90] After the War Councils, they would be deported to forced labor in the French colonies as a reminder that they were just like those savages that the Empire was trying to civilize.

On December 16, 1871, Michel confessed during her trial that she has initiated the fires, which the pétroleuses seemed to have provoked. What was at the stake during the process and her condemnation was the performativity of fear, an emotion that led Michel to regard herself through a conservative lens as being repulsive, "ugly," "with a high sloping forehead, a large nose, a very wide mouth with a thin upper lip and pouting lower lip, skinny arms and legs, a deep voice, and robust gestures and movements."[91] As the symbol of the Paris Commune, Michel's fearful female body became an impossible one, while coming into being as the reversal of late-nineteenth-century gender expectations about what it meant "to feel like a natural woman."[92]

Pétroleuses, suffragettes, viragos, Femi-Nazis. All those terms reveal to what extent feminists are still today identified with emotional terrorists, whose bodies incite fear because they represent what seems to be the horrific: the liberation of female sexual desire.[93] In spite of their fictional nature, the pétroleuses have never completely disappeared from society. They are resurrected each time conservatives invoke their name in order to reactivate past stories about fearsome female bodies. As a famous twenty-first-century pétroleuse, Viriginie Despentes, reminds us, working-class women still persevere today in regarding their own bodies with abjection, as if they were exhibited like animals at the *Jardin des Plantes*.

> I am writing as an ugly one for the ugly one. . . . Of course, I would not write what I write if I were beautiful, so beautiful that I turned the head of every man that I met. It is a member of the lower working-class that I speak for, that I spoke yesterday and I am speaking for today. . . . We have always existed.[94]

Notes

This chapter is the result of the research conducted within the projects *Le temps des cerises: Les ambulancières de la Commune de Paris*, which was funded by the University of Geneva's Department of Community Medicine (MIMOSA award 2014) and *Ces femmes qui ont fait l'humanitaire: une histoire genrée de la compassion de la Guerre franco-prussienne à la Seconde Guerre Mondiale* (SNSF Professorship award 2017).

1. Sara Almukhtar, Jeremy Ashkenas, Larry Buchanan, Troy Griggs, Jasmine C. Lee, Sergio Peçanha, Jugal K. Patel, and Anjali Singhvi, "The Path of Terror along a Crowed Boulevard in Barcelona," *New York Times*, August, 17, 2017.

2. Christina Caron, "Heather Heyer, Charlottesville Victim, Is Recalled as a 'Strong Woman,'" *New York Times*, August, 13, 2017.

3. On fear, see Joanna Bourke, *Fear: A Cultural History* (London: Virago, 2005); and James Aho, ed., *Facing Fear: The History of an Emotion in Global Perspective* (Princeton, N.J.: Princeton University Press, 2012).

4. For a psychoanalytic interpretation of fear, see Sigmund Freud, *The Uncanny* (London: Penguin, 2013); and Julia Kristeva, *Powers of Horror: An Essay on Abjection* (1980), trans. Leon S. Roudiez (New York: Columbia University Press, 1982).

5. Slavoj Zîzek, *Against the Double Blackmail: Refugees, Terror and Other Troubles with the Neighbors* (London: Penguin, 2016).

6. Judith Butler, *Gender Trouble: Feminism and the Subversion of Identity* (New York: Routledge, 1990), 182.

7. Sara Ahmed, *The Cultural Politics of Emotions* (New York: Routledge, 2004), 63–81. For further reading, see Al Gore, "The Politics of Fear," *Social Research* 71, no. 4 (2004): 779–98; and Judith Butler, *Precarious Life: The Powers of Mourning and Violence* (London: Verso, 2004).

8. On terror and terrorism within the French revolutionary tradition, see Sophie Wahnich, *In the Defence of Terror: Liberty or Death in the French Revolution*, trans. David Fernbach (London: Verso, 2012).

9. Edith Thomas, *The Women Incendiaries* (1963), trans. James Atkinson and Starr Atkinson (Chicago: Haymarket, 2007), 166. More recent publications about the women of the Paris Commune include Kathleen B. Jones and Françoise Vergès, "Women of the Paris Commune," *Women's Studies* 14, no. 5 (1991): 491–503; Gay L. Gullickson, *Unruly Women of Paris: Images of the Commune* (Ithaca, N.Y: Cornell University Press, 1996); Marisa Linton and Christine Hivet, "Les femmes et la Commune de Paris de 1871," *Revue historique* 298, no. 603 (1997): 23–47; and Carolyn J. Eichner, *Surmounting the Barricades: Women in the Paris Commune* (Bloomington: Indiana University Press, 2004).

10. Thomas, *Women Incendiaries*, 166–67.

11. Patricia Pia-Célérier, "Les Pétroleuses de la Commune de Paris ou le Mythe Terroriste," *Romance Quarterly* 42, no. 2 (1997): 93–98. See also David Horn, *The Criminal Body: Lombroso and the Anatomy of Deviance* (New York: Routledge, 2003).

12. See Piroska Nagy's contribution to this volume (chapter 7). For further reading about the political dimensions of emotions, such as pain, see Rob Boddice "Introduction: Hurt Feelings?," in *Pain and Emotion in Modern History*, ed. Rob Boddice (Houndmills: Palgrave Macmillan): 1–15.

13. On the Dark legend of the Commune, see Robert Tombs, *The Paris Commune 1871* (Abingdon: Routledge, 2013), 198. An example of this historiographical tradition is François Furet, *Revolutionary France 1770–1880* (Oxford: Blackwell, 1988), 500–506.

14. About the Red legend of the Paris Commune, see Karl Marx, *The Bürgerkrieg in Frankreich* (Leipzig: Franke's, 1871).

15. Coline Cardi and Geneviève Pruvost, eds., *Penser la violence des femmes* (Paris: Découverte, 2012).

16. About the notion of emotional body, see the editors' introduction to this volume. On emotional practices, see Monique Scheer, "Are Emotions a Kind of Practice (And Is That What Makes Them Have a History?): A Bourdieuian Approach to Understanding Emotion," *History and Theory* 51 no. 2, (2012): 193–220; Fay Bound Alberti, "Emotion Theory and Medical History," in *Medicine, Emotion and Disease, 1700-1950* (Basingstoke: Palgrave Macmillan, 2006): xviii–xxvvi; and Jo Labanyi, "Doing Things: Emotion, Affect, and Materiality," *Journal of Spanish Cultural Studies* 11, nos. 3–4 (2010): 223–33.

17. On past histories of French female revolutionaries, see Dominique Godineau, "Violences politiques," in *Penser la violence des femmes*, 67–74; and Dominique Lagorgette, "La violence des femmes saisie par les mots: 'Sorcière,' 'Tricoteuse,' 'Vésuvienne,' 'Pétroleuse'; Un continuum toujours vivace?," in *Penser la violence des femmes*, 375–87.

18. Bourke, *Fear*, 354–55.

19. Ahmed, *Cultural Politics*, 62.

20. Kristeva, *Powers of Horror*, 1–6; Butler, *Gender Trouble*, 175–83 ; and Ahmed, *Cultural Politics*, 82–100.

21. The title of this section is inspired by Edward Albee's script, *Who's Afraid of Virginia Woolf? A Play* (New York: Scribner, 1962), which was first presented at the Billy Rose Theatre.

22. On the Paris Commune, see Alistair Horne, *The Fall of Paris: The Siege and the Commune 1870-71* (London: Penguin, 1965); Jacques Rougerie, *La Commune de 1871* (Paris: Press Universitaires de France, 1997); and John Merriman, *Massacre: The Life and Death of the Paris Commune of 1871* (New Haven, Conn.: Yale University Press, 2014).

23. On everyday war experiences during the Siege of Paris, see Bertrand Taithe, *Defeated Flesh. Welfare, Warfare and Modern War in the Making of Modern France* (Manchester: Manchester University Press, 1999), 9–12.

24. On resentment as an emotion that allows us to create social groups, see Dolores Martín-Moruno, "On Resentment," in *On Resentment: Past and Present*, ed. Bernardino Fantini, Dolores Martín-Moruno, and Javier Moscoso (Newcastle upon Tyne: Cambridge Scholars, 2013), 1–16.

25. On the National Guard, a citizen militia formed by untrained men, see Dale Clifford, "The Quest for Direct Democracy: The National Guard and the Siege of Paris, 1870–1," *Historical Reflections/Réflexions historiques* 4, no. 1 (1977): 45–65.

26. About the origins of the French working-class movement, see William H. Sebel, "Artisans, Factory Workers, and the Formation of the French Working Class, 1789–1848," in *Working-Class Formation: Nineteenth-Century Patterns in Western*

Europe and the United States, ed. Ira Katznelson and Aristide R. Zolberg (Princeton, N.J.: Princeton University Press, 1986), 45–71.

27. On the episode of the cannons at Montmartre, see Gaston da Costa, *La Commune vécue: 18 mars-28 mai, 1871* (Paris: Librairies-imprimeries réunis, 1903–1905), 1:12; Prosper-Olivier Lissagaray, *Histoire de la Commune* (Paris: Dentu, 1871), 108–10; Louise Michel, *La Commune* (Paris: Inkbook, 2012), 178; and Adolphe Thiers, *Memoirs of M. Thiers* (London: Allen, 1915), 124.

28. On the different political factions involved in the Paris Commune, see Charles Rihs, *La Commune, 1871: Sa structure et ses doctrines* (Paris: Seuil, 1973), 85–108.

29. Michel, *Commune*, 178.

30. Roger Petersen and Evangelos Liaras, "Countering Fear in War: The Strategic Use of Emotion," *Journal of Military Ethics* 5, no. 4 (2006): 317.

31. The exact number of people executed during the bloody week continues to be controversial. I follow here the estimation proposed by Jacques Rougerie, *Paris insurgé: La Commune de 1871* (Paris: Gallimard, 1995), 113. See also Robert Tombs, "How Bloody Was *La semaine sanglante* of 1871? A Revision," *Historical Journal* 55, no. 3 (2012): 679–704.

32. About the places in which the bloody week took place, see Colin Jones, *Paris: Biography of a City* (London: Penguin, 2004), 325. On the Communards' Wall as a site of memory, see Franck Frégosi, "La 'montée' au Mur des Fédérés du Père-Lachaise," *Archives de sciences sociales des religions* 155 (2011): 165–89.

33. Louise Michel, *Louise Michel devant le 6e conseil de guerre: Son arrestation par elle-même, dans une lettre au citoyen Paysant* (Paris: Salle des dépêches du citoyen, 1880), 4. An English translation has been prepared by Bullitt Lowry and Elizabeth Ellington Gunter in Louise Michel, *The Red Virgin: Memoirs of Louise Michel* (Birmingham: University of Alabama Press, 1981), 85.

34. On performativity in the courtroom, see Caroline Braunmühl, "Theorizing Emotions with Judith Butler within and beyond the Courtroom," *Rethinking History* 16, no. 2 (2012): 221–40.

35. On Louise Michel's red legend, see Edith Sellers, "The Red Virgin of Montmartre," *Fortnightly Review*,1 (1905): 202–304; Edith Thomas, "Louise Michel, la vierge rouge," *Miroir de l'histoire* 100 (1958): 509–15; and Xavière Gauthier, *La vierge rouge: Biographie de Louise Michel* (Paris: Chaleil, 1999).

36. For more information on the women's police records, see the archives of the *Préfecture de la Police de Paris*: André Léo (Ba 1008), Anna Jaclard (Ba 1124), Louise Michel (Ba 1183). On women's testimonies, see Victorine Brocher, *Souvenirs d'une morte vivante* (Paris: Delesalle, 1909); and Louise Michel, *Je vous écris de ma nuit: Correspondance générale de Louise Michel (1850–1904)* (Paris: Editions de Paris, 1999).

37. On ambulance women, see Dolores Martín-Moruno, "*Le temps des cerises*: Ambulance Women in the Paris Commune," *Bulletin of the UK Association for the History of Nursing*, 3 (2014): 44–56; and David A. Shafer, "Plus que des *ambulancières*: Women in the Articulation and Defence of their Ideals during the Paris Commune (1871)," *French History* 7, no. 1 (1993): 85–101.

38. Béatrix Excoffons, "Portrait d'une pétroleuse," in *Mémoires de femmes, mémoire du people*, ed. Louis Constant (Paris: Maspero, 1979), 92–97; Martin Phillip Johnson, "Citizenship and Gender: The Légion des Fédérées in the Paris Commune of 1871," *French History* 8, no. 3 (1994): 276. See also Quentin Deluermoz, "Des communardes sur les barricades," in *Penser la violence des femmes*, 106–9.

39. Commmune de Paris, "Appel aux citoyennes de Paris," in *Reimpression du Journal Officiel de la République Française sous la commune* (Paris: La Commune, 1871), 225. Some posters announcing the recruitment of ambulance women are preserved at the *Bibliothèque Nationale de France* in Commune de Paris, *Affiches du comité central de la garde nationale et de la Commune de Paris* (Paris: BNF, 1871), 4 vols.

40. About women's organizations during the Commune, consult the *Archives du Service historique de la défense*, "Comités des femmes," 22.

41. Amies et Amis de la Commune de Paris, *La Commune: l'action de femmes* (Paris: Les Amis de la Commune de Paris, 2006).

42. About Michel's ideas concerning the abolition of prostitution, see Edith Thomas, *Louise Michel*, trans. Penelope Williams (Montreal: Black Rose, 1980), 89.

43. André Léo, "Aventures de neuf ambulancières à la recherche d'un poste de dévouement," *La Sociale: Journal quotidien du soir* 3 (May 6, 1871). It can be consulted at the International Institute of Social History, Lucien Descaves's Papers, as well as the BNF (Paris).

44. Pierre-Joseph Proudhon, *La justice dans la révolution et dans l'église: Onzième étude; Amour et Marriage* (Brussels: Office de Publicité, Montagne de la Cour, 1860), 162.

45. About how fear works aligning women's bodies, see Ahmed, *Cultural Politics*, 70–71.

46. Michel, *Red Virgin*, 81.

47. On the role of public and journalism, see Gian Marco Vidor, "The Press, the Audience, and Emotions in Italian Courtrooms (1860s–1910s)," *Journal of Social History* 51, no. 2 (2017): 1–24.

48. On the Italian Positivist school, see Dolores Martín-Moruno, "Pain as Practice in Paolo Mantegazza Science of Emotions" in *History of Science and the Emotions*, ed. Otniel Dror, Bettina Hitzer, Anja Laukötter, and Pilar León-Sanz, *Osiris* 31, no. 1 (2016): 137–62.

49. Cesare Lombroso, *Criminal Man* (1896); trans. Nicole Hahn rafter and Mary Gibson (Durham, N.C.: Duke University Press, 2006), 78.

50. On emotions as objects and agents integral to scientific practices, see Paul White, "Focus: The Emotional Economy of Science," *Isis* 100, no. 4 (2009): 792–97.

51. Lombroso, *Criminal Man*, 78.

52. Ibid., 82.

53. Angelo Mosso, *Fear* (1884); trans. E. Lough and F. Kiesow (London: Longmans, Green, and Co., 1896), 108.

54. Lombroso, *Criminal Man*, 75.

55. Ibid., 284.

56. Michel was a Romantic poet whose work has been qualified as mediocre. For more information, see Thomas, *Louise Michel*, 265.

57. Lombroso, *Criminal Man*, 284.

58. Ibid., 284–85.

59. Michel, *Red Virgin*, 86.

60. On ugliness and Louise Michel, see Patrice Higonnet, *Paris: Capital of the World* (2002), trans. Arthur Goldhammer (Cambridge, Mass.: Harvard University Press, 2005), 109.

61. On abjection as gender trouble and emotional trouble, see Catherine Lutz, "Feminist Theories and the Science of Emotion," in *Science and Emotions after 1945: A Transatlantic Perspective*, ed. Frank Biess and Daniel M. Gross, 357.

62. Michel, *Red Virgin*, 84.

63. Cesare Lombroso and Guglielmo Ferrero, *Criminal Woman, the Prostitute, and the Normal Woman* (1923), trans. Nicole Hahn Rafter and Mary Gibson (Durham, N.C.: Duke University Press, 2004), 66.

64. On a gendered historical perspective about hysteria, see Sabine Arnaud, *On Hysteria: The Invention of a Medical Category between 1670 and 1820* (Chicago: University of Chicago Press, 2015); and Janet L. Beizer, *Ventriloquized Bodies: Narratives of Hysteria in Nineteenth-Century France* (Ithaca, N.Y.: Cornell University Press, 1993).

65. Vicenzo Ruggiero, *Understanding Political Violence: A Criminological Approach* (Maidenhead, U.K.: Open University Press), 40–41.

66. On the influence of Lombroso in the development of discourses about female hysteria in late-nineteenth-century France, see Mark S. Micale, "Discourses of Hysteria in Fin-de-Siècle France," in *The Mind of Modernism: Medicine, Psychology and the Cultural Acts in Europe and America, 1880–1940*, ed. Mark S. Micale (Stanford, Calif.: Stanford University Press, 2004), 80. See also, Catherine Glazer, "De la Commune comme maladie mentale," *Romantisme* 15, no. 48 (1985): 63–70.

67. Lombroso, *Criminal Man*, 75.

68. On the legalization of divorce and free unions during the Paris Commune, see James McMillan, *France and Women: Gender, Society and Politics* (London: Routledge, 2000), 133.

69. Bourke, *Fear*, 335.

70. Kristeva, *Powers of Horror*, 1.

71. Maxime du Camp, *Les convulsions de Paris* (Paris: Hachette, 1878–1880) 2:401–3. See also Maxime du Camp, *Paris, ses organes, ses fonctions et sa vie dans la seconde moitié du XIXe siècle* (Paris: Hachette, 1875), t. 6, 318.

72. Lombroso, *Criminal Woman*, 66.

73. Gabriel Tarde, *L'opinion et la foule* (Paris: Alcan, 1909), 195. The quotation is also cited by Daniel Pick, *Faces of Degeneration: A European Disorder, 1848–1918* (Cambridge: Cambridge University Press, 1989), 93. See also Fae Bauer and Serena Keshavjee, eds., *Picturing Evolution and Extinction: Regeneration and Degeneration in Modern Visual Culture* (Newcastle upon Tyne: Cambridge Scholars, 2015).

74. Kristeva, *Powers of Horror*, 11.

75. Michel, *Red Virgin*, 87.

76. Michel, *Red Virgin*, 73.

77. On the term "war on terror" as coined by U.S. president George W. Bush after September 11, see Richard A. Clarke, *Against All Enemies: Inside America's War on Terror* (New York: Free Press, 2004).

78. Eliane Sciolino, "Bombings in Madrid: The Attack; 10 Bombs Shatter Trains in Madrid, Killing 192 People," *New York Times*, March, 12, 2014.

79. Giles Tremlett, "ETA or al-Qaida? 192 killed and 1,400 Injured in Train Bombings," *Guardian*, March, 12, 2014.

80. For a critical view about the Spanish democratic transition, see Thierry Maurice, *La transition democratique: L'Espagne et ses ruses mémorielles (1976–1982)* (Rennes: Presses Universitaires de Rennes, 2013); and Guillem Martínez et al., ed., *CT o La cultura de la transición* (Barcelona: Debolsillo, 2012).

81. Sylvia Revello, "Terrorisme ou les multiples vies d'un mot," *Le Temps*, August, 22, 2017.

82. Gullickson, *Unruly Women*, 168–70; and Merriman, *Massacre*, 139–70.

83. About the fires, see Jean-Claude Caron, *Les feux de la discorde: Conflits et incendies dans la France du XIXe siècle* (Paris: Hachette, 2006).

84. Gullickson, *Unruly Women*, 171.

85. Michel, *Red Virgin*, 79.

86. Ibid., 73.

87. Ibid., 73.

88. Ibid., 73. On abject bodies, see Judith Butler, *Bodies that Matter: On the Discursive Limits of Sex* (New York: Routledge, 1993), v.

89. Michel, *Red Virgin*, 72.

90. John Hutchinson, *Champions of Charity: War and the Rise of the Red Cross* (Boulder, Colo.: Westview, 1996), 204.

91. "Louise Michel," *Encyclopaedia Britannica*, https://www.britannica.com/biography/Louise-Michel.

92. Butler, *Gender Trouble*, 3.

93. Delphine Gardey and Iulia Hasdeu, "Cet obscur sujet du désir: Médicaliser les troubles du la sexualité féminine en Occident," *Travail: Genre et Sociétés* 34 (2015): 73–92.

94. Virginie Despentes, *King Kong Theory* (2006), trans. Stéphanie Benson (New York: Feminist, 2010), 2.

PART IV

Humanitarian Bodies in Action

The last part of the book deals with the performative effects of emotions in the making of humanitarian bodies from the nineteenth century to the present.[1] Most specifically, it focuses on the evolution of humanitarian emotions, such as sympathy, empathy, and compassion, and retraces their transnational circulation crossing borders, connecting people, and shaping movements of solidarity around the globe.[2] From this perspective, bodies appeared as a complex web of relations established between victims, caregivers, international agencies, political powers, and the general public.

Emerging as a vague neologism, humanitarianism has been interpreted as a "revolution in moral sentiments," which would only become synonymous with an emergency-relief operation in the late nineteenth century—namely, after the creation of the Red Cross movement.[3] In spite of its noble and selfless origins, the spirit of capitalism has been a central force in the emergence of a "humanitarian sensibility."[4] We do not forget that its main purpose is to touch the public by affective means in order to raise funds. To achieve this, the humanitarian business has as its core strategy the dissemination of narratives and images.

In the 1980s, Thomas Laqueur already defined humanitarian narratives as those that "speak in an extraordinarily detailed fashion about the pains and death of people" and, thereby, are able to engender compassion in the reader as a kind of moral imperative.[5] Since Henri Dunant's *A Memory of Solferino* (1862), those narratives have been used as way of mobilizing the public's compassion, which may be considered—according to Bertrand Taithe—as "the humanitarian feeling par excellence" because of its connections with relief workers' action.[6]

Beyond narratives, photographs have become essential materials with which to reveal the power of emotions, as they have had material consequences within the history of humanitarianism and international politics.[7] Susan Sontag's *Regarding the Pain of Others* has recently inspired scholars such as Heidi Fehrenbach and Davide Rodogno to thinking about the morality of sight.[8] Indeed, for a long time, ethical and politics dilemmas had been at the heart of practices, such as looking at distant suffering. As Hannah Arendt explained, the spectacle of violence is always ruled by a "politics of pity" because the relation between the fortunate viewers and the unfortunate victims engenders political inequalities.[9] Indeed, humanitarian emotions led us irremediably to question ourselves about why the pain of certain people has become visible while others' sufferings have been silenced in public opinion.[10]

Echoing these reflections, this section explores narratives during the Spanish Carlist Wars, the visual culture of disaster, and the concept of compassion fatigue.[11] In chapter 9 Jon Arrizabalaga examines the uses of narratives and their entanglements with humanitarian intervention carried out by the Spanish Red Cross (SCR) during the Carlist Wars (1872–76). Even though the SCR was created as a neutral agency to provide relief in international conflicts, the SCR intervened during that war to help soldiers on both sides. The letters, articles, and pamphlets written by prominent activists such as Nicasio Landa and Concepión Arenal became a means to circulate and promote a new kind of compassion among the public in order to launch healthcare initiatives. Arrizabalaga concludes that by turning compassion into humanitarian action, the SRC appeared as a new emotional body able to reconcile the Two Spains.

In chapter 10 Emma Hutchison explores the construction of emotional bodies from a visual perspective, which understands the creation of audiences as a changing affective process. Hutchison analyses the performative effects of looking at images of pain. Furthermore, she argues that the visualization of suffering is performative, as it provokes an emotional response in the viewer. A historical approach to the representation of others' pain also demonstrates that the audience's responses—namely, empathy and compassion—has been related to the shifting conceptions of pain since the nineteenth century.

Finally, Bertrand Taithe examines, in chapter 11, compassion fatigue as a performative emotion that has shaped humanitarian agencies as emotional bodies since the late nineteenth century. The history of this concept, which has been used as both a metaphor and a medical term, demonstrates that different understandings of it have framed humanitarian organizations and individuals in very different ways. In particular, Taithe analyses the meanings and effects of speaking about compassion fatigue of the public, the agencies, and the caregivers, and how humanitarian organizations have slowly incorporated mechanisms to protect its workers against compassion fatigue's pernicious effects.

Notes

1. On transnational history see Durba Ghosh, "New Directions in Transnational History: Thinking and Living Transnationally," in *New Directions in Social and Cultural History*, ed. Sasha Handley, Rohan MacWilliam, and Lucy Noakes (London: Bloomsbury, 2018), 191–212.

2. See Emma Hutchison, *Affective Communities in World Politics: Collective Emotions After Trauma* (Cambridge: Cambridge University Press, 2016); and Bertrand Taithe "Empathies, soins et compassions: Les émotions humanitaires," in *Histoire des émotions: De la fin du XIXe siècle à nos jours*, ed. Alain Corbin, Jean-Jacques Courtine, and Georges Vigarello (Paris: Sous-sol, 2017), 364–81.

3. Michael Barnett, *Empire of Humanity: A History of Humanitarianism* (Ithaca, N.Y.: Cornell University Press, 2011), 49.

4. Thomas L. Haskell, "Capitalism and the Origins of the Humanitarian Sensibility," *American Historical Review* 90 no. 2, pts. 1 and 2 (1985): 339–61, 547–66.

5. Thomas W. Laqueur "Bodies, Details, and Humanitarian Narratives," in *The New Cultural History*, ed. Lynn Hunt (Berkeley: University of California Press, 1989), 176.

6. Bertrand Taithe "'Cold Calculation in the Faces of Horrors?' Pity, Compassion, and the Making of Humanitarian Protocols," in *Medicine, Emotion and Disease, 1700—1950*, ed. Fay Bound Alberti (London: Palgrave Macmillan, 2006), 79–99.

7. To go further on humanitarian communication strategies, see Valérie Gorin, "Advocacy Strategies of Western Humanitarian NGOs from the 1960s to the 1990s," in *Humanitarianism and Media: 1990 to the Present*, ed. Johannes Paulmann (New York: Berghahn, 2018), 201–21.

8. Heidi Fehrenbach and Davide Rodogno, eds., *Humanitarian Photography: A History* (Cambridge: Cambridge University Press, 2016).

9. Hannah Arendt, *On Revolution* (1963) (Hardmonsworth: Penguin, 1990), 59–114.

10. Luc Boltanski, *Distant Suffering: Morality, Media and Politics*, trans. Graham Burhell (Cambridge: Cambridge University Press, 1999); Didier Fassin, *Humanitarian Reason: A Moral History of the Present*, trans. Rachel Gomme (Berkley: California University Press, 2012); and Roland Bleiker, David Campbell, and Emma Hutchison, "Imaging Catastrophe: The Politics of Representing Humanitarian Crises," in *Negotiating Relief: The Dialectics of Humanitarian Space*, ed. Michele Acuto (Oxford: Oxford University Press, 2013), 47–58.

11. Susan D. Möller, *Compassion Fatigue: How the Media Sell Disease, Famine, War and Death* (New York: Routledge, 1999).

9. Performing Compassion in Wartime

Humanitarian Narratives in the Spanish Civil Wars of the 1870s

JON ARRIZABALAGA

SINCE THE BEGINNING of the new century, the relationships between war and emotions like fear, mourning, brutalization, enthusiasm of young soldiers, joy or pleasure in killing, and resentment have been considerably explored.[1] Yet these are by no means the only collective emotions that extreme situations like wars unleash among human beings. They compete with other emotions, such as compassion toward victims and their sufferings. In past and present times, this emotion has moved many people to empathize with victims' individual fate and to seek their relief.

From the mid-eighteenth century on, particularly in Europe and North America, compassion toward others' suffering gradually became a central issue in the public sphere. It influenced social reform debates and policies in areas as disparate as the abolition of slavery, the improvement of living conditions in slum districts, the confinement of the insane, prisoners, and beggars, the relief of indigents, the education of women and children, and the concern for the survival of "primitive peoples." Thomas Haskell first labeled this new form of active compassion as "humanitarian sensibility." More recently, scholars like Luc Boltanski and Bertrand Taithe have also discussed it.[2]

This humanitarian sensibility became apparent, among other ways, through "humanitarian narratives" that, according to Laqueur, describe particular suffering and offer a model for precise social action. This suffering, he writes, "pertains to the personal body, not only as the focus of pain but also as the common bond between those who suffer and those who would help and as the object of the scientific discourse through which the causal links between an evil, a victim, and a benefactor are forged."[3]

In contrast to other areas where humanitarian sensibility had appeared earlier, its penetration in the sphere of war did not become ostensible until the mid-nineteenth century, when, spurred by the growing demands of the modern warfare, national military health services went through deep reforms. Then, it was part of a renewed impetus given by many varied philanthropic initiatives during the Second Industrial Revolution and the colonial expansion of the European powers.[4] The international movement of the Red Cross (hereafter RC) became the most successful organization in promoting humanitarianism by claiming compassion for the victims of war.[5]

The story of the RC's founding is well known. It goes back to the initiative taken by five prominent citizens of Geneva calling for an international conference to be held there in October 1863. Its objective was to study the establishment of relief societies to help national armies improve their capacity to care for soldiers wounded in modern wars. The RC's main instrument was its ability to mobilize civil volunteers of both sexes, trained during peacetime in specific relief tasks. These volunteers formed part of a single, albeit rather decentralized, organization for each nation-state connected to the international association. Their humanitarian activities were legally protected by the neutral status of these organizations with regard to the contenders on either side. Those states signing the *Convention pour l'amélioration du sort des militaires blessés* in August 1864—better known as the Geneva Convention—were obliged to guarantee the immunity of the RC's personnel and material means as well as any individual or premises under the protection of the RC flag.[6]

Spain was one of the participant states at the conference of experts held at Geneva in 1863, joining the Convention of Geneva in 1864. The Spanish Red Cross (hereafter SRC) developed slowly until the end of the 1860s, when the outbreak of the Franco-Prussian War (1870–1871) caused it to revive as it implemented different relief initiatives for the victims of that war. Yet its true baptism of fire happened with the outbreak of the Second Carlist War (1872–1876). This was the last of a series of civil confrontations in nineteenth-century Spain bringing the Liberal government army face to face with the insurrectional supporters of a legitimist cause led by the Carlist pretenders to the Spanish throne under the pretext of a dynastic litigation. The new, bloody confrontation happened during the so-called Democratic Sexennium (1868–1874), a period of serious political instability subsequent to the abdication of Queen Isabel II and including four successive regimes—namely, the monarchy of Amadeo of Savoy, the First Spanish Republic, a failed unitarian republic, and, finally, the Bourbon Restoration under Alfonso XII. It was then that the SRC fully deployed its relief activities, even though the Geneva Convention did not then apply to civil wars.

This chapter explores the humanitarian narratives written during the Second Carlist War by two major leaders of the Spanish Red Cross (SRC) at the time: the medical officer and first general inspector of the SRC, Nicasio Landa, and the lawyer, social reformer, and first secretary of the SRC's Central Section of Ladies, Concepción Arenal. By humanitarian narratives, we understand here those reflected in a variety of primary sources (letters, reports, articles), which will be analyzed with regard to their similarities and differences as well as the following four issues: their publics, purposes, and strategies; their choices as to who deserved humanitarian relief; the manifestations of concern for the physical and emotional well-being of sick and wounded combatants in different stages (frontline care, field and rearguard hospitals) and transfer procedures (stretchers, ambulance coaches) of humanitarian relief; and the diverse actors providing this relief—all with a view to assessing to what extent these narratives of war relief aimed at and contributed to performing the population's compassion toward the victims of civil wars and to strengthening emergent humanitarian bodies such as the SRC.[7]

Building Humanitarian Narratives at War

There is a considerable number of humanitarian narratives apropos of the Second Carlist War, even though most of them were written by few actors, notably the SRC leaders Nicasio Landa and Concepción Arenal. Both of them always aimed to engage the compassion of their readers. Yet their styles were very different with regard to reaching the various sectors of their male and female audiences. Indeed, Landa's narratives were predominantly (albeit not exclusively) intended for male readers and mainly focused on showing practical solutions for a wide range of problems through technological innovations either instrumental or logistic, with an emphasis on the humanitarian modus operandi.

In contrast, Arenal's narratives were particularly addressed to female readers in their potentially double role as collateral victims and humanitarian actors; her narratives were stylistically sophisticated with a more intimate touch, mostly consisting of moving stories with happy endings, thanks to a range of humanitarian initiatives. Nevertheless, both personalities had a common purpose in writing these humanitarian narratives—namely, spreading the RC's mission in Spain to educate the citizenry in the values of war humanitarianism, stimulate active compassion toward the victims of war, and broaden the social base of humanitarian volunteers.

A liberal Catholic and polyglot, the medical officer Nicasio Landa (1830–1891) was fascinated with scientific advancement, its technological achievements, and its contribution to social progress. After having been the representative of the Spanish Ministry of War (and the single Spanish participant) in the 1863 expert conference of aid societies organized by the "Committee of the Five" (later better known as the ICRC) at Geneva, he became a tireless humanitarian activist for the rest of his life. Moreover, Landa was the first general inspector of the SRC between 1864 and 1876, served as commissioned observer in the Franco-Prussian War (between August and September 1870), and led the SRC's action during the Carlist War (1872–1876) from Pamplona—where he was attached to a military garrison—and at the head of energetic provincial committee of the SRC in Navarre. From 1876 to the late 1880s he was actively involved in the *Institut de Droit International*—an institution aiming, among other things, to build a corpus of international war law that could legally reinforce the interventions of the ICRC and other humanitarian organizations in violent conflicts.

Among the great many sources, including Landa's humanitarian narratives, I have paid particular attention to three: Landa's letters in *La Caridad en la Guerra*—the official gazette of the SRC, which he had founded in Pamplona in 1870 on the occasion of his trip to the Franco-Prussian War;[8] his *Muertos y heridos* (Dead and Wounded), a long account dedicated to Concepción Arenal describing the "pains and misfortunes suffered by innocent victims" in the Carlist War as well as the relief of medical intervention implemented by the SRC;[9] and his report of an innovative elastic suspension system for stretchers adaptable to oxcarts and wagons, which he addressed to the Spanish military medical authorities in the middle of the war, asking them to authorize its adoption by the SRC.[10]

A social and liberal Catholic strongly influenced by Krausism,[11] the lawyer Concepción Arenal (1820–1893) was an active defender of abolitionism and social reform in Spain through many philanthropic initiatives among the poor, for women in prisons, in women's education, and for relief to war victims. During the Carlist War, she fully devoted herself to the SRC, even running the war hospital maintained by its women's central committee at Miranda de Ebro, Burgos (in the rearguard of the active Northern front) for half a year in 1874. In addition to the gazette *La Caridad en la Guerra*, Arenal used *La Voz de la Caridad* (1870–1883), a journal of social welfare and prisons she co-founded and edited with Antonio Guerola, to publish her main works regarding the war; she offered it to the SRC Ladies' Section as its official gazette during the most crucial period of the conflict.

There, she anonymously condensed in seven "Letters from a hospital" her most moving humanitarian experiences leading the Miranda war hospital during nearly six months—between June and November 1874.[12] Arenal's letters often exude antiwar criticisms in terms both moral and sociopolitical. It is no wonder that the political authorities prevented the publication of one of her letters.[13] She also used *La Voz de la Caridad* to first publish *Cuadros de la Guerra* (Scenes of the War), a series of twenty-four articles that were later collected as a book.[14] Written about the same period as her letters, these articles aimed to be a personal chronicle of war disasters through successive scenes—some of them set inside hospitals—telling of the sufferings and death of victims, civil and military, and describing different humanitarian relief actions.

Who Deserved Humanitarian Relief?

The benefits of the Geneva Convention (1864) were only applicable to soldiers of regular armies who were sick or wounded in wars between those nation-states that had signed it. The fact that the Carlist War was a civil conflict caused the Geneva Committee to refrain from being involved. However, this did not prevent the SRC's volunteers from deploying their humanitarian aid on the battlefields. For this purpose, they mobilized not only solidarity in Spain and elsewhere but also all their capacity to influence those spheres of Spanish political power that would provide the required legal framework to protect their interventions. They achieved this aim thanks to a surprising and successful initiative by the Navarrese committee of the RC in the Spanish Parliament on February 21, 1870, on the occasion of the parliamentary debates over a new law of public order, a major sticking point between moderate and the progressive Liberals in nineteenth-century Spain. And the new law of 1870, which would be in force until a revised one was approved in 1933, conferred extraordinary constitutional faculties implementable in the event of suspension of guarantees by authorities either civil (in case of state of alert) or military (in case of state of war).

Members of the Parliament were being asked to consider within the new law two Geneva Convention guarantees applicable only to wounded soldiers in international wars—namely, that wounded combatants in case of rebellion or sedition were also exempt from punishment, and that those providing medical aid to them were not to be hindered in their task. In the section concerning "state of war," within the law passed on April 24, 1870, there was no mention of pardon for rebels or seditionists, yet its Article 22 did say that those "individuals belonging to legally established philanthropic associations for aid to the wounded" could not be considered seditious or rebels. This legal protection was unique in European comparative law at the time.[15]

Two years and eight months after its approval, in the face of a foreseeable resurgence of civil hostilities, the SRC's committee in Navarre invoked the new law of public order in a circular letter addressed to the leaders of its local and provincial sections over Spain; the SRC's national standing committee later ratified the circular. Allegedly, this law protected the "exercise" of SRC's "philanthropic mission" by providing the "rescue procedures seemingly most adequate for the kind of war threatening this country, without prejudice to its [SRC's] far-reaching ability to act on what its charity prescribes as most advisable in each particular case." The circular admitted that the observance of the Geneva Convention could not be demanded in "civil strifes" (*luchas intestinas*), yet the Navarrese committee appealed to military honor and patriotism, affirming that "it is expected that its [the Convention's] charitable provisions will serve as a rule to every honorable military man since a fellow countryman, though having an opposing opinion, cannot be treated worse than a foreign invader."[16] As Landa himself claimed, "if the Navarrese committee had striven to relieve its brothers in Germany and France, how could it not be prepared to aid those of its own tribe, the Navarrese!"[17]

Both features, the legal clause and the moral argument appealing to a common fatherland, were enough (while the war lasted) to reasonably safeguard the SRC's activities under the principle of neutrality. As the Navarrese committee emphasized, the SRC was open to "every person of good will, whatever their social position or political opinions, provided their record of morality and honor offers guarantees that they will not misuse our badges to the detriment of neutrality."[18] On the other side, the ambient pressure in favor of humanitarian values in war, along with their political convenience in acquiring international recognition as belligerents, caused the Carlist insurgents also to take up this and other principles of the Geneva Convention, with the result that they too promoted an aid society, *La Caridad*, acting in parallel with the RC.

Thus, it is not surprising that Landa was campaigning for compassion toward every sick or wounded combatant, with no distinction of side or military rank. He emphasized that "love of mankind" was a synonym of Christian charity, far beyond the slanders emanating from both sides, and he identified wounded soldiers with martyrs, since Christian charity conferred a sacred condition on every sufferer.[19] Landa's campaign for spreading the

RC's mission is pointedly illustrated in an expressive passage in his account "Dead and Wounded," witnessing a situation in the Sierra of Urbasa, Navarre, on June 19, 1872, when the war had just begun. After having fallen on the battlefield, a wounded Carlist combatant called Pedro Irigaray (PI)—indeed, a deserter from the regular army who had joined the insurrection—had the following exchange with some charitable women (W) looking after him:

[PI:] [Where am I?]
[W:] In Zudaire.
[PI:] Of which party are those who have brought me here?
[W:] They are those of the Red Cross, along with our doctor Francisco G[uitarte].
[PI:] But I want to know [*the patient added, compelled by his condition as a deserter*] who are in charge here, the Carlists or the Liberals?
[W:] Keep calm because only charity is commanding here; here there are only Brothers.[20]

It is clear that humanitarian interventions in the Carlist War were basically directed toward sick and wounded combatants by dealing with first-aid tasks and evacuation to field hospitals (*hospitales de sangre*) as much as their further transfer to rearguard hospitals, either military or civil, and usually fitted out *ex professo* for convalescence. Yet the healthcare provided tended to prioritize attention to the wounded rather than the ill and gave officers and other commanders special care not supplied to ordinary soldiers. It is not, therefore, surprising that Arenal addressed appeals to denounce any discrimination between sick combatants and to level social criticism of the soldiers' bad living conditions in campaign as a very relevant cause of disease and death, just as, in a similar way, Florence Nightingale had done. She also attacked arbitrariness and classism in the way soldiers (in contrast to officers and commanders) were looked after. Finally, Arenal, who defended the value of individual human life, praised the anonymous poor soldiers' courage and other moral strengths in facing pain and death, though she was quick to question soldiers' typical acceptance of their fate. Let me give some expressive examples of this.

At the request of Landa, who was concerned after hearing of "charitable hospitals where only the wounded were admitted," Arenal devoted the fifteenth entry in her "Scenes of the War" series to the sick soldier. She qualified him as an "obscure and neglected victim of the war" because he was discriminated against by military officers and commanders, by hospital visitors, and even by some donors of humanitarian aid, despite the fact that the RC flag protected the former as much as the latter. Having already in an earlier text wondered whether tough (*sufridos*) soldiers were not so much needed as brave (*valientes*) ones,[21] and having stated that "being wounded is not necessarily evidence of more bravery than being unwounded," Arenal argued as follows:

> It is enough to consult any statistic, and compare the military men wounded and dead due to disease in peacetime and wartime, to understand that war victims are the majority of those succumbing to disease. Let us add that diseases cause more victims than bullets in every lasting fight, if there are no great means, much intelligence and restless solicitude to prevent military men in campaign from falling sick and being looked after once they have fallen."[22]

In one of her letters "from a hospital," Arenal again emphasized the idea that the soldier who has died of disease was "one of the many war victims who will never appear as such because he died neither on the battlefield nor as a result of wounds." She personalized this idea in the death of a young man called Hilario Fuentes, who, by being "badly dressed and fed," lacked the "iron nature necessary to resist life in the camps." She contrasted the hard living conditions of troops in campaign with the carefulness of the humanitarian aid that the poor soldier had received before and after his death:

> Carefully looked after, he received the assistance of science, the solace of religion; he lacked neither the prayers of a priest, nor the tears of a woman: what sad consolation for his poor mother, but we are unable to send her anything else."[23]

In another scene of the war, Arenal referred to a soldier convalescing from war wounds and infected with smallpox, who had been transferred from an RC field hospital to "a rather worse" one intended for infectious patients. She pointed out that its ward for "contagious patients" (*sala de virolentos*) was a "horrible focus of infection" where the sick soldiers were "neither looked after nor watched." Moreover, according to military regulations, soldiers could not be taken care of in private houses "unless their ailments allow them to present themselves every day for consultation"—in contrast to officers, who could "recover wherever they want."[24]

Once more, in a third scene, Arenal insisted on the classism of military regulations, reporting an evacuation from a military hospital of two hundred convalescent soldiers in order to make room for others in more serious condition. She denounced the fact that it had been undertaken, in the middle of the summer at the hottest time of the day, by carts rather than by the nearby train. And she wondered why, if this railway had been operational some days before "to transfer the generals," what had been available "for healthy commanders" could not be now used "for wounded soldiers."[25] In her determination to defend the individual dignity of anonymous common soldiers who were looked after by the SRC, Arenal stated that "many whom we might teach to read are teaching us to suffer—which is indispensable knowledge in this valley of tears." She praised the "great moral superiority" in the "fight with physical suffering" that these "ignorant men, more inferior to us with regard to intelligence," showed when facing the "terrible proofs of disease by merely resigning themselves, without noise and apparently without effort, to evils that might discourage us."[26]

Furthermore, in another passage she contrasted the disparate appreciation that military commanders and humanitarian volunteers made of casualties involving soldiers in campaign. To the former all was limited to mere numbers, so that losing two soldiers in exchange for taking a town was "insignificant," while to the latter any individual casualty was already excessive. A detailed report of the lesions and sufferings of two wounded soldiers who had recently been admitted to the RC hospital at Miranda—one of them having just died and the other in terrible death throes—enabled her to illustrate the humanitarian viewpoint—hers.[27] She wrote the following emotive account:

> In addition to the tears any compassionate woman might shed on seeing men departing for combat [then imminent at the nearby town of Laguardia], in this hospital there are the falling tears of a mother who sees her son among the combatants. And in the case of his death in the field, there would be just *one casualty*, a loss meaning nothing for the world. Yet it would be all for the poor mother who saw him disappear from view with such anxiety, who looks at the overcast weather thinking that he will get wet, who sees the lands on the other side of the Ebro [River] wondering whether they will be soaked in his blood.[28]

However, Arenal's appreciations of the capacity for suffering in silence revealed by the soldiers at the Miranda hospital not only included her praise. She could not hide her ambivalent feelings about their silence ("at first sight this way of suffering comforts, but it distresses when one analyzes it"), complaining that she never heard "the crying out of a soul that demands an explanation of the cause of his misfortune." And she blamed this conformism not on the superficial native evils like "race," "Christian resignation," "pagan stoicism," or "Muslim fatalism," but on "ignorance, lack of an elevated spirit as well as of the knowledge of law and the principles of justice."[29]

Moving Population toward Compassion

One of the main motives of Landa's and Arenal's narratives was to disseminate the RC's mission in the bloody Carlist War by arousing the citizens' compassion and extending the social basis of its humanitarian volunteers.

Let us look at some examples that illustrate the narratives of both actors at this point as well as their mutual differences.

The peculiarities of Landa's strategy to reinforce the citizens' adherence to the RC's cause might be best seen in the report he sent to the SRC's permanent commission as early as June 1872. It consisted of the description of a carefully prepared and ritualized intervention of an "expeditionary ambulance" sent from Pamplona to Echarri-Aranaz (about forty kilometers away and with a railway station) to bring aid to thirteen soldiers and a Carlist combatant who had been seriously injured in a skirmish. The content of the report on the aid supplied to this reduced group of victims was intended to spread the news of the RC's good humanitarian practices in order to move the population toward compassion. The redoubling effect that the account might have had on the subscribers and other readers of *La Caridad en la Guerra*—the official gazette of SRC—should not be underestimated.

According to Landa, in the town hall of Echarri-Aranaz a small field hospital had been improvised under the neutral RC flag. Maintained by the "charitable spirit of its inhabitants" and led "with the greatest wisdom" by the local doctor who appears not to have even been an RC member at the time, the hospital took in all the wounded. The ambulance volunteers immediately dealt with "the treatment and aid both moral and material to the wounded." The following day, having set up a district committee in Echarri and another in the neighboring town of Bacaicoa, they organized the evacuation of those—ten people—whose condition permitted it, first on stretchers as far as the railway station and then in a "[train] wagon with beds" to Pamplona. Having anticipated by telegraph the news of the arrival at their destination, their reception and further transfer to the military hospital was organized with the greatest solemnity and display of humanitarian resources:

> There was a parade of ten people of the Committee [of Pamplona's RC] . . . and forty charitable brothers who brought the stretchers. When the train arrived, the wounded were offered a soft drink and were put on the stretchers, each volunteer bringing a sunshade provided by the ladies of Pamplona to protect them from the hot sun. The retinue got underway with the flag of the ambulance flying at the front. Each stretcher was carried by four men and guarded by one or two hospitable [RC male members]; and a carriage for those wounded who could be seated [and for] the ambulance equipment brought up the rear. . . . A numerous public crowded in silent respect all along the way, sympathizing with the victims of the war and blessing the Christian work of the Red Cross.[30]

For her part, Arenal began, most significantly, her letters "From a hospital" by providing a Goyaesque picture of the horrors of war, where she sketched a sizeable group of mothers saying goodbye to their youngest sons.[31] She had witnessed the scene from the train in the station of Pozáldez, a town on her way from Madrid to Miranda, to take charge of the RC hospital. Arenal began by regretting her lack of artistic talent to "paint all the colors brought about by war to make it as odious . . . as deserved," as well as neither having "a decisive vote in any academy" nor being a "rich protector of the arts" to offer a "prize to the best picture representing *the mothers of Pozáldez*." She then gave a naturalistic declaration of the principles that should prevail in the artist to stir up the active compassion of her readers:

> The genius would be there, not to idealize, but to re-create the reality. Pain should not be painted in an embellished and outlined way, nor matrons with correct shapes, rosy cheeks and elegant dresses. Pozáldez's mothers were dark, disheveled, tattered, horrible to those eyes that, like a mirror, impassively reproduces the images, though, transfigured by pain, they had the sublime beauty that disdains forms and colors because it comes from the heart and touches it.[32]

Arenal devoted another letter to stimulating female voluntary work in the war hospitals of the RC, contesting two erroneous perceptions of the risks of this work for their health.[33] On the one hand, she considered as "entirely unfounded" the "fear of catching any disease or jeopardizing one's health as a result of living in an unhealthy atmosphere" in any hospital whenever there are "cautions and adequate cleaning," as was the case of the hospital she led at Miranda. Allegedly, it had "better hygienic conditions" than "most bedrooms in Madrid," because care was taken that its "assistants go out to the country for fresh air from time to time . . . and their lives are methodical and perfectly adjusted to the rules of hygiene." On the other hand, she defended the infinitely beneficial effects of compassion for the "health of the soul" given that seeing "this great amount of alien suffering" not only made resignation easier in the case of their own, but also increased "appreciation for the good things whose value is highlighted by whoever is deprived of them." Moreover, she claimed that "every trouble and hardship" were fully compensated for by the evident and tangible good that was done. In evoking the satisfaction caused by the chance to act as a mother to the sufferers, Arenal was appealing to an essentialist vision of female emotions, on the assumption that maternity as a natural feature made women able to look after others:

> The care taken to provide medicines, cleanliness, substantial food and gentle kindness, replace carelessness, abandon, untidiness, surliness, and the material and moral consequences are immediate and visible. What a satisfaction to see all the good, that would not be done without us, and to serve as a mother to those calling her in their suffering![34]

Here and in other passages Arenal mocked the "happy people" whose escape "from the spectacles of suffering that may disturb their happiness" seemed to her "natural" but not "reasonable," and she attacked "so many bored and unhappy people who suffer in a futile way."[35] She ended by praising altruism as a modus vivendi:

> Given a certain state of the soul, the purpose of being happy is no less absurd than that of looking young when a body declines. Living for others is the one way to find any happiness for oneself. People who are stale, bored, hopeless are those who have not said: *If I cannot be happy, I want to be useful*, so that they have neither converted their existence into an instrument for good, nor received it indirectly when it is impossible to receive it directly.[36]

Caring for the Sick and Wounded in Campaign

The recent experience of the Franco-Prussian War (1870–1871) favorably influenced the deployment of the SRC's humanitarian aid to wounded and sick combatants in the last Carlist War. Indeed, it provoked the earliest mobilization of solidarity in the SRC, and the interventions by the Geneva Committee and the French and Prussian national societies of the RC on that occasion offered an excellent model. This can be understood from three letters Nicasio Landa sent at the end of August 1870 during his trip to the war front, where he was commissioned as the SRC's general inspector.

In his letter from Basel, Landa referred to his visit to the "Agency" that the Geneva Committee had established there as an "advanced point for international aid," giving a detailed description of the functioning and competencies of this "office of correspondence and consignment." He observed that this agency, within its managerial tasks of war correspondence, was in charge not only of the communications "of the relief committees of the belligerent countries as well as with those neutral and vice versa" but also of the correspondence "of the wounded who were writing from foreign hospitals to their families, and vice versa."

This service, which Landa qualified as the "greatest and of inestimable moral value," had been supplemented with the new task, recently taken over by the agency, of ensuring that families' money reached their relatives who were wounded abroad.[37] We do not know to what extent the SRC's logistics allowed replication of such an efficient correspondence service during the Carlist war. It is known, however, that its permanent commission, at the proposal of its Navarrese committee, agreed to adopt "because of its utility and economy" two models of "postal cards, one to give information about the condition of the wounded to their families, and another for the publishable correspondence of the Association." The first of these models was reproduced in the SRC's bulletin.[38] No wonder, then, that the Carlist relief association *La Caridad* used *El Cuartel Real*—the insurgents' official press organ—to keep Carlist families acquainted with the whereabouts of their combatant relatives taken into different hospitals under its flag, in order to conveniently manage the collective emotions among the insurgents.

The third of these letters came from Karlsruhe and dealt with the organization and deployment of humanitarian help by German associations of the Red Cross. It focused on those resources that were established in that "theater of war" by the national society of the Great Dukedom of Baden, one of the twelve states that first signed on to the Geneva Convention in 1864.[39] On this occasion, one of Landa's main points of attention was a large rearguard hospital—four hundred beds—that the Baden RC had established in an old engine shed. He showered praise on its functioning in terms of medical as well as moral and material care, with particular emphasis on the "beneficial influence" that the "presence of educated women" had on hospitals such as these. Among them, he drew attention to the "young ladies from the best families of Karlsruhe who, enlisted in the committee, come by turns to stand guard [as nurses] under the direction of other ladies." All of them, he added, "hide either their luxury or poverty under a blue-striped apron, and take great pains to carry out with neither ostentation nor fuss, along with the Sisters of Charity and the Deaconesses, the humblest and even most disgusting tasks."[40]

In this point, Landa echoed the favorable opinion of the French lawyer and politician Édouard Laboulaye (1811–1893) on women's role in a U.S. model hospital Laboulaye had visited during the American Civil War. Landa agreed with Laboulaye that women make it possible for a "hospital not to be for the soldier just another kind of barrack but an extension of a domestic household. . . . I observe that at every bedside there is a trestle frame which serves to place a card portrait so that each patient can gaze at the image of his loved one beside him. Who, if not a woman, would think of adding such a detail to the ordinary furniture of a hospital!"[41] Years after, multiple reminiscences of German war hospitals could be found as inspiring the organization of the RC hospitals during the Carlist War. It became clear when Landa was turning to evoke Laboulaye's ideal, but particularly when seeing the crucial role women were then playing in achieving it. Indeed, Landa claimed that this ideal had already been reached in the hospital he had opened in Miranda and left in the hands of the Ladies' Section of the Madrid RC:

> Some days ago I visited it, and found that the ideal had been accomplished. Walls and beds were so white, floors so clean, servants so attentive, and patients so happy that the beneficial influence of the loving and compassionate sex is, of course, obvious. When I governed this hospital, I looked for its cleanliness without ever achieving its current neatness; I tried hard to keep order and discipline even by resorting to threat and moral punishment. Today, without needing any of this, the house is a mansion of peace and calm; certainly, I had flown the flag of the Red Cross above the building, but the angels of charity still did not cover it with their wings. Indeed, a man's voice is tough, even when he begs, while a woman's is sweet, even when she reprimands. Certainly, there are important things that are learned neither by talent nor by money, but by affection that only you [the ladies of Madrid Red Cross] can achieve.[42]

According to Arenal, Landa had had to overcome great material and logistic difficulties to hastily fit out the Miranda war hospital with eighty to ninety-five beds "to take in the most serious patients, who were literally in the street mud." The city was a rail junction "of certain strategic relevance" in the context of the northern front of the Carlist War. For her part, Arenal did not hide her unavoidable difficulties in getting either "Sisters of Charity, French or Spanish, or [Sisters] of Hope or Servants of Mary" to take care of it. This should be put into the context of a time when the incomprehension toward, if not open opposition and serious calumnies against, the SRC's activities and particularly those implemented by its Ladies' Section was particularly notable.[43] In order to fill this void, she had resorted to "charitable women" whose compassion was contributing to the creation of collective bodies like the SRC, feeling themselves united by a humanitarian ideal in their war relief tasks with sick and wounded soldiers, beyond the insuperable factional differences of their combatant relatives:

> J. and M. have come to bring their tireless activity and endless charity to this house with the help of some young ladies from the town. Being the two most assiduous [nurses] and never missing at the time of handing out the food, they have one, her father, and the other, her brother, with the Carlists; yet they look after the soldiers of the Republic as the most natural and simple thing by sublimely ignoring the merit of their action. The other nurses have a son and two brothers in the Republic's army; and while hate encourages one against the other, charity unites these women who disregard every meanness, every mistake, and every crime of the parties at arms.[44]

Arenal vindicated the positive "influence of benevolent feelings, even in the middle of a war which signifies hate and resentment together." An anthropological optimism led her to claim that "the strength of love resists everything, even defeat," as shown by the soldiers' esteem for any general who manifested "any affection" toward them. In any case, she wanted to emphasize the model behavior of the soldiers in the hospital at Miranda, as they responded to the good treatment they were receiving there:

> Here there are neither regulations, nor severe discipline, nor physicians with stripes and medals, nor any sort of fear; and it is notable the good behavior of the soldiers. More than a hospital, it seems like a convent because of the silence: neither a row, nor a dispute, nor disrespect to the women, the physician, the chaplain father, nor misappropriation of other people's possessions. On the contrary, how many proofs of gratitude and consideration, and even of gentlemanliness and tenderness in rough men, some of whom, when leaving, say their thanks with eyes moist! In the middle of the war that, as it goes on, generates in the armies so many bad things, how can the patients in this hospital be so good? Because they are treated well. It is the saddest thing that in ruling mankind, there is so little recourse to the use of *love*—so great and noble, and always obeyed.[45]

Again, Arenal's humanitarian narrative contrasted greatly with that of the report Landa wrote as a major physician and the SRC's general inspector, proposing a new system of elastic suspension for stretchers he had developed. Landa addressed it to his military superiors nine months before the end of the Carlist War, with the aim of getting its approval for use in the SRC's ambulances.[46] His objective was to improve the way in which the wounded were transported, particularly in its longest and most grueling stage, from the first-aid hospitals in the field to the permanent ones in safe territory, in such a way that minimized suffering. Having contrasted, during the war in Spain, modern transportation systems in "ambulance coaches, train wagons and hospital-ships" with the too-usual hard reality of wooden carts of animal traction, Landa presented the new suspension system of his invention as "solid, simple and cheap." He had designed it in collaboration with a machine manufacturer at Pamplona after having studied similar suspension systems developed in other western countries. He had even tried out the new device on his own bones and those of some friends, lying on the suspended stretchers on a cart running "over thick roots and roughnesses in a poplar grove close to Pamplona." Landa claimed that his device would dramatically improve the comfort of any wounded transferred on even the humblest cart, and that it was easily adaptable to most sophisticated systems of sanitary transport. Significantly, among his arguments to persuade his military superiors to approve the new suspension system, he evoked in a moving way the real conditions of sanitary transport in Spain in wartime:

I have been able to appreciate the sum of suffering that one or two days in a cart can impose on a wretched wounded soldier, who only endures them because of his eagerness to arrive at a hospital or to reach his family. I will never forget the sad moment when a man with a fractured limb, unable to tolerate any longer the torture of an oxcart, begged me to leave him abandoned in a ditch by the road.[47]

Conclusion

The SRC's intervention in the Spanish civil wars of the 1870s—mostly the Second Carlist War—provides a good case study to explore from a history of emotions perspective, notably because it can offer new, complementary insights into the role humanitarian narratives played on performing compassion for war victims in nineteenth-century Europe. In this way, women's humanitarian action in these civil wars notably contributed to shape a gendered conception of compassion for them. From its inception, the SRC developed humanitarian narratives that shared a mission and values common to the rest of the RC international movement, though they were gradually directed toward the specific demands of humanitarian relief in civil confrontations rather than following the RC's original script of helping sick and wounded soldiers in international wars. Despite the Geneva Committee's inhibition to intervene in civil wars, the Geneva Convention had permeated the humanitarian imagination of wide sections of Spanish elites and the general population to the point that both sides agreed to respect the terms of the Geneva Convention, and their mutual agreement worked reasonably well.

Narratives of the SRC's leaders like Concepción Arenal and Nicasio Landa were quite successful in bridging the ideological and political gap between the two sides bloodily confronting each other, though their styles and targets were rather different, each revealing strong gendered relations. Indeed, Landa's narratives were associated with a practical or instrumental reason, while Arenal's accounts mostly referred to private lives and, hence, emphasized female emotions at a time when they had not usual access to the public sphere, so that women were mostly able to make politics through the private sphere. In any case, both of them contributed to the building, with its pluses and minuses, of a single emotional community around common humanitarian practices and values in wartime, beyond the social fracture that fueled, and at once was fueled by, those civil conflicts.

Promoting active compassion for the victims of war and providing sick and wounded combatants with humanitarian help through successive stages and by different transfer procedures was a central issue in both humanitarian narratives. And they also coincided in assigning women a crucial role in the physical and emotional care of combatants' bodies at war hospitals on the alleged basis of the "beneficial influence of the loving and compassionate sex." Through their humanitarian actions in these civil wars, women contributed to shaping a gendered conception of compassion for war victims.

In brief, the performative effects of Arenal's and Landa's humanitarian narratives on the population's emotions in the face of these civil wars—and, specifically, the last Carlist War—contributed not a little to "civilizing" these bloody conflicts by reframing them into the practices and values derived from the Geneva Convention of 1864. Both narratives were rather successful in mobilizing compassion among the people, creating the material conditions for a new humanitarian body in which the "two Spains" remained unified over the civil conflict. To what extent the emotions enacted in these care regimes influenced policy beyond the end of the Carlist War is uncertain; however, the SRC ended this war so completely exhausted that it was unable to catch its breath again until twenty years later, on the occasion of the Cuban War of Independence of 1895–1898.

Notes

This contribution is the result of ongoing research within the framework of the projects funded by the Spanish Government: "Military Health Services, War Medicine, and Humanitarianism in Nineteenth-Century Spain" (HAR2011-24134), and "Relief Action and Medical Technologies in Humanitarian Emergencies, 1850–1950: Agencies, Agendas, Spaces, and Representations" (HAR2015-67723-P [MINECO/FEDER]). I am particularly indebted to Dolores Martín-Moruno for offering her expertise and guidance on this topic, and to Annie Oakes for her precious help with the English style of the article.

1. See Joanna Bourke, *Fear: A Cultural History* (London: Virago, 2005); Jay Winter, *Sites of Memory, Sites of Mourning: The Great War in European Cultural History* (Cambridge: Cambridge University Press, 2014); George L. Mosse, *La brutalisation des sociétés européennes: De la Grande Guerre au totalitarisme* (Paris: Hachette Littérature, 2000); Michael C. C. Adams, *Living Hell: The Dark Side of the Civil War* (Baltimore, Md.: Johns Hopkins University Press, 2014); Joanna Bourke, *An Intimate History of Killing: Face-to-Face Killing in Twentieth-Century Warfare* (London: Granta, 1999); Marc Ferro, *Resentment in History* (Cambridge: Polity, 2010); Javier Ordoñez, "Artificial Hatred," in *On Resentment: Past and Present*, ed. Bernardino Fantini, Dolores Martín-Moruno, and Javier Moscoso (Newcastle: Cambridge Scholars, 2013), 223–39; Beatriz Pichel, "French Resentment and the Animalization of the Germans during the First World War," in Fantini, Martín-Moruno, and Moscoso, *On Resentment*, 241–55.

2. Thomas L. Haskell, "Capitalism and the Origins of the Humanitarian Sensibility," *American Historical Review* 90, nos. 2 and 3, pts. 1 and 2 (1985): 339–36, 547–66; Luc

Boltanski, *Distant Suffering: Morality, Media and Politics* (Cambridge: Cambridge University Press, 1999); Bertrand Taithe, "'Cold Calculation in the Faces of Horrors?' Pity, Compassion and the Making of Humanitarian Protocols," in *Medicine, Emotion and Disease, 1700–1950*, ed. Fay Bound Alberti (London: Palgrave Macmillan, 2006), 79–99.

3. Thomas Laqueur, "Bodies, Details and the Humanitarian Narrative," in *The New Cultural History*, ed. Lynn Hunt, (Berkeley: California University Press, 1989), 177–78.

4. James Crossland, *War, Law and Humanity: The Campaign to Control Warfare, 1853–1914* (London: Bloomsbury, 2018).

5. John F. Hutchinson, "Rethinking the Origins of the Red Cross," *Bulletin of the History of Medicine* 63, no. 4 (1989): 557–78; John F. Hutchinson, *Champions of Charity: War and the Rise of the Red Cross* (Oxford: Westview, 1996).

6. Guillermo Sánchez-Martínez, "Enemies by Accident, Neutral on the Rebound: Diversity and Contingency at the Birth of War Humanitarianism, 1862–1864," *Asclepio* 66, no. 1 (2014): 28, doi:10.3989/asclepio.2014.02.

7. On how narratives could achieve things by performing emotions, see Jo Labanyi, "Doing Things: Emotion, Affect, and Materiality," *Journal of Spanish Cultural Studies* 11, nos. 3 and 4 (2010): 223–33.

8. Nicasio Landa, *La Caridad en la Guerra* 1, no. 7 (Ginebra, August 26, 1870): 1–2; 1, no. 8 (Basilea, August 28, 1870): 1, no. 2 (Karlsruhe, August 31, 1870): 2; 1, no. 9 (Basilea, August 28, 1870): 1–2.

9. Guillermo Sánchez and Jon Arrizabalaga, eds. *Nicasio Landa: Muertos y heridos, y otros textos* (Pamplona: Pamiela, 2016), 135–255.

10. See Jon Arrizabalaga and J. Carlos García-Reyes, "Innovación tecnológica y humanitarismo en el traslado de heridos de guerra: El informe de Nicasio Landa sobre un nuevo sistema de suspensión elástica de camillas (Pamplona, 29 mayo 1875)," *Manguinhos* 23, no. 3 (2016): 887–97.

11. Named after the German philosopher Karl Christian Friedrich Krause (1781–1832), Krausism was a universal and idealistic philosophical system combining monotheism and pantheism, advocating doctrinal tolerance and academic freedom from dogma. It was very influential in nineteenth-century Spain and inspired the Institución Libre de Enseñanza (founded in 1876), an educational project that had a significant impact on renewing Spanish intellectual and cultural life from the Restoration to the Civil War.

12. Concepción Arenal, *Artículos sobre beneficiencia y prisiones: Tomo II* (Madrid: Librería de Victoriano Suárez, 1900), 461–69 (1st letter); 478–87 (2nd letter); 494–501 (4th letter); 512–18 (5th letter); 519–28 (6th letter); 541–48 (7th letter).

13. For antiwar remarks, see Arenal, *Artículos sobre beneficiencia*, 463–69 (1st letter); 486–87 (2nd letter); 516–17 (5th letter); 541–42 (7th letter). The censored 3rd letter appears to have never been published. For the reference to its prohibition, see p. 494 (4th letter).

14. Concepción Arenal, *Cuadros de la guerra carlista* (Ávila: La Propaganda Literaria, 1880). My quotations come from a later edition of this work (Madrid: Librería de Victoriano Suárez, 1913).

15. For the text of the new law of public order, see *Gaceta de Madrid* (April, 24, 1870): 1.

16. *La Caridad en la Guerra* 4, no. 34 (1873): 6.

17. Sánchez and Arrizabalaga, *Nicasio Landa*, 148.

18. *La Caridad en la Guerra* 4, no. 34 (1873): 7.

19. Landa, "Muertos y heridos," 203.

20. Ibid., 161.

21. Concepción Arenal, "La caridad en la guerra y la justicia en la caridad," *La Voz de la Caridad* 100 (May 1, 1874): 54.

22. Arenal, *Cuadros*, 123–29.

23. Arenal, *Artículos sobre beneficiencia*, 486.

24. Arenal, *Cuadros*, 41–47.

25. Ibid., 51–62.

26. Arenal, *Artículos sobre beneficiencia*, 481.

27. Ibid., 514–17.

28. Ibid., 517–18. Relationship between tears and female emotions have been suggestively studied by Ute Frevert, *Emotions in History: Lost and Found* (Budapest: Central European University Press, 2011), 98–99.

29. Arenal, *Artículos sobre beneficiencia*, 524–25.

30. *La Caridad en la Guerra* 3, no. 29 (1872): 3. For another account of this episode in Landa's *Muertos y heridos*, see Sánchez and Arrizabalaga, *Nicasio Landa*, 163–65.

31. Arenal, *Artículos sobre beneficiencia*, 461–69.

32. Ibid., 464.

33. Ibid., 478–87.

34. Ibid., 483.

35. Ibid., 484 and 545–46.

36. Ibid., 484–85.

37. Landa, [letter from Basel, August 28, 1970], *La Caridad en la Guerra* 1, no. 8 (1870): 1–2.

38. *La Caridad en la Guerra* 4, no. 43 (1873): 4, 16.

39. Landa, [letter from Karlsruhe, August 31, 1870], *La Caridad en la Guerra* 1, no. 8 (1870): 2; I/9 (1870): 1–2.

40. Landa, [letter from Karlsruhe, August 31, 1870], *La Caridad en la Guerra* 1, no. 9 (1870): 1.

41. Ibid. Landa's inspiration source here appears to have been Laboulaye's *Paris in America* (New York: Scribner, 1863), esp. chapter 26 ("The Charity Hospital"), 267–68. Laboulaye's description refers to the "Providence Hospital," a hospital of New England directed by Mrs. Hope, "doctor in medicine and professor of hygiene" (267).

42. *La Época*, June 21, 1874. The phrase "loving and compassionate sex" (*sexo*

amante y compasivo) appears to have actually been Landa's rephrasing of Arenal's "charitable and loving sex" (*sexo piadoso y amante*) two years before. See *La Voz de la Caridad* 52 (May 1, 1872): 49.

43. J. Carlos García-Reyes, Guillermo Sánchez-Martínez, and Jon Arrizabalaga, "Movilización patriótica, medicina de guerra y humanitarismo: La Cruz Roja española en los conflictos civiles del Sexenio Democrático," *Estudos do Século XX*, 12 (1992): 85–86.

44. Arenal, *Artículos sobre beneficiencia*, 467.

45. Ibid., 527–28.

46. Arrizabalaga and García-Reyes, "Innovación tecnológica" (the text of Landa's manuscript report at pp. 891–93).

47. Landa, *Memoria descriptiva*, 1875, 1v–2r; Arrizabalaga and García-Reyes, "Innovación tecnológica," 892.

10. Humanitarian Emotions through History

Imaging Suffering and Performing Aid

EMMA HUTCHISON

INTERNATIONAL HUMANITARIANISM is more prominent than it has ever been throughout history. In the past half-century, human rights issues, such as refugee law and policy, and a broad scope of humanitarian agenda—from a "right of relief" after disaster to a growing "right of protection"—have intertwined to create a normative framework important to domestic and international governance, legitimacy, and order.[1] An ethic of "saving strangers"—the imperative for individuals, governments, and nongovernmental organizations to reach out to suffering others in times of hardship and need—has, at least institutionally, never been stronger.[2]

As significant as humanitarian principles and actions have become, the course and factors that have influenced—and continue to influence—the conception and rise of international humanitarianism are yet to be fully understood.[3] A range of social science and humanities scholarship contributes considerably to appreciating the contemporary politics and ethics at stake.[4] But only a few studies look back across humanitarianism's broader social and cultural origins to better grasp how humanitarianism is enacted today and may continue to transform in the future.[5]

One pervasive and crucial yet, so far, not thoroughly appreciated aspect of humanitarianism stands out in particular: emotions. Emotions have been considered fundamental to humanitarian narratives and practices since their inception. Historians, for instance, speak of the guilt and shame,[6] the "arousing sympathy,"[7] and the "irresistible compassion"[8] that so moved people in modern times, they rethought ideas of cruelty and sought to eradicate human hardship. In this sense, scholars hint that the history of humanitarianism can be conceived of through an increasingly organized ethic of "compassion across boundaries."[9] But while emotions are seen to pervade humanitarian sentiments, motivations, and actions, we know surprisingly little about how the emotions and bodily affects felt in response to experiencing and, in particular, to witnessing suffering have functioned to shape and support the rise of humanitarianism.

This chapter thus begins to address this shortcoming. I chart the emergence, progress, and prospects of humanitarianism through examining the pervasive emotional underpinnings of humanitarian actions. I start from the seemingly commonsensical assumption that emotions—how individuals and communities feel when faced with others' suffering, and how emotions have evolved over time—are key to the development of global humanitarianism. I argue—and demonstrate—that the history and contemporary practice of humanitarianism can be viewed in part through a lens of changing emotional meanings and moral significance attributed to pain.[10] While pain was historically perceived to be propitious to religious salvation, the increased awareness of and capacity to treat pain in modern times made it unpalatable. Pain was transformed into something to be pitied. Where possible and deemed necessary, it was to be alleviated and rallied against. Both affective and moral, this shift precipitated significant humanitarian reforms and the gradual expansion of a number of humanitarian customs and norms, from the abolition of slavery to decolonization and discourses of human rights, and from laws of war to the creation of humanitarian organizations such as the Red Cross and World Health Organization.

This chapter examines the linkages between the shifting emotional meanings attributed to pain and ensuing humanitarian responsibilities both conceptually and empirically. Conceptually, I discuss a range of literatures on what I call "humanitarian emotions," showing that they are performed as a consequence of witnessing pain. In particular, I show how these emotions have shifted over time to procure and elevate humanitarianism to the prominent place it now occupies.[11] At stake here are the "emotional bodies" of audiences, and specifically the performative aspects of the affects and emotions through which audiences make sense of suffering and mobilize humanitarian agency in response. To put it differently, as Dolores Martín-Moruno and Beatriz Pichel suggest in their introduction, I engage with how the everyday felt practice of emotions is implicated in the changing codes, norms, and institutions within societies.[12]

Empirically, I examine historical representations and contemporary media images of suffering. Visual representations—be they sketches of cruel, inhumane practices of slavery during modern times, emerging photographs of atrocity, deprivation and disadvantage in the nineteenth century, or the proliferation of media and aid images following calamities of the last century—are particularly crucial because they have long been perceived to poignantly convey the nature of pain and suffering.[13] Images of suffering both communicate and enable audiences to enact emotions. They are social and material artefacts that are both constituted by and, in turn, constitutive of how we feel about our own and others' suffering.[14] In this way, it is the interwoven performativity of images and emotions that are at stake: images are a medium through which the affective sensibilities that abet humanitarian actions—historically through to today—are practiced.[15] Tracing the history and performativity of visualizing pain thus illuminates the connections between emotions, changing meanings of suffering, and the humanitarian mobilizations that have been historically enacted.

The Origins of Humanitarianism: Emotions and Shifting Conceptions of Suffering over Time

While the most significant humanitarian advances might appear to have occurred in the past one hundred years, humanitarianism is by no means a contemporary invention. Compassionate ethics and politics did not spring simply from the great wars and emancipatory waves of decolonization in the twentieth century.[16] Between two and three centuries old, the humanitarianism movement as an ethic of "organized compassion" possesses a longer, complex history.[17]

This section traces the origins of humanitarianism back to the modern, Enlightenment era.[18] I focus on how social and medical advances during the eighteenth and nineteenth centuries precipitated a fundamental shift in how pain was considered. The emotional meaning and significance of pain changed dramatically. Suffering was traditionally considered virtuous, but during this period there came to be a "new repugnance and disgust in the face of pain" from which a humanitarian sensibility emerged.[19]

Historically, Western Christian societies perceived of pain as an inescapable and, therefore, redemptive human phenomenon. Considered key to spiritual salvation, suffering was situated as a positive experience; pain was seen as part of a process of religious recovery that would help to "perfect the spirit."[20] As Elizabeth Clark puts it, the "bleeding body . . . was both a confirmation and a link to divinity."[21] If encountered, pain and suffering were hence to be stoically, even if unpleasantly, endured: "suffer in this life," people believed, "and you would not be suffering in the next." Today, the notion that pain once served a higher-order, almost utilitarian purpose is still captured in the well-known aphorism: "No pain, no gain." Pain as a punitive measure—a philosophy still practiced in both Western and non-Western societies—is a further example of the former redemptive value of suffering.[22] In this sense, a kind of noble experiencing of bodily pain governed the emotional and moral meaning of suffering. Pain possessed strategic value.

However, during the eighteenth and nineteenth centuries the understanding of pain as a pathway to spiritual enlightenment came into question. Pain came to be seen less as an unavoidable human experience and instead as something that fell under human control. This shift was triggered in part by the development of modern medical practices that sought to alleviate the discomforts of illness and surgery. Haunted by their patients' suffering, physicians and surgeons, it was said, became "men of feeling"[23] and so searched to discover techniques that quelled patients' distress. Pain became not merely distasteful but "loathsome and unacceptable."[24] Practices of relieving pain—at first in surgery but increasingly in everyday life—were correspondingly transformed into a "blessing rather than a defect."[25]

This heightened capacity to alleviate pain, particularly from the mid-eighteenth century, fundamentally changed understandings of what it meant to suffer. As pain became more treatable, and preventable, it was transformed from a constructive life experience leading to spiritual growth into an abhorrent one. Importantly, with this shift, a moral transformation was also taking place: the new sensitivity toward pain cultivated changed modes of affective reasoning and moralizing about suffering. A reformist humanitarian spirit and agenda emerged. Slowly, people began to reconsider their attitudes toward suffering, particularly, and crucially, the suffering experienced by traditionally derided social groups, including the impoverished, the ill and insane, and criminals—although foremost here was arguably the suffering of slaves.[26] Prevailing ideas and customs about cruelty, human dignity, and what constituted humane-ness and the humane treatment of others were rethought.[27] Discourses of "humanity" emerged, as did, eventually, conceptualizations of "human rights."[28]

But this changing conception of pain and what pain meant in terms of moral responsibilities to suffering individuals was not simply an instrumental transformation: it was deeply emotional. To encounter pain, to give pain meaning, is always an encounter with emotions.[29] Meanwhile, the experience and meaning of emotions shifts through time and space: emotions are social and cultural; they are constituted and transform within cultural environments as well as through history.[30] Hence, in this respect, how we perceive of pain and think we ought to respond (emotionally and politically) is contextual; it is contingent upon how we have been socialized to *feel* about suffering.[31]

The affective dynamics associated with encountering bodies in pain are in this way crucial: emotional transformations underlie the development of newfound humanitarian sensibilities, narratives, and mobilizations. As Thomas Laqueur points out, humanitarian narratives and practices can be conceived of as the enactment of the "the common bond between those who suffer and those who would help," which is steeped in how we each feel when witnessing others' suffering.[32] Humanitarianism is, in other words, about the affective bonds between bodies.

The expanded awareness of pain's effects and the heightened ability to prevent suffering functioned to promote a newfound sympathy for suffering. To adopt Arlie Russell Hochschild's conception of emotions, sympathy at the sight of suffering gradually became a "feeling rule," overturning previous indifference or even apathy for the suffering other.[33] Put differently, to feel compassion when faced with others' suffering gradually came to define what it meant to be human and "humane."[34] To have sympathy for suffering strangers was to have humanity; to be "coldly indifferent to suffering" was to be seen as "less than human."[35] Sympathy consequently became an expected emotional custom and virtue.

Visualizing Suffering and the Historical Emergence of Humanitarian Emotions

What were the mechanisms through which these key affective and moral shifts took place? How was it that individuals grew more aware of the abhorrent, unnecessary nature of suffering? How did the meaning of humanitarianism shift from a potentially laughable to a laudable phenomenon—and, how was it that others' suffering became something that was felt for, emotionally, by witnesses? Part of the answer lies, I suggest, in representations—in the writings, the word of mouth, and a range of visual practices through which an awareness of pains' effects was circulated.

Representations of pain in modern times were instrumental to suffering's changing emotional awareness. During the late eighteenth century and particularly the nineteenth century, numerous complementary narratives of suffering began to flourish: novels, poems, memoirs, journalistic accounts, and other forms of artistic, aesthetic engagement such as sketches, paintings by leading artists, caricatures, cartoons, and even silverwork, cameos, and other jewelry. Through such representations suffering groups were brought to light as they had never been before.[36] And, crucially, these representations took on a performative function: they reshaped what it meant to both experience and witness pain. Representations mobilized and enabled audiences to enact a new culture of "spectatorial sympathy" and humanitarian sensibility.[37]

Visual representations were particularly powerful.[38] Graphic sketches, paintings, caricatures, and (from the nineteenth century on) photographs highlighted the emotional dimensions of pain in ways that textual narratives arguably could not. Some of the most famous art during this time is especially known for how it emotionalized suffering and sought to play on viewers' imagination and empathy.[39]

Two genres of images were especially influential. The first was early imagery—sketches, primarily, but also other art forms—of brutal practices associated with the slave trade and ownership.[40] The second comprised images of the suffering of other neglected social groups, mostly of women, children, the poor and destitute, and the sick.[41]

Consider the first: imagery that cultivated sympathy for the cruelty and suffering inflicted upon slaves. In these images, black slaves were predominantly depicted as victims situated within a controlling, domineering white society.[42] Various stereotypes typically associated with victimhood—prominently race and gender—were employed in these representations.

One example of such an image is the influential 1792 historic caricature "The Abolition of the Slave Trade" by Isaac Cruikshank (fig. 10.1). Cruikshank's sketch belongs to an emerging genre of caricatures at the time that portrayed the atrocities at the heart of the commercial slave trade. Viewed through a contemporary lens, the scene depicted is no doubt distressing and deeply emotional. However, in the eighteenth century, sketches such as Cruikshank's were crucial in beginning to raise awareness and to cultivate wider public sympathy for the cruelties inflicted upon slaves. This particular sketch depicts a case in which a captain of a slave ship (Kimber) was accused of murdering a young slave girl who refused to dance naked on his ship's deck. In the sketch the girl is almost completely naked, strung up to be whipped. She hangs by her foot, her face away from the viewer. Her torturers, clothed in formal attire of the day, watch on, grinning. Although she is upside-down, the young girl's hands are on her head, bringing to mind her agony, her physical distress and degradation—perhaps also her pleas for clemency.

Like much other early abolitionist imagery, Cruikshank's rendering prompts viewers to witness and (as was the case in this instance) reconsider the treatment of slaves both from a distance and through the eyes of the white perpetrators.[43] Looking away from the viewer, the young girl is not

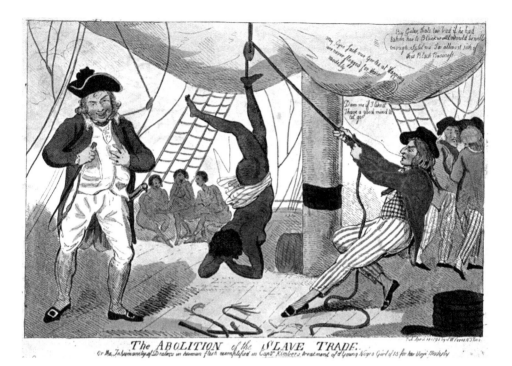

Figure 10.1: "The Abolition of the Slave Trade; or, The inhumanity of dealers in human flesh exemplified in Capt'n Kimber's treatment of a young negro girl of 15 for her virgin modesty." Attributed to Isaac Cruikshank, 1792.

only physically but also metaphorically faceless: she is every slave, but she is also no slave. Through her facelessness and anonymity, she is devoid of her personhood, the inherent individualism we each possess precisely because of the uniqueness of our face.[44] A particular emotional power politics thus comes into play: the loss of her unique self enables viewers to imagine her pain as not simply *her* pain but as a *universal* pain: that of every slave. This similarly encourages a universalizing form of sympathy for the plight of all slaves. By contrast, the perpetrator's actions appear as the actions of a few: their faces and glee in clear view shift the viewer toward emotional abjection (rather than identification) with white slave traders.

The famous abolitionist medallion crafted by Josiah Wedgwood, one of Britain's most famous potters, in 1787 is a further example of influential slave imagery. Both a piece of jewelry and propaganda, Wedgwood's image was originally intended to be worn by abolitionists as a means of identification.[45] But more than half a century later Wedgwood's image and specifically its

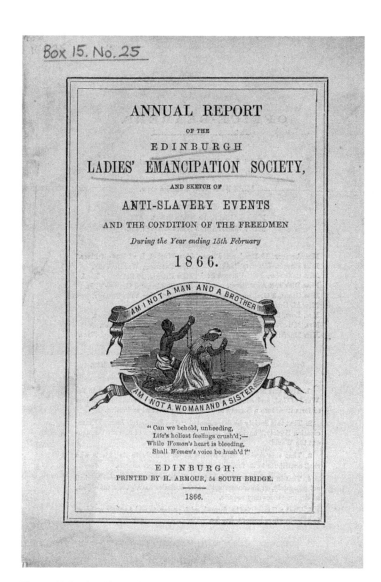

Figure 10.2: "Am I Not a Man and a Brother?" Medallion crafted as part of antislavery campaign by Josiah Wedgwood, 1787. Shown here is an adaption of Wedgwood's original medallion, which was published on the cover of the Annual Report of the Edinburgh Ladies Emancipation Society, 1866.

appeal to a common humanity and a humane sympathizing prompted it to resonate widely. The image went on to carry a recognizable humanitarian symbolism: it became the official medallion of the British Anti-Slavery Society in 1795 and continued to be central throughout the campaign to abolish slavery, well into the 1800s.

While very different in nature and social status, the suffering endured by women, the destitute and disadvantaged, and the sick also became an emerging genre of humanitarian imagery. Consider, for example, changing perceptions of women's suffering.

Throughout history women's suffering had been largely disregarded. Historically, the "perfect lady," it was said, was one who would "suffer and be still."[46] Women were expected to endure egregious forms of pain—foremost, childbirth—as silently and as unbeknownst to others as was possible. Some argue that if women's pain was publicized, it frequently became an object of a voyeuristic sensationalism, sexual lust, and even, at times, laughter.[47] However, in the eighteenth century the growth of humanitarian sentiments slowly put a stop to formerly unquestioned social customs surrounding women's experiencing of pain.[48] Through images that documented various forms of gender abuse, women's suffering became a further source of the growing humanitarian sympathy.

Nonetheless, in both of these genres—while very different in the suffering represented—recurring frames and tropes were employed that became markers of humanitarian sympathy. I highlight two in particular.

Foremost, and first, involves the depiction of sufferers as victims. Sufferers were portrayed as voiceless and powerless. Through their abject pain or their explicit pleas for consideration, sufferers appeal to audiences emotionally through a victimhood that increasingly necessitated compassionate feelings. Suffering bodies took on new meanings: bodies in pain—whether it was slaves enduring previously unfathomed atrocities or other marginalized groups—became "emotional bodies" in ways they may not have been previously conceived of. And it was because of the very emotionality of the suffering body that pain and cruelty became repulsive, something to prevent and guard against, and a key inspiration and catalyst for newfound humanitarian sensibilities.

Moreover, and second, particular tropes emerged that defined, more than others, the very idea of a victim. Slaves (black men and women alike), mothers and children, and children alone were distinguished and portrayed as inherently needy bodies. They were bodies that viewers were encouraged to feel for and empathize with because of their perceived helplessness, disadvantage, and need. Marginalized groups thus became humanitarian objects precisely because they lacked power and a perceived ability to help themselves.

In sum: historic humanitarian imagery can be seen to both reflect and be constitutive of the dramatic shift and cultivation of early modern humanitarian emotions. In this sense, early representations of suffering took on a performative function: visual imagery in particular prompted audiences to enact compassionate emotions that were central to humanitarian sentiments. Humanitarianism's emergence and growth must therefore be understood as much more than the ideas, customs, and practices through which it became manifest. Expanding humanitarian awareness and, eventually, institutions was at least in part a product of and further constitutive of the changing ways that emotions associated with suffering were felt and performed bodily with audiences. The origins of humanitarianism in this way illuminate the central theme at stake in this collection: how the performativity of emotions can have tangible empirical—social, normative, and institutional—effects. Indeed, humanitarian ideals, customs, and actions were made possible precisely because of the imagery and ensuing emotions through which suffering took on new meanings.

Emotions, Images, and Contemporary Humanitarianism

The emotional dimensions of witnessing suffering through images remain essential to contemporary humanitarianism.[49] By drawing attention to catastrophe and suffering, in often graphic and emotionally distressing ways, images help to summon necessary humanitarian actions. Some scholars even go as far as to suggest that images are fundamental to summoning intervention or aid. Denis Kennedy, for instance, contends that images have become the "public face" of humanitarianism: "images of suffering are a means towards a set of humanitarian ends."[50] Michael Barnett and Thomas Weiss likewise claim that "the humanitarian sector lives on the adage of one picture is worth a thousand words. . . . The more graphic the image and the more it screams innocent victim, the more effective it will be in mobilizing compassion, action, and money."[51]

Understood here is that imagery can be instrumental in communicating humanitarian meanings and enabling collective feelings about distant disaster. Images mobilize a social, collective, and highly politicized vision of often far-away, incomprehensible crisis and prompt viewers to enact a range of emotions and to help in response.

At the same time, emotions associated with humanitarian imagery are often seen to present a significant "humanitarian dilemma."[52] The types of images that most effectively solicit solidarity in times of human need and garner the most humanitarian assistance are also those that enact what is termed a "politics of pity."[53] A politics of pity suggests that while audiences feel grievous and deep sympathy for the suffering before them, they still remain quietly and safely detached. Philosopher Hannah Arendt was one of the first to delineate this emotional-political dynamic. For Arendt, pity meant "to be sorry without being touched in the flesh."[54] Pity, in other words, is perceived to maintain a distance between viewer and victim and, in doing so, fosters viewers' incapacity or unwillingness to engage in a deeper, potentially more reflective form of empathic identification or understanding. A hierarchy between viewer and victim is created.

Significant here is that the images most likely to mobilize humanitarianism are also those that focus on victims' vulnerability and dependence. Such imagery typically relies on and replicates a number of ethically problematic stereotypes, foremost those associated with racial and cultural difference, gender, and age. There is, for instance, a general assumption that certain kinds of images—"wide-eyed . . . sad-eyed" emaciated children, helpless refugees, and pleading mothers—are more helpful in raising humanitarian awareness.[55] Sufferers are as such framed not as resilient actors but as vulnerable and disempowered victims; they are shown dwarfed by destruction and stricken by shock. Sufferers wait, passive and powerless, for the arrival of aid, instead of actively helping themselves and their communities. Suffering individuals and communities are thereby disempowered and appropriated through imagery; bodies in pain become objects of viewers' pity.

These visual humanitarian dynamics are often discussed as a more recent phenomenon, yet when viewed through the lens of historical imagery, they can be seen to have historically embedded social and emotional origins. Indeed, I suggest that contemporary humanitarian frames and their affective resonances are in part a product of the post-Enlightenment legacies surrounding the representation of suffering.[56] One trend in particular is central: like the slave imagery discussed earlier, contemporary images tend to bring disaster into focus through the use of frames that disempower sufferers, rendering them helpless and needy. Humanitarian imagery achieves this by depicting sufferers as vulnerable, struck down by tragedy, devoid of agency, and dependent. Employing these frames is powerful, as it harks back to time-honored humanitarian tropes that provide audiences with easily recognized points of emotional (sympathetic) identification.

Consider, for instance, tropes typically employed to depict contemporary humanitarian disaster and ensuing human need. Arguably the most classic—as well as stereotypical and readily identifiable—humanitarian symbol is the image of the mother and child. Political geographer Kate Manzo even

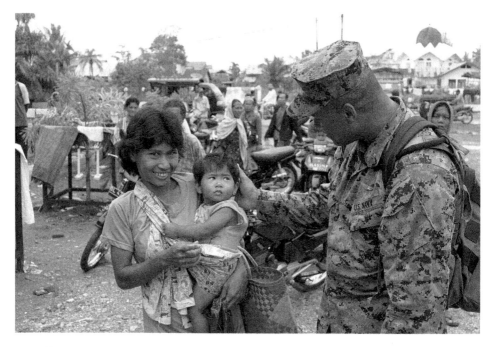

Figure 10.3: Head Surgeon of the Combined Support Group-Indonesia, U.S. Navy Lieutenant Commander Loring Issaac Perry, takes a moment to comfort an Indonesian woman and her child who lost everything they had during the tsunami in the city of Meulaboh on the island of Sumatra, Indonesia. Photograph by Pfc. Nicholas T. Howes, USMC, January 1, 2005.

goes as far as to claim that so commonplace and emotionally compelling are images of women together with children in disaster discourses that the mother-and-child image has come to be understood as an international "symbol of distress," as a marker of charity and humanitarianism.[57] Figure 10.3, a photograph taken in the days after the 2004 Asian tsunami catastrophe, is a characteristic illustration.

In this image we see a mother and child—who go nameless while, as is all too common, the army medic does not—presented as grateful beneficiaries of aid. They stare up seemingly happily at the camera. The mother's calm air together with the army medic's caring gesture signals a gratitude for the assistance and aid. However, mother-and-child images are typically far more graphic. Mothers are portrayed in visible distress; they are captured distraught in their grief over dying or dead children. Much of the emotional and cultural symbolism of the mother-and-child image emerges from the essentialized, stereotypical notion of motherhood, specifically that motherhood is a female role.[58] As Liisa Malkki explains, the image of mother and child presents something that is perceived to go to the heart of humanity and to be in some form evident within all cultures, a "sentimentalized, composite figure—at once feminine and maternal, childlike and innocent."[59] But there is also more to this visual pattern: a lack of power and a cry for help to those who have the ability to deliver. Women are portrayed as passive—powerless and prone to the circumstances surrounding them. Women and women's social roles after disaster are thus presented in a singular light that highlights and links a traditional familial domesticity with a sense of fragility and vulnerability.

It is precisely through the gender stereotype that is implied—that is, the inferred sense of feminine passivity, dependence, and emotionality—that compassionate, humanitarian emotions can be so readily mobilized. For some, this emotional appeal and resonance of the mother-and-child image is derived directly from a historically significant affective symbol: the pieta.[60] The Madonna mourning the loss of her child, as depicted in figure 10.4, is the quintessential and arguably universally recognized icon of compassion and grief.

Some scholars, moreover, have shown that through gendered frames disaster is in this way frequently "feminized."[61] The excessive use of feminine gender stereotypes shapes how viewers come to consider the respective humanitarian situation more generally. Women come to represent all sufferers, who then, too, become perceived with a corresponding sense of stricken powerlessness—the very opposite of the resilience required to help themselves.

Another closely associated trope that is frequently employed consists of images that depict the immediate catastrophe and almost singularly present survivors/sufferers as passive recipients rather than active participants in humanitarian aid processes. In these images, victims are presented as powerless and submissive—they are dependent and humanitarian receivers, akin the politics of pity outlined earlier. They appear totally reliant on the distribution of foreign aid (rather than, for instance, helping themselves, or even helping Western aid workers to distribute aid). It also seems that while victims are in need, the Western relief workers are "saving the day"; the relief workers are the "white knights," so to speak.[62] Of course, this might in some instances be the case, in relation to victims' day-to-day survival, but when used repeatedly, this type of imagery helps to mobilize the idea that victims are unable to help themselves. Western relief workers are in contrast the active agents; their giving hands indicate assurance and control.

The passive/active dichotomy in this style of imagery is significant in that it functions to convey both the urgent situation and seeming dependence of survivors while simultaneously prompting the viewer to identify with

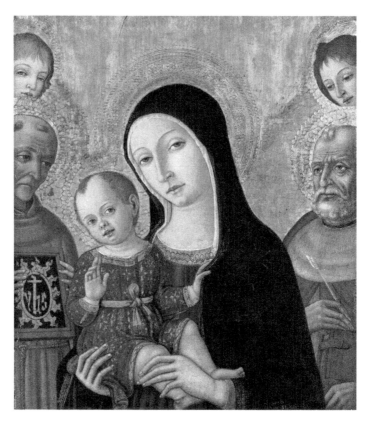

Figure 10.4: "The Madonna and Child with Saints Bernardino of Siena and Jerome, behind them Two Angels." Matteo di Giovanni, 1435–1495.

the aid workers. A type of superior (and masculine) Western mindset is created, meaning that existing perceptions of the developing world's passivity and dependence are both invoked and in turn reconstituted. How such imagery suggests a type of paralysis or inability to respond can be seen as instrumental to generating an understanding of victims as disempowered and, consequently, reliant on overseas aid. A social relationship that is based in a colonial—as well as a cultural and racial—gaze is in this way perpetuated.[63] Graphic photographs of distressed faces embody a sense of desperation and communicate a sense of victims' powerlessness that functions to affirm wider and historically constituted aid discourses that maintain hierarchical humanitarian relations between the Western and developing world.[64] But it is also through such framing that particular emotional dispositions and associated humanitarian meanings begin to emerge. Specifically, this style of humanitarian imagery—promoting colonial understandings of developing world others—constructs victims as objects of sympathy and encourages audiences to engage with the disaster through a politics of pity.

To reiterate, a politics of pity suggests that while audiences feel sympathetic toward the suffering visualized, it is an emotional dynamic that enables audiences to simultaneously remain detached.[65] A hierarchy between viewer and victim is created, as it is here in these images. Images that overwhelmingly focus on victims' vulnerability and dependence—most notably through the combined prevalence of women and/or children and racial difference—implicates pity by positioning pleading victims in relation to a sympathetic and empowered viewer. A politics of pity is fostered not only upon perceptions of victims' dire needs but the confluence of perceptions of cultural difference and humanitarian need. Victims thus become subsumed into the dominant North/South humanitarian discourse that privileges spontaneous and short-lived bursts of public agency toward distant vulnerable others, such as the solidarity that is typically mobilized in the wake of devastating natural disasters.

Emotional dispositions that have for long been associated with the ensuing humanitarian solidarity are in this way—through prevailing imagery—consolidated. Contemporary images, whether they are in the media or from the vast array of humanitarian NGOs—typically depict crises and human need in a manner that corresponds with a moral emphasis on pity and sympathy for the suffering other—a moral code that has distinguished Western politics and ethics since modern times. So much is this the case that some scholars even contend Western audiences are more distinguished by a perceived moral obligation to feel emotions such as pity than they are by actually acting upon such emotions for the long- or even short-term betterment of the distant others they are supposedly feeling for.[66]

This is not, however, to claim that sympathy and pity are the only emotions and affects that are implicated with and help to mobilize humanitarian actions. While the representations and tropes I highlight here—stereotypes employed to communicate victimhood and human need—have been long established, other frames and meanings increasingly proliferate and have become important to the global humanitarian order. Indeed, scholars problematize these singular humanitarian frames in an effort to identify representations that implicate perceivably more reflective emotions and meanings, such as empathy, compassion, indignation, and even guilt.[67]

Emotions, Performativity, and the Transformation of Humanitarian Practices

Humanitarianism as a moral desire and political imperative is intrinsically linked to images of suffering and the associated, historically shifting emotional meanings attributed to pain. During modern times, what it meant to endure pain and to suffer underwent a radical transformation. Suffering became abhorrent. Consequently, the moral norms and social customs around pain also changed. Suffering became something to feel for rather than something to ignore or to laugh at or forget. But this does not mean that sympathy for suffering was unconditional.[68] While an emotional culture of sympathy for suffering grew, how audiences are emotionally attached and consequently feel for others has always been (and always will be) bound by culture and context, time and space.

Significant in this respect is that emotions and affects—how bodies connect emotionally—shift and change over time. Here, the visualization of suffering played and continues to play an equally important performative role. Images are fundamental to shaping and reshaping audiences' emotional experiences of suffering and the types of humanitarian meanings and mobilizations that ensue.

Yet, as this chapter has shown, the images and emotions that have typically led to humanitarian meanings and agency perform a precarious paradox. While dominant imagery—throughout history from the time of slavery into the present day—enable audiences to enact emotions such as pity, sympathy, and compassion, it does so through visually performing (and replicating) a range of gender and racial stereotypes and hierarchies. Such stereotypes hinge on the power of the viewer and perceiver and relegate the sufferer. The affects and emotions that ensue from such imagery are thus are also a form of hierarchy: prevailing emotional norms and regimes are born from a position of privilege—whether this be of gender or of cultural or geographic distance. Some scholars take this even further. David Kennedy writes of humanitarianism's "dark side."[69] Humanitarian sentiments and emotions are partial and selective and have been used through history to justify political projects that paradoxically perpetuated violence and injustice. Sympathy, the emotion perceived to lie at the heart of humanitarianism's rise, is also, on the one hand, considered key to bestowing suffering subjects with humanity, while, on the other hand, sympathy is perceived to simultaneously objectify and dehumanize the very suffering subjects it supposedly embraces.[70]

Pointing to the problematic historical legacy and the undersides of humanitarian politics is not to devalue the humanitarian impulse and political imperative altogether. Rather, it is to emphasize that the humanitarian order, no matter how noble and well intentioned, is inevitably linked to power.[71] The emotional registers and norms that underpin humanitarian actions are, moreover, not exempt from such power. However, understanding the performativity of emotions—and conceiving of emotions as practices that bodies "do"[72]—provides critical tools to reflect upon and to potentially reimagine the interwoven performativity of images, emotions, power, and humanitarianism. Crucially, conceiving of emotions as bodily practices that are stimulated in conjunction with the world around us also tells us that such emotions can be reshaped; emotions "can be engines of conversion."[73] Emotions can transform the meanings of the very representations they emerge from, thereby making "emotions themselves the causes of their own transformation."[74] Emotions can therefore themselves be forms of agency that transform how we think about others' suffering and ensuing humanitarian mobilizations.

Crucial here are the forms of representation through which suffering comes to be known and perceived of. How suffering is visualized, spoken of, written about—how our own and others' pain is narrated—can trigger emotions and evoke a concomitant form of humanitarian responsibility. This is why it is essential for us to be mindful of the history of visualizing suffering and the emotional origins and legacies that are left behind. How human suffering and hardship has been historically represented—and is imaged today—is central to the types of emotional and moral meanings that the respective suffering acquires. As a phenomenon intimately connected to these emotional and moral meanings, humanitarianism can be seen to be at least partially contingent upon and performed through the images used to depict human hardship.

Notes

This chapter emerges from my Australian Research Council (ARC) Discovery Early Career Research Award (DE180100029) project on emotions and the politics of humanitarianism, as well as research conducted through a University of Queensland Foundation Research Excellence Award and as an associate investigator in the ARC Centre of Excellence for the History of Emotions. The chapter was presented as a keynote address at the ARC Centre of Excellence of the History of Emotions, "Emotions, Media, History" Symposium at the University of Adelaide. Thank you to all who attended and commented, and especially to those who contacted me personally—Tom Clark, Eric Parisot, and Kathryn Temple—for helpful feedback. For further insight and discussion, I would also like to thank the editors, Dolores Martín-Moruno and Beatriz Pichel, as well as Michael Barnett, Roland Bleiker, Lorenzo Cello, Constance Duncombe, Tim Dunne, and Luke Glanville.

1. Michael Barnett, *Empire of Humanity: A History of Humanitarianism* (Ithaca, N.Y.: Cornell University Press, 2011); Alex J. Bellamy, "A Death Foretold? Human Rights, Responsibility to Protect and the Persistent Politics of Power," *Cooperation and Conflict* 50, no. 2 (2015): 286–93.

2. Nicholas J. Wheeler, *Saving Strangers: Humanitarian Intervention in International Society* (Oxford: Oxford University Press, 2000).

3. See Michael Barnett, *The International Humanitarian Order* (Milton Park, U.K.: Routledge, 2010), 177.

4. It is impossible to list all the works that explore the present as well as historical ethical and political dynamics of humanitarianism. Some influential works across the field include: Barnett, *Empire of Humanity*; Lynn Hunt, *Inventing Human Rights: A History* (London: Norton, 2007); Samuel Moyn, *The Last Utopia: Human Rights in History* (Cambridge, Mass.: Harvard University Press, 2010); Davide Rodogno, *Against Massacre: Humanitarian Intervention in the Ottoman Empire 1815–1914* (Princeton, N.J.: Princeton University Press, 2012).

5. The history of humanitarianism is, however, a growing field of study, with scholars from a range of disciplines examining various aspects—from key social movements, the roles of women, and the violence of both slavery and colonialism—that led to humanitarianism's development and rise. Notable studies in these directions include: Emily Baughan and Bronwen Everill, eds. "Empire and Humanitarianism," *Journal of Imperialism and Commonwealth History* 40, no. 5 (2012); Didier Fassin, *Humanitarian Reason: A Moral History of the Present* (Berkeley: University of California Press, 2012); Abagail Green, "Humanitarianism in Nineteenth Century Context: Religious, Gendered, National," *Historical Journal* 57, no. 4 (2012): 1157–75; Karen Halttunen, "Humanitarianism and the Pornography of Pain in Anglo-American Culture," *American Historical Review* 100, no. 2 (1995): 303–34; Peter Stamatov, *The Origins of Global Humanitarianism: Religion, Empires, and Advocacy* (Cambridge: Cambridge University Press, 2013).

6. Ruth Leys, *From Guilt to Shame: Auschwitz and After* (Princeton, N.J.: Princeton University Press, 2007).

7. Richard Ashby Wilson and Richard D. Brown, "Introduction," in *Humanitarianism and Suffering: The Mobilization of Empathy*, ed. Richard Ashby Wilson and Richard D. Brown (Cambridge: Cambridge University Press, 2009), 10.

8. Norman S. Fiering, "Irresistible Compassion: An Aspect of Eighteenth-Century Sympathy and Humanitarianism," *Journal of the History of Ideas* 37, no. 2 (1976): 195–218.

9. Barnett, *Empire of Humanity*, 19; see also Rebecca Gill, "Networks of Concern, Boundaries of Compassion: British Relief in the South African War," *Journal of Imperial and Commonwealth History* 40, no. 5 (2010): 827–44.

10. Here I draw upon and expand pioneering works of scholars such as Margaret Abruzzo, Rob Boddice, Joanna Bourke, Elizabeth Clark, Norman Fiering, Lynn Hunt, and Javier Moscoso.

11. I note at the outset that there are significant phenomenological distinctions

at stake in the terms "emotions," "feelings" and "affect." These distinctions are the subject of often intense debate; however, the following broad conceptions can be drawn. Feelings are thought to be bodily sensations felt physically. Emotions, then, are perceived to be the conscious manifestations of bodily feelings. Affect, meanwhile, is a broader realm of moods, dispositions, and attachments that are typically theorized to be nonconscious and precognitive and is thus outside of representation. In this chapter I predominantly use the term "emotion"; however, I take an approach that sees feelings, emotions, and affect as interwoven, insofar as they are all constituted, regulated, and can be transformed within social environments.

12. Implicit here is an understanding of emotions as practices that emerge from bodily dispositions conditioned within social, cultural, and historical contexts. See Monique Scheer, "Are Emotions a Kind of Practice (And Is That What Makes Them Have a History)?," *History and Theory* 51, no. 2 (2012): 193–220.

13. Ulrich Baer, *Spectral Evidence: The Photography of Trauma* (Cambridge, Mass.: MIT Press, 2001).

14. Heide Fehrenbach and Davide Rodogno, "Introduction: The Morality of Sight," in *Humanitarian Photography: A History*, ed. Heide Fehrenbach and Davide Rodogno (Cambridge: Cambridge University Press, 2015), 5; Green, "Humanitarianism in Nineteenth Century Context," 1160; Halttunnen, "Humanitarianism," 303–34; Matthew Norton, "Narrative Structure and Emotions Mobilization in Humanitarian Representations: The Case of the Congo Reform Movement, 1903–1912," *Journal of Human Rights* 10, no. 3 (2011): 311–38.

15. Articles that discuss the performativity of material objects in conjunction with the everyday practice of emotions/affects include: Karen Barad, "Posthumanist Performativity: Toward an Understanding of How Matter Comes to Matter," *Signs: Journal of Women in Culture and Society* 28, no. 3 (2003): 801–31; Katie Barclay, "New Materialism and the New History of Emotions," *Emotions: History, Culture, Society* 1, no. 1 (2017): 161–83.

16. See in this volume Jon Arrizabalaga, "Performing Compassion in Wartime: Humanitarian Narratives in the Spanish Civil Wars of the 1870s," and Bertrand Taithe, "Compassion Fatigue: The Changing Nature of Humanitarian Emotions."

17. Barnett, *Empire of Humanity*, 50. This is even though the term "humanitarian" was only first enunciated in 1844. See also Margaret Abruzzo, *Polemical Pain: Slavery, Cruelty, and the Rise of Humanitarianism* (Baltimore, Md.: Johns Hopkins University Press, 2011), 1–15; Barnett, *Empire of Humanity*, 19; Thomas Haskell, "Capitalism and the Origins of Humanitarianism," *American Historical Review* 90, nos. 2 and 3, pts. 1 and 2, (1985): 339–61, 547–66.

18. Many scholars trace the origins of humanitarian emotions, such as sympathy, compassion, and pity, to this period. Samuel Moyn, for instance, calls the Enlightenment era the "age of feeling" in which (a post-1750) sentimentalism was fostered. See Samuel Moyn, "Empathy in History: Empathizing with Humanity," *History and Theory* 45, no. 3 (2006): 399.

19. Halttunnen, "Humanitarianism," 318.

20. Joanna Bourke, *The Story of Pain: From Prayer to Painkillers* (Oxford: Oxford University Press, 2014).

21. Elizabeth B. Clark, "'The Sacred Rights of the Weak': Pain, Sympathy, and the Culture of Individual Rights in Antebellum America," *Journal of American History* 82, no. 2 (1995): 471.

22. Abruzzo, *Polemical Pain*, 2.

23. Fiering, "Irresistible Compassion," 212; Haltunnen, "Humanitarianism," 303 and 310.

24. Haltunnen, "Humanitarianism," 310.

25. Steven Bruhm cited in Haltunnen, "Humanitarianism," 310.

26. For linkages with early photographic practices of visualizing children, see (in this volume) Leticia Fenández-Fontecha, "The Language of Children's Pain (1870–1900)."

27. See Abruzzo, *Polemical Pain*, 10–14; Clark, "Sacred Rights of the Weak," 469; Fiering, "Irresistible Compassion," 195–97 and 209–13.

28. Lynn Hunt, *Inventing Human Rights: A History* (New York: Norton, 2007).

29. Rob Boddice, "Introduction: Hurt Feelings?," in *Pain and Emotion in Modern History*, ed. Rob Boddice (Basingstoke: Palgrave Macmillan, 2014), 6.

30. A wide assemblage of humanities and social science scholarship now abides with this approach to emotions. Across history, see for instance Peter N. Stearns and Carol Z. Stearns, "Emotionology: Clarifying the History of Emotions and Emotional Standards," *American Historical Review* 90, no. 4 (1985): 813–36; Barbara Rosenwein, *Emotional Communities in the Early Middle Ages* (Ithaca, N.Y.: Cornell University Press, 2006). In anthropology and sociology, see Catherine A. Lutz, *Unnatural Emotions: Everyday Sentiments on a Micronesian Atoll and Their Challenge to Western Theory* (Chicago: University of Chicago Press,1988); Arlie Russell Hochschild, *The Managed Heart: Commercialization of Human Feeling* (Berkeley: University of California Press, 2012).

31. David B. Morris, *The Culture of Pain* (Berkeley: University of California Press, 1991), 20.

32. Thomas W. Lacqueur, "Bodies, Details, and the Humanitarian Narrative," in *The New Cultural History*, ed. Lynn Hunt (Chicago: University of Chicago Press, 1989), 177.

33. Hochschild, *Managed Heart*, 56–63.

34. Abruzzo, *Polemical Pain*, 10–14; Fiering, "Irresistible Compassion," 196. To be clear, "humane" in this context is referring to the morally and socially acceptable treatment of others, including marginalized and traditionally outcast social groups, such as slaves.

35. Fiering, "Irresistible Compassion," 196 and 212.

36. Hunt's *Inventing Human Rights* and Lacquer's "Bodies, Details, and the Humanitarian Narrative" provide comprehensive overviews of different types of genres and representational frames adopted by human rights and humanitarianism advocates.

37. Haltunnen, "Humanitarianism," 307; Wilson and Brown, "Introduction," 19.

38. While visual imagery is particularly important, especially in modern times when literacy rates were not high, the role of images is interwoven with other narrative styles in various periods. For linguistic (poetic and fiction) narratives, for instance, see Hunt, *Inventing Human Rights*, and Lacquer, "Bodies, Details, and the Humanitarian Narrative."

39. A famous example is one of J. M. W. Turner's most celebrated works, "Slave Ship: Slavers Throwing Overboard the Dead and Dying, Typhoon Coming On," painted in 1840. For a summary of the artwork and its significance in the abolitionist movement see: http://www.mfa.org/collections/object/slave-ship-slavers-throwing-overboard-the-dead-and-dying-typhoon-coming-on-31102.

40. See, for instance, Stephen Best, "Neither Lost nor Found: Slavery and the Visual Archive," *Representations* 113, no. 1 (2011): 150–63; Maurie McInnis, *Slaves Waiting for Sale: Abolitionist Art and the American Slave Trade* (Chicago: Chicago University Press, 2011); Nicholas Mirzoeff, *The Right to Look: A Counterhistory of Visuality* (Durham, N.C.: Duke University Press, 2011), 48–116; Marcus Wood, *Blind Memory: Visual Representations of Slavery in English and America 1780–1865* (London: Manchester University Press, 2000).

41. See Heide Fehrenbach, "Children and Other Civilians: Photography and the Politics of Humanitarian Image-Making," in Fehrenbach and Rodogno, *Humanitarian Photography*, 165–99; Laura Mulvey, *Visual and Other Pleasures* (Basingstoke: Palgrave, 1989); Carolyn Taylor, "Humanitarian Narrative: Bodies and Detail in Late-Victorian Social Work," *British Journal of Social Work* 38, no. 4 (2008): 680–96.

42. Wood, *Blind Memory*, 215–19.

43. See Wood, *Blind Memory*, 160–61; and Sharon Sliwinski, "Human Rights," *Visual Global Politics*, ed. Roland Bleiker (Milton Park, U.K.: Routledge, 2018).

44. Jenny Edkins, *Face Politics* (Milton Park, U.K.: Rouledge, 2015).

45. Mary Guyatt, "The Wedgwood Slave Medallion," *Journal of Design History* 13, no. 2 (2000): 93–94.

46. Martha Vicinus, ed., *Suffer and Be Still: Women in the Victorian Age* (Bloomington: Indiana University Press, 1972).

47. Simon Dickie, *Cruelty and Laughter: Forgotten Comic Literature and the Unsentimental Eighteenth Century* (Chicago: Chicago University Press, 2011); Haltunnen, "Humanitarianism and the Pornography of Pain," 315–17.

48. This is not to say, however, that a fascination with women's pain—and, in particular, the idea that a woman in pain is provocative and alluring—was overturned. Perpetuating women's suffering may have outwardly become increasingly a social taboo, yet today a culture of sensationalizing women's pain continues.

49. See, for example, Michael Barnett and Thomas G. Weiss, *Humanitarianism Contested: Where Angels Fear to Tread* (Milton Park, U.K.: Routledge, 2011), 118–20; Juha Käpylä and Denis Kennedy, "Cruel to Care? Investigating the Governance of Compassion in the Humanitarian Imaginary," *International Theory* 6, no. 2 (2014): 255–92.

50. Denis Kennedy, "Selling the Distant Other: Humanitarianism and Imagery;

Ethical Dilemmas of Humanitarian Action," *Journal of Humanitarian Assistance* 6, no. 2. (2009): 255–92.

51. Barnett and Weiss, *Humanitarianism Contested*, 119.

52. Kennedy, "Selling the Distant Other," 255–92; Anne Vestergaard, "Humanitarian Branding and the Media: The Case of Amnesty International," *Journal of Language and Politics* 7, no. 3 (2008): 472, 490.

53. A "politics of pity" was first delineated by philosopher Hannah Arendt. See Hannah Arendt, *On Revolution* (London: Penguin, 1990). For articulations that discuss the links with humanitarian imagery, see Barnett and Weiss, *Humanitarianism Contested*, 119–20; Luc Boltanski, *Distant Suffering: Politics, Morality and the Media*, trans. Graham Burchell (Cambridge: Cambridge University Press, 1999), 8 and 155; Lilie Chouliaraki, "Post-Humanitarianism: Humanitarian Communication beyond a Politics of Pity," *International Journal of Cultural Studies* 13, no. 2 (2010): 110–12.

54. Arendt cited in Tristan Naylor, "Deconstructing Development: The Use of Power and Pity in the International Development Discourse," *International Studies Quarterly* 55, no.1 (2011): 177–97.

55. See, for example, Debbie James Smith, "Big-Eyed, Wide-Eyed, Sad-Eyed Children: Constructing the Humanitarian Space in Social Justice Documentaries," *Studies in Documentary Film* 3, no. 2 (2009): 159–75; Anke Strüver, "The Production of Geopolitical and Gendered Images through Global Aid Organizations," *Geopolitics* 12, no. 4 (2007): 680–703.

56. Following passages draw my previous work, most notably Emma Hutchison, "A Global Politics of Pity? Disaster Imagery and the Emotional Construction of Solidarity after the 2004 Asian Tsunami," *International Political Sociology* 8, no. 1 (2014): 1–19.

57. Kate Manzo, "Imaging Humanitarianism: NGO Identity and the Iconography of Childhood," *Antipode* 40, no. 4 (2008): 649–51.

58. See Linda Åhäll, "Motherhood, Myth and Gendered Agency in Political Violence," *International Feminist Journal of Politics* 14, no. 1 (2012): 103–20; Laura Briggs, "Mother, Child, Race, Nation: The Visual Iconography of Rescue and the Politics of Transnational and Transracial Adoption," *Gender and History* 15, no. 2 (2003): 183–84.

59. Liisa Malkki, "Speechless Emissaries: Refugees, Humanitarianism, and Dehistoricization," *Cultural Anthropology* 11, no. 3 (1996): 388.

60. About the project led by David Campbell, "Imaging Famine," see http://www.imaging-famine.org, accessed May 2018; Michelle Bogre, *Photography as Activism: Images for Social Change* (New York: Focal, 2012), 47.

61. Margaret Kelleher, *The Feminization of Famine: Expressions of the Inexpressible?* (Durham, N.C.: Duke University Press, 1997); Saskia Sassen, "Women's Burden: Counter Geographies of Globalization and the Feminization of Survival," *Nordic Journal of International Law* 71, no. 2 (2002): 255–74.

62. Anne Orford, *Reading Humanitarian Intervention: Human Rights and the Use of Force in International Law* (Cambridge: Cambridge University Press, 2003), 165–66.

63. See Roland Bleiker and Amy Kay, "Representing HIV/AIDS in Africa: Pluralist

Photography and Local Empowerment," *International Studies Quarterly* 51, no. 1 (2007): 144–46.

64. On the hierarchical nature of humanitarian aid see, for example, Chioke I'Anson and Geoffrey Pfeifer, "A Critique of Humanitarian Reason: Agency, Power, and Privilege," *Journal of Global Ethics* 9, no. 1 (2013): 49–63; Antonio Donini, "The Far Side: The Meta Functions of Humanitarianism in a Globalised World," *Disasters* 34, supp. 2 (2010): 220–37; Sheila Nair, "Governance, Representation and International Aid," *Third World Quarterly* 34, no. 4 (2013): 630–52.

65. See also Boltanski, *Distant Suffering*; Chouliaraki, "Post-Humanitarianism," 110–12.

66. Lilie Chouliaraki, "The Theatricality of Humanitarianism: A Critique of Celebrity Advocacy," *Communication and Critical/Cultural Studies* 9, no. 1 (2012): 2; Keith Tester, *Humanitarianism and Modern Culture* (University Park: Pennsylvania State University Press, 2010).

67. See, for instance, Carolyn Pedwell, *Affective Relations: The Transnational Politics of Empathy* (Milton Park, U.K.: Palgrave Macmillan, 2014).

68. See Boddice, "Introduction: Hurt Feelings?," 1–15.

69. David Kennedy, *The Dark Side of Virtue: Reassessing International Humanitarianism* (Princeton, N.J.: Princeton University Press, 2004).

70. Lynn Festa, "Humanity Without Feathers," *Humanity: An International Journal of Human Rights* 1, no. 1 (2010): 4–5 and 16; Amit S. Rai, *Rule of Sympathy: Sentiment, Race, and Power 1750–1850* (New York: Palgrave, 2002), xiv–xv.

71. Michel Foucault, *Discipline and Punish: The Birth of the Prison*, trans. Alan Sheridan (New York: Vintage, 1995).

72. Labanyi, "Doing Things: Emotions, Affect, and Materiality," *Journal of Spanish Cultural Studies* 11, nos. 3 and 4 (2010): 223–33; Scheer, "Are Emotions a Kind of Practice?," 193–220.

73. Rosenwein, *Emotional Communities*, 18–19.

74. Ibid., 197.

11. Compassion Fatigue

The Changing Nature of Humanitarian Emotions

BERTRAND TAITHE

IT IS DIFFICULT to trace the first references to fatigue—emotional, moral, and physical—in the humanitarian context. Early humanitarians were concerned with the organized struggle against slavery or the defense of aboriginal people under threat of extermination, and they witnessed horrors and sufferings to an unbearable degree.[1] In their campaigns they represented very graphically the sufferings of their wards and appealed to emotional responses matching the disarray they confessed experiencing.[2] En-plotting sufferings through a humanitarian narrative proved indeed one of the surest ways of bringing readers to tears and of lighting a cause.[3] The translation of sufferings into a narrative was to make sense of the plights of often voiceless multitudes and to confirm their humanity because of their suffering as sentient beings.[4] In the humanitarian narratives sufferings differed from bodily pain because they referred to grieving and agonies of a moral nature as well as more physical and often incommunicable bodily agonies. To experience pain through the writings of a humanitarian was not within the remit of text; to share in suffering was. That distinction was often made, and the earliest humanitarian texts bring to the forefront the sufferings of the victims and also, by sympathy or because of their own exertion, that of their helpers.

Mental sufferings and over-exertions were always part of the humanitarian narrative and—from the late nineteenth century onward—so was the notion of fatigue. The notion of fatigue is closely related to other notions of bodily productivity and effort efficiency developed at the turn of the twentieth century.[5] While in many ways this notion has a precise physical and medical meaning, it also has a corresponding set of metaphorical meanings—all these interpretations have been part of the history of humanitarianism. They relate to the representation of bodily endeavor on behalf of humanity, and fatigue engages profoundly with the core issues at the heart of humanitarian work.

More controversially, this chapter argues that at every stage of its history, the concept of compassion fatigue, whether it intended to describe a physical bodily reality and clinical cases or was intended as a metaphor, served political and organizational purposes for humanitarians. In this sense compassion fatigue performed a key role in the debates on the nature of humanitarian work, its effect on humanitarians, their emotions and their bodies, in a manner this chapter roughly sketches. Responding to its challenge became a preoccupation of humanitarians and their organizations. Compassion fatigue in its various guises emerged in biographies, histories and self-narratives, reports on activities, and myriad other official and private writings.[6] In all these writings, compassion fatigue, as a concept, portrayed and evoked different things—allegedly from a purely descriptive standpoints—but it also performed specific roles. It explained and justified failure and alone could evoke the incommensurable emptiness left behind, after compassion. As a descriptor of emotions it performed a key role to explain or justify behavior, shape or condition responses to genuinely observable symptoms, or allow causes and consequences to be defined by embodied emotions.

Humanitarian history is not one of successive forms of the same emotional response to human sufferings but rather an aggregation of different forms of social and political responses to distant sufferings. Compassion fatigue relates to this history in the sense that it is evoked to explain the failings of humanitarians or of their supporters in face of insurmountable odds. Over a long period, humanitarianism developed greatly from short-term relief appeals, on the one hand, and long-standing organizations on the other. Some were extraordinarily successful but short lived—for instance, the famine and war relief appeals organized by Lord Sutherland's Stafford House Committee in the United Kingdom in the 1870s, which were often endorsed as the Lord Mayor funds.[7] With the exception of the Red Cross movement initiated in 1863 and operational from 1866 and 1870 onward,[8] most humanitarian work remained intimately linked to the world of charities, including hospitals and hospices, missionary dispensaries and schools, soup kitchens, and orphanages. The growth of voluntary organizations has been chartered incompletely, but the interwar period undoubtedly witnessed the growth of specific organizations such as Save the Children who sought to address children's sufferings at home and abroad.

The long Cold War, which we might say began with the Russian famine of 1921, was particularly favorable to the growth of voluntary organizations, which later became known as nongovernmental organizations, or NGOs.[9] This long period was the genesis of all the leading organizations known today and brought into frequent and rich interaction states and organizations, diplomats, and military personnel with volunteers and enthusiasts. Endlessly reinvented and reincarnated, the humanitarian sector nevertheless remains part of the same charity marketplace in which a famine in Niger competes for funds and public support with research in rare diseases.[10] Since 1989 humanitarian organizations have begun to understand themselves as a system—running alongside a renewed United Nations and its services. Paradoxically, this period of immense growth has also been the period during which states have taken the largest stakes in the financing and even policy shaping of the humanitarian world.[11] Ironically, even as the humanitarian system became increasingly disincarnated and some say dehumanized, compassion fatigue and burnout arose as the ultimately alienating forms of the humanitarians' overcommitment.

Widely understood and felt, perceptible in human encounters, compassion fatigue nevertheless seldom featured explicitly in policy or organizational structures until the 1980s at the earliest. In the 1980s and 1990s humanitarian NGOs then imported within their structures the concepts of debriefing and psychological support from the military in order to support staff and organizations.[12] Compassion fatigue affected both individuals in their bodies and organizations in their structures. It wasted people and causes alike. The deployment of psychiatric staff in humanitarian emergencies was intimately tied to settlements of refugees, with refugee camps inviting humanitarian organizations to support the psychological demands of their work and take care of refugees' mental health. Yet, insofar as it is possible to ascertain it exactly, psychiatric and psychological specialists were not deployed in the field until 1988 and the Armenian earthquake.[13] When humanitarians became more aware of psychiatric needs among their patients and "beneficiaries," they also engaged more profoundly with their own mental and physical exhaustion. The history of compassion fatigue is thus interweaving the sources produced around humanitarian aid, and the performativity of compassion fatigue—throughout myriad narratives—has also shaped humanitarian agencies as emotional bodies.

Part One: Humanitarian Excess

The origins of humanitarianism are complex and deeply rooted in religion, idealism, internationalism, and new philosophies of altruism of the early-nineteenth-century philosophy and sociology, with none of them accounting for all the complexities of the multitude of human endeavors to address sufferings. A narrower understanding of humanitarianism not as a philosophical or political worldview but as the descriptive category has been used to make sense of those who work in relief efforts for sufferers of disasters, wars, displacement, and violence in all its manifestations. To ameliorate the fate of individuals usually entails the transfer and distribution of goods, money, resources, and support. Compassion or solidarity is often raised as the explanation for the process that leads some individuals to act when others turn away. The emotional dimension of humanitarianism is therefore central to its identity, but this emotion is profoundly encoded culturally.

The classicist David Konstan, for instance, argues that pity was produced by a "cognitive assessment" that had to override repulsion or the fear of misfortune.[14] The Christian theme of compassion and sympathy (the act of feeling *about* another person) became a central theme in eighteenth-century philosophy.[15] Not to express or experience sympathy and pity would signal a nonhuman predisposition and would challenge morality. Yet too much sympathy would also denote a form of pathology revealing the inability to measure what one can and cannot do, a form of self-centered wallowing in grief.[16] The psychological work that had ensued from Charles Darwin's 1872 *Expression of the Emotions in Man and Animals* defined the boundaries of normal and abnormal sympathy.

Though related, pity and compassion are not synonymous. Cultural historians have argued that a shift toward the freer portrayal of emotions became a central dimension of a textual and visual sensibility that made the bed of the growth of humanitarian compassion.[17] Texts, cultural historians have argued, enable us to do more than chart the appearance of terms of compassion; they became, according to them, the central mechanism through which compassion might appear and act as a moral imperative. Thomas Laqueur argued thus that literature detailing narratives of suffering constituted the heart of "the humanitarian narrative" of the late Enlightenment. Beyond sympathy, empathy (feeling *with* another person) would have transformed these narratives into manifestos, eliding political and social responses among the readers.[18] There is strong evidence that humanitarian texts multiplied and diversified and that, soon, they were joined by complementary visual narratives that induced further emotional responses. These new texts developed, if not invented, new forms of affect invested with moral responsibilities. New feelings entailed new actions and new gestures—physical responses as well as new social engagements. The humanitarian narrative was one widely shared across the full spectrum of charitable works. While historians have tended to separate missionary work abroad from conversion work at home, charity work in the urban centers from humanitarian relief work, this distinction would not have made any sense to Victorian volunteers or the public, which supported indiscriminately small and large organizations according to their affective responses. The development of the press in the 1840s and 1850s and of visual material from photographs in the 1870s and 1880s facilitated the representation of sufferings worldwide and the matching calls for relief.

The main beneficiaries of this "media" boom were not merely new organizations such as the Red Cross but also old or even ancient enterprises such as the missionaries who experienced a revival in the late nineteenth-century. Missionaries developed their own print media and were considerably involved in the denunciation of colonial atrocities and local forms of savagery. They initiated some of the most effective association of photography and humanitarian work, defining an affective vocabulary that still has much currency today.[19] Nevertheless, there were differences. By the 1870s the words *humanitarian* and *humanitarianism* had a variety of meanings, some legal, some related to idealism.[20] In Britain and France these were largely negative terms and signaled a propensity toward a sentimentalist and ineffectual approach to suffering,[21] at odds with rational charity. Within the charitable world there had been a campaign toward an unsentimental, efficient management of human and financial resources that would redefine compassion away from unbridled excesses. Those who intended to respond to extremes of sufferings inflicted by wars, from Florence Nightingale to Henry Dunant, proposed a compassionate rationality that would direct resources and people where they would be most needed following the iron rules of medical and bureaucratic triage.[22]

Many of these calls and directives toward more professional and rational management were in response to a great danger humanitarians had either witnessed or imagined. This danger entailed the risk to the self-compassionate work. Dunant described the frantic and ultimately pointless efforts of his associates answering spontaneously, but in a disordered crowd, the needs of wounded soldiers scattered on the battlefield of Solferino. Nightingale criticized the neglect and systemic violence that discouraged and undermanaged medical relief work entailed. Both challenged the manner in which individuals might engage in humanitarian work if led by their affect alone rather than their expertise and training.[23]

There is a blatant paradox in these early dogmatic theoreticians of humanitarian work when they rejected the more spontaneous, yet more "authentic" forms of volunteering, in favor of more systematic approaches leaving little to the expression of character. This tension between volunteering and professionalizing humanitarian work remains at the heart of humanitarianism since its origins because it is dynamic and productive: volunteerism and the affective responses are necessary to the vitality and growth of institutions that then embody this urge in the shape of a bureaucracy. Yet volunteers have always had a stake in differentiating themselves from amateurs. Early humanitarians were keen to highlight their own courage and perseverance in stark contrast with the fumbling efforts of amateurs or the cowardice of often locally recruited staff: doctors working under Russian fire, berated the flight of most of their Ottoman staff; Dunant feared for the mental health of some of his Solferino collaborators or mocked the cowardice of his coach driver.[24] Missionaries had presented their own endeavor to face insurmountable odds in eschatological terms and with the full acceptance of sacrifice and martyrdom. More secular approaches to humanitarian work shied away from stating explicitly this reliance on god or providence but raised similarly messianic expectations.[25]

Humanitarians had to face danger and risk and occasionally celebrate the ultimate sacrifice of some of their co-workers,[26] but the efficient delivery of their task required the scientific management of their effort and the avoidance of overexertion. Fatigue in this early humanitarian context represented the waste of effort or the inability to face the reality of extremes of suffering. The sometimes counterintuitive modes of triage among sufferers offered the possibility to rationalize work in such a manner as to deliver the most effective succor. This triage logic implied a reining in of emotions and a profound subversion of its mechanics of horror. The most gravely wounded might not make it to the operating table—the dying might have to be given only palliative care.

This meant neglecting the more pitiful sights in favor of those who might benefit the most from care; it meant excluding entire categories of pain. In charitable work in the United Kingdom this meant turning away from the morally deficient toward more innocent or hopeful cases. Focusing relief on children rather than old alcoholics was a rational application of this approach.[27] Few would challenge the rationale of scientific relief work proposed by clearing house organizations like the Charity Organization Society or the Guild of Help.[28] Causes with less appealing subjects—venereal disease victims or sick prostitutes, for instance—experienced the reluctance of the public to hear their plea for help.[29]

In a competitive fundraising environment, the constant concern was that charity occupied a specific and limited financial space in family budgets. Money spent on the *Titanic* disaster victims might cost London hospital dearly in 1912; the Bengal famine might damage the fundraising efforts of local Manchester orphanages. The metaphor of fatigue applied to a heavily pressured public constantly solicited for additional support and exposed to competing causes. The exhaustion of charity was a fiction in the late Victorian era. While historians of the gift tend to agree that families spent a reasonably stable portion of their income for various favorite or more spontaneous causes,[30] the financial basis of giving expanded with the economy and fundraisers constantly rose to the challenge by developing new and exciting methods of fundraising. Many of these methods took physical pleasures as a medium to convince the public to contribute to causes: consuming bazaars, spectacles and shows, music concerts, and sporting events all in the name of humanity enabled the public to share in the demands of compassion while enjoying themselves or advancing their own networks.[31]

Humanitarian narratives participated in this culture of sharing and mediated participation. The books and narratives slotted neatly in the travel literature of the era and often made similar references to adventures and excitement. Where these narratives engaged with physical and moral demands it was to emphasize how character and discipline enabled humanitarians to transcend the difficulties of their exhausting endeavor. Fatigue was the domain of the weak and rudderless when it came to the delivery of aid. It was a plausible excuse for failed fundraising, but it remained unwarranted in facts when the whole voluntary sector was concerned. At both levels, fatigue served a metaphorical purpose in contrast with the new energy unleashed on the sufferings of the world by Victorian and Edwardian humanitarians. Being a humanitarian, like Vincent Kennett Barrington, a gentleman, sportsman, and administrator of major humanitarian campaigns in the 1870s, was to be the embodiment of an ideal in which emotions drove a finely tuned body through work which would destroy a lesser human being.[32] The indefatigable humanitarian of this high Victorian period was not necessarily masculine, but humanitarianism could combine virility and affect to redefine how emotions might drive men through the twin perils of discouragement and physical exhaustion.

Part Two: The Caregiver Fatigued

Nevertheless, observations of the exhaustion of the caregivers did not disappear and could not be transcended by mere efforts of the will. In the 1940s the notion of compassion fatigue, in the sense of the exhaustion of the compassionate helpers, was reinterpreted as a psychiatric category in its own right. As a psychiatric disorder the term was coined in the 1940s for the excessive exertions of overly charitable hospital workers. The classic early cases referred to the sufferings of nurses who, incapable of leaving their patients' side, had to be restrained for their own sake and medically treated.[33] Wartime psychiatric reports, which have dwelled longest on the idea of compassion fatigue in the immediate aftermath of major battles of World War II, identified this exhaustion still in the continuation of character failings, as the opposite of leadership—affecting men and women in positions of responsibility—accountable for the suffering of their subordinates; these individuals collapsed in a heap of self-pity caused by the great pity they had for others. In this utterance the body blow of compassion is genuinely one that—like an emotional shell shock—blurs the boundaries between self and environment—their body was overwhelmed by surrounding sufferings. The relationship between compassionate trauma and trauma became a central explanatory pattern for compassion fatigue.[34]

The notion of secondary stress disorder[35]—the imprint of someone else's stress through compassion as defined more recently in the work of Charles Figley[36]—is not therefore some new or the fanciful extension of the concept of stress disorder[37] but stands as a new configuration of the compassionate overexertion Dunant described. In itself it is an essential component of humanitarian compassion—it represents its share of danger and it defines the boundaries of self-denial in humanitarian situations.

Much of the pressure of this caregiver fatigue coming from within the medical literature advocated greater discipline and strong monitoring of the staff's mental health. This notion fed from the analysis of trauma among war patients, on the one hand, and from the realization that it might be, on the other hand, a case of "secondary traumatic stress disorder," the contagious effects of sufferings on those who seek to assist.[38] Compassion fatigue as secondary trauma was clinically demonstrated from the 1950s in the United States and was observed in a multitude of locations. While the Victorian discourse on character no longer sufficed to explain away the failing of otherwise exceptionally professional staff, organizational explanations were put forward to understand why some individuals became more sensitive than others to the sufferings of their patients.[39] Paradoxically, this approach also emphasized the responsibility of the employer when, in the humanitarian context, the terms of employment were often muddled by constant references to the spirit of volunteering.

Herbert Freudenberger described burnout itself in his 1974 study of aid volunteers working on the delivery of healthcare in cases of extreme social deprivation.[40] The differentiation between volunteer and mercenary work relied here on notions of commitment rather than expertise—expertise, training, or professionalism were not under scrutiny. The effects of excessive affective commitment were burnout. Burnout was defined as "emotional exhaustion, a process of depersonalisation and reduced productivity" affecting primarily volunteers and social and healthcare workers.[41] Some went as far as to argue that these workers developed their work as an "obsessive passion" that made them more prone to the phenomenon of burnout (particularly when associated with the circumstances of expatriate humanitarian life and its poor hygiene).[42] The exclusive embodiment of one passion and one emotion at the expense of a more balanced range of affects was becoming the Achilles' heel of organizations running on enthusiasm and emotion.[43]

Despite its origins, the adoption of the concept of burnout in the humanitarian sector was gradual at an institutional level.[44] Humanitarian agencies and organizations reluctantly came to the realization that they owed their staff the same duty of care as workers in hospitals and medical structures.[45] Unlike earlier character failings of individuals, burnouts were deemed the stuff of bad human resource management (itself an innovation in voluntary organizations of the 1990s) or indeed due to the absence of psychological support.[46] This definition of fatigue hollowed out the human factor in intense humanitarian work[47] and privileged instead the organizational menace burnout represented for any organizations.[48]

When in the 1980s the demands of psychiatric help for refugees was raised as a new humanitarian mandate, it fed from new research on trauma and in particular the idea of a posttraumatic stress disorder condition which might affect entire populations of refugees and also, albeit indirectly, their helpers.[49] Humanitarian debriefings from fieldwork were documented unevenly in different organizations in the 1980s, despite clear signs that some staff suffered considerably in the strenuous circumstances of underresourced humanitarian work. Debriefing became more generalized throughout the 1990s and the symptoms of "burnout" were defined clearly to describe fatigued individuals.

Yet compassion fatigue could refer to a range of other practices that would not allow brushing away individual responsibilities and allowed a more negative focus on the humanitarians themselves. Despite attempts to clearly separate burnout (a cumulative overwork pressure on affect that could be solved by rest or new employment) and compassion fatigue by assimilation to the suffering of others (and excess of compassion leading to mimetic suffering and secondary traumatic stress),[50] the term came to be employed to explain a range of bad practices, particularly in healthcare facilities under duress. From the 1980s onward, compassion fatigue became the explanation for poor medical behavior and inuring to the pain of others. In particular, scandals in mismanaged structures that put more emphasis on targets and speediness of treatment were blamed on a culture of callousness brought about by compassion fatigue. Through the acceptance of triage logic based on financial considerations, it was feared, the care worker might experience a form a detachment that would turn the calculation and its cold logic into the expression of humanitarian aid. This excessive detachment and its calm but hurried and ultimately indifferent distribution of relief then, in turns, would negate compassion, and, authors argue, lend itself to shortcuts, further economies of scale, and "bad practice." The quasi-psychotic detachment of this form of compassion fatigue meant that sufferers remained functional. Unlike the apathetic and detached, the exhausted or exalted, or even the unhinged sufferers of compassion fatigue, the staffs alienated by compassion fatigue brought about in this modernist environment were accused of keeping their neglect almost invisible to the sight of observers. Yet their profound subversion of humanitarian values was, it was alleged, a more radical and dangerous challenge to humanitarian work.

This third meaning of compassion fatigue, more common in the press[51] than in scientific literature, is particularly salient in negative reporting of large and dysfunctional medical structures such as elements of the British National Health Service. In this particular context compassion fatigue and burnout refer to the collapse of compassion itself—not the collapse of the compassionate body, but a purely psychological collapse of his or her ability to empathize meaningfully with people in their care.[52]

Since the 1860s at least, the entire economy of empathy on which humanitarian work relied has been represented in crude terms: volunteers exuding a limited amount of compassion might eventually fall prey to their own empathy and become patients in turn. The shift in the late twentieth century toward a fully clinical diagnosis (as opposed to the denunciation of behavioral aberrations) has shifted emphasis from individuals to organizations precisely at a time when NGOs developed the human resources and concerns of large international organizations. These concerns included duty of care concerns that, while present in law since the late nineteenth century for most employers, were widely ignored in the voluntary sector. Compassion fatigue in its different guises put the priority clearly on reforming institutional structures and on reinforcing control mechanisms around volunteers and employees. It is unclear, however, if these shifts reflected the growth of institutional structures or merely encouraged them.

A wider concern with the status of victim across society in a postheroic age—as Fassin and Rechtman argued—might cut across many other activities and social roles beyond humanitarian work. Yet the fact that burnout was primarily identified in the 1970s as a specificity of the overexerted volunteers and that so much of the psychological literature of the 1990s and 2000s has been devoted to humanitarian workers, reveals a more profound association between humanitarian workers and these now organizational concepts of compassion fatigue and burnout.

Part Three: The Exhaustion of Giving

If burnout gradually acquired a fundamental place in the management of staff, its equivalent and predecessor, compassion fatigue, became more commonly metaphorical, and the bodies it referred to were social bodies rather than individuals dispensing care. Equally dangerous from the point of view of humanitarian aid construed as the distribution of goods and relief would be the exhaustion of sympathy converted in resounding cash. Monetarist logic has long permeated the humanitarian sector's understanding of its finances. It is common to read that each charity or disaster-fund relief competes for the limited resources of the giving public. The history of the gift, like its anthropology, challenges this logic, which, if it can be proved right at a micro level—some fundraising will fail and some needs remain unanswered—is demonstrably contradicted overall by the public's ability to reinvent giving on a different scale according to the circumstances. Yet compassion fatigue has often been waved as an excuse by fundraisers competing in a brutal marketplace.[53] Like much of the rest of the capitalist market economy, the charity market is both an imagined world of expansive consumption—susceptible to be expanded by the invention of new needs, forms, and social interaction (for instance, social media or mobile phones)—and a fiercely competitive one in which products might find themselves suddenly obsolete.

Yet its communication techniques are unlike those of most products sold on the basis of aspiration and desire. At a superficial level humanitarian selling techniques bear witness to the same process of secondary stress—in which the victims of suffering are simultaneously pitiable and abject. This troubled desirability of abjection arose simultaneously in the new humanitarian campaigns of the late nineteenth century when Mgr. Lavigerie, archbishop of Algiers, sought funds for the malnourished orphans of the great Algerian famine by emphasizing their readiness to feed themselves with excrements and even corpses.[54] Similar tropes of abjection and exploitation whereby the object of charity was simultaneously repulsive and corrupted and a helpless victim, were regularly deployed in Western Europe for the converted sinner or the fallen.[55] Much like pornography might induce indifferent and perverted social and sexual encounters—the pornography of pain, Karen Halttunen argued,[56] might by the sheer accumulation of images (and the focus here is on images rather than text in the late twentieth and twenty-first centuries) turn off or, if not repulse, *bore* a public unable to appreciate the difference between hyper-real violence (the games or the films) and documented atrocities.

From the 1970s onward, followers of Susan Sontag have argued that humanitarians have gradually inured the wider public to the horrors of the world. Luc Boltanski in the early 1990s and Susan Moeller in the late 1990s developed the arguments of the critique.[57] Sontag argued (though she later recanted some of these views) that images of pain belonged to a pornographic register that gradually eroded their truth.[58] Sontag pointed out the performative affect that exposure to repetitive and reiterative images of sufferings might entail. Historians of humanitarian photography have more recently echoed this point.[59] Thus, they point out, images of Biafra echoed those of Congo and emaciated children of previous wars and conflicts. While some have argued that this repetitive imagery erodes the significance or the human reality of what is represented, their repetition owes primarily to their perceived effectiveness in humanitarian fundraising campaigns.[60] That images from the Biafra war are now widely known to have been thoroughly instrumentalized by a cynical regime desperate for public support and international recognition, does not affect their role in stimulating new organizations (such as Concern in Ireland)[61] and significant public support.[62] That support did not materialisze into the political support the Biafrans were looking for, but it stimulated profoundly the European humanitarian market. Arguably, these images contributed to what Paulmann defines as a humanitarian conjuncture during which new and old forms of humanitarian work become reinvigorated.[63]

From the 1970s response to famine in Bangladesh to Band Aid, analysts of humanitarian communication have focused on two allegedly new phenomena: the role of celebrities as mediators for emotions in the face of horror[64] and more graphic representations of horror. The specialist of British journalism Susan Franks in particular argued for the significance of the reporting of the 1984 Ethiopian famine and defined it as a turning point;[65] others have focused on the media and entertainment mediation which Band Aid represented.[66]

Far from representing a case of compassion fatigue, these episodes were the apex of successful media campaigns making use of television to bring home distant sufferings and the plight of those attempting to alleviate them. It is significant that in his famous BBC reporting Michael Buerk asked an exhausted nutrition nurse how she felt—much to her surprise, as she confessed in a later program.[67] The journalist needed to find a "human interest," a woman able to convey her personal emotional response in the middle of a major humanitarian crisis precisely because the crisis was so significantly beyond comprehension.[68] In this the journalist followed well-established rhetorical devices employed by charities and humanitarians since the late nineteenth century by bringing to the forefront a singular object of compassion, a focal point of affect onto which spectators might focus rather than experience discouragement in the face of overwhelming sufferings.[69] The television media was itself not new to affective displays, and medical charities had long used the telethon to increase awareness and raise funds for difficult causes. The original telethon dated from the early days of mass television in North America (1949) and was exported gradually around the world, reaching France in the 1980s and growing to cover a wider range of issues and fundraising campaigns.[70] The format of the telethon combined heartfelt appeals, reportage, and entertainment over a long period of continuous broadcast and lent itself to specific fundraising events such as disaster relief appeals.[71] This use of television built on innovative practices by humanitarian organizations from the 1950s and 1960s. In particular, World Vision proved a pioneer of humanitarian communication and advertising on television.[72]

While one could seriously revise the claims to innovation that these television practices entailed—many of the forms it took were building on media work from the late Victorian and interwar periods—there was undoubtedly a new scale of theatrical performances at the heart of their spectacle. The systematic recourse to celebrity mediators whose role was to experience "genuine" emotions on behalf of the spectators enabled new embodiments of compassion.[73] Celebrities' responses associated the spectators in their feelings and were meant to induce an outpouring of spontaneous generosity. Beyond the spectacle of recipients and beneficiaries of the charity, the spectators would be able to watch their alter ego, onstage, enacting for them their own emotions.

Though these methods were overwhelmingly successful at raising funds for a variety of causes such as forgotten diseases or crises, they have also suffered from the demands they make on media programming, and their edge has been dulled over the years by sheer repetitiveness. They became seasonal events. Over the same period, brutal images, such as the iconic picture taken by the south African photographer Kevin Carter of a starving child and a rotund vulture, brought into question the ethics of representations of suffering.[74] The 1990s academic critique of humanitarian communication strategies (which John Taylor and Susan Moeller argued, for example) alleged that the public would be increasingly repelled by images of suffering due to their repetitive horror. At ethical and practical levels, critiques of the

1990s challenged the effectiveness of communication strategies based on crude images of suffering. Humanitarian agencies responded to these largely unsubstantiated claims by developing more sophisticated ethical stances on what was permissible and not permissible in terms of visual communication. Yet even scant examination shows that their marketing departments continued to use stock imagery, which still fit in a long tradition going back to the Indian famines of the late nineteenth century.

The critical reprobation of compassionate imagery raised the specter of compassion fatigue, but marketing specialists denied its reality in practice. Meanwhile the media continues to employ very similar images to raise awareness, resurrecting periodically a compassionate body from its shallow grave. Far from being the tool of communication for humanitarians, the media produced and managed the greatest fundraising campaigns of the early 2000s. The most salient example was, of course, the Tsunami fundraising campaign of 2006, criticized by some humanitarians such as *Médecins Sans Frontières* (MSF) for failing to recognize that the raised funds exceeded needs at a time when food crises in Africa failed to bring in significant amounts.[75]

Ironically, the most vehement critiques were also some of the most proficient communicators of sufferings. From the 1980s onward some NGOs imported American techniques of direct fundraising; MSF, for instance, managed to increase year after year the proportion of income directly raised from the public. In contrast, the humanitarian sector in general has tended to increase its dependence on state donors—such as USAID or ECHO, acting for the United States or the European Union, and SIDA or DFID for the Swedish and British governments. The massive increase of funding of the humanitarian sector disguised its increased reliance on nonvoluntary funding and on its alignment with political and foreign policy objectives devoid of emotional content.[76]

Taking institutional money could remove the need to make passionate and compromising calls to emotions. In this sense, compassion fatigue served a critical purpose in the sense that it enabled some humanitarians to reconsider their own tradition of representation and facilitated some distancing from media coverage—yet it did not affect the baseline. There is a paradox, therefore, in this growing concern for public opinion and feelings toward sufferings when most humanitarian organizations chose to grow their institutional fundraising away from the public. This type of fundraising based on tenders and bid processes is radically opposed to emotional responses and further distances the emotional dynamic of organizations from that of their volunteers and employees.

Conclusion

This chapter argues that compassion fatigue has haunted the humanitarian enterprise since its inception and that it has served a multitude of purposes when it has been evoked by humanitarians and their critiques. The compassion fatigue of bumbling amateurs enabled the early organizers of international humanitarian aid to reinforce their calls for the professionalization and systematization of aid. This drive toward a more effective and affectively restrained humanitarianism has become a leitmotif of the humanitarian sector from Florence Nightingale until the Sphere Project's attempt to define global standards, launched in 1997.[77] Compassion fatigue and burnout has, nevertheless, continued to be the plight of humanitarian staff. It is only since the 1970s that this concern has made more urgent the need for humanitarian organizations to consider their responsibilities and manage their staff.

The final and more vulgar interpretation of compassion fatigue is related to two key aspects of humanitarian communication and self-imagining: its ethics of communication and its ability to raise funds.[78] There is no evidence over recent years that humanitarians have suffered financially from their overcrowded marketplace and from the saturation of pornographic images of pain. Evoking compassion fatigue seems to have justified seeking funding from other sources than the public and shifting volunteer organizations toward becoming the willing orderlies of the state. Thus the extraordinary blossoming of humanitarian organizations in the 1990s and early 2000s seldom relied on public fundraising.[79] The first definition of compassion fatigue served the logic of cold compassion and the urge to develop solidarity in an organized and bureaucratic form, while the second, its mirror opposite at first sight, explained away the poor practices that bureaucratic order might create and the pathologization not only of the world in which care workers exhaust themselves but also the pathologization of themselves. Finally, the vulgar understanding of compassion fatigue serves as memento mori for the humanitarian dream.

Notes

1. Amalia Ribi Forclaz, *Humanitarian Imperialism: The Politics of Anti-Slavery Activism, 1880–1940* (Oxford: Oxford University Press, 2015); Alan Lester and Fae Dussart, *Colonization and the Origins of Humanitarian Governance: Protecting Aborigines across the Nineteenth-Century British Empire* (Cambridge: Cambridge University Press, 2014).

2. Karen Halttunen, "Humanitarianism and the Pornography of Pain in Anglo-American Culture," *American Historical Review* 100, no. 2 (1995): 303–34; Mar-

ianne Noble, "The Ecstasies of Sentimental Wounding in Uncle Tom's Cabin," *Yale Journal of Criticism* 10, no. 2 (1997): 295–320.

3. Karen Halttunen, "Humanitarianism," 303–34.

4. Roselyne Rey, *The History of Pain* (Cambridge, Mass.: Harvard University Press, 1995); Fay Bound Alberti, ed., *Medicine, Emotion and Disease, 1700–1950* (Basingstoke: Palgrave Macmillan, 2006).

5. See Anson Rabinbach, *The Human Motor: Energy, Fatigue and the Origins of Modernity* (Oakland: University of California Press, 1990), and more recently Steffan Blayney, "Industrial Fatigue and the Productive Body: The Science of Work in Britain, c. 1900–1918," *Social History of Medicine*, https://doi.org/10.1093/shm/hkx077.

6. Jo Labanyi, "Doing Things: Emotion, Affect and Materiality," *Journal of Spanish Cultural Studies* 11, no. 3–4 (2010): 223–33.

7. In Britain the Lord Mayor or Mansion House funds were sponsored by the City of London Mayor but were not genuinely organized by Mansion House. For a full exploration of the elite and demotic forms of fundraising in Victorian England, see Sarah Roddy, Julie-Marie Strange and Bertrand Taithe, *The Charity Market and Humanitarianism in Britain, 1870–1912* (London: Bloomsbury, 2018); Sarah Roddy, Julie-Marie Strange, and Bertrand Taithe, "Humanitarian Legitimacy, Fraud and Self-Regulation: A Tale from the Archives?" *Disasters* 39, no. 3 (2015): 188–203.

8. Caroline Moorehead, *Dunant's Dream: War, Switzerland and the History of the Red Cross* (London: HarperCollins, 1998); Bertrand Taithe, *Defeated Flesh: Welfare, Warfare and the Making of Modern France* (Manchester: Manchester University Press, 1999).

9. Johannes Paulmann, "Conjunctures in the History of International Humanitarian Aid during the Twentieth Century," *Humanity: An International Journal of Human Rights, Humanitarianism, and Development* 4, no. 2 (2013): 215–38; Michael Barnett, *Empire of Humanity: A History of Humanitarianism* (Ithaca, N.Y.: Cornell University Press, 2011).

10. David Jefferess, "Humanitarian Relations: Emotion and the Limits of Critique," *Critical Literacy: Theories and Practices* 7, no. 1 (2013): 73–83; Gorm Rye Olsen, Nils Carstensen, and Kristian Høyen, "Humanitarian Crises: What Determines the Level of Emergency Assistance? Media Coverage, Donor Interests and the Aid Business," *Disasters* 27, no. 2 (2003): 109–26.

11. ALNAP, "The State of the Humanitarian System," accessed, April, 22, 2016, http://www.alnap.org/what-we-do/effectiveness/sohs

12. Louis Crocq, "Histoire du Debriefing," *Pratiques Psychologiques* 10, no. 4 (2004): 291–318.

13. Robert Henley, Randall Marshall, and Stefan Vetter, "Integrating Mental Health Services into Humanitarian Relief Responses to Social Emergencies, Disasters, and Conflicts: A Case Study," *Journal of Behavioural Health Services and Research* 38, no. 1 (2011): 132–41.

14. David Konstan, *Pity Transformed* (London: Duckworth, 2001), 12.

15. Norman S. Fiering, "Irresistible Compassion: An Aspect of Eighteenth-Century

Sympathy and Humanitarianism," *Journal of the History of Ideas* 37, no. 2 (1976): 195–218.

16. Konstan, *Pity Transformed*, 22–23.

17. Thomas Laqueur, "Bodies, Details and the Humanitarian Narrative," in *The New Cultural History*, ed. Lynn Hunt (Berkeley: University of California Press, 1989), 176–204; Carolyn Taylor, "Humanitarian Narrative: Bodies and Detail in Late-Victorian Social Work," *British Journal of Social Work* 38, no. 4 (2008): 680–96.

18. Richard Ashby Wilson and Richard D. Brown, *Humanitarianism and Suffering: The Mobilization of Empathy* (Cambridge: Cambridge University Press, 2009); Anne-Claude Ambroise-Rendu, and Christian Delporte, *L'indignation: Histoire d'une émotion, XIXe-XXe siècle* (Paris: Nouveau Monde, 2008).

19. Kevin Grant, "The Limits of Exposure: Atrocity Photograph in the Congo Reform Campaign," in *Humanitarian Photography: A History*, eds. Heide Fehrenbach and Davide Rodogno (Cambridge: Cambridge University Press, 2015), 64–88; Dean Pavlakis, *British Humanitarianism and the Congo Reform Movement, 1896–1913* (Farnham, U.K.: Ashgate, 2015); Christina Twomey, "Framing Atrocity: Photography and Humanitarianism," *History of Photography* 36, no. 3 (2012): 255–64.

20. Fritz-Joachim von Rintelen and Herbert W. Schneider, "Positivism, Humanitarianism, and Humanity," *Philosophy and Phenomenological Research* 11, no. 3 (1951): 413–17.

21. Frank T. Carlton, "Humanitarianism, Past and Present," *International Journal of Ethics* 17, no. 1 (1906): 48–55.

22. Guillaume Lachenal, Céline Lefève, and Vinh-Kim Nguyen, eds., *La Médecine du Tri: Histoire, éthique, anthropologie* (Paris: PUF, 2014).

23. Charles E. Rosenberg, "Florence Nightingale on Contagion: The Hospital as Moral Universe," in *Healing and History*, ed. Charles E. Rosenberg (New York: Science History, 1979), 116–36; Sandra Holton, "Feminine Authority and Social Order: Florence Nightingale's Conception of Nursing and Health Care," *Social Analysis* 15 (1984): 59–72.

24. Henry Dunant, *A Memory of Solferino* (Geneva: ICRC, 2016), 64–65 and 80.

25. Bertrand Taithe, "Mourir pour des idées humanitaires: Sacrifice, témoignage et travail humanitaire 1870–1990," in *Mourir pour des Idées*, ed. Caroline Cazanave (Besançon: PUB, 2008), 239–54.

26. The cult of sacrifice among humanitarians remains nevertheless and arguably has experienced a revival since the 1990s. The case of Sergio Vieira de Mello was a recent exemplar of this revival. Samantha Power, *Chasing the Flame: Sergio Vieira de Mello and the Fight to Save the World* (London: Penguin, 2008).

27. Bertrand Taithe, Julie-Marie Strange, Sarah Roddy, "The Charity-Mongers of Modern Babylon: Bureaucracy, Scandal, and the Transformation of the Philanthropic Marketplace, c. 1870–1912," *Journal of British Studies* 54, no. 1, (2015): 118–37.

28. Brian Harrison, "Philanthropy and the Victorians," *Victorian Studies* 9, no. 4 (1966): 353–74; Charles Mowat, *The Charity Organisation Society, 1869–1913: Its Ideas and Work* (London: Taylor and Francis, 1961); Francis Michael Longstreth Thomp-

son, "Social Control in Victorian Britain," *Economic History Review* 34, no. 2 (1981): 189–208; Keith Laybourn, *The Guild of Help and the Changing face of Edwardian Philanthropy: The Guild of Help, Voluntary Work and the State, 1904–1919* (Lewiston, N.Y.: Mellen, 1994).

29. Bertrand Taithe, "Consuming Desires: Prostitutes and Customers at the Margins of Crime and Perversion in France and Britain, c. 1836–1885," in *Gender and Crime*, ed. M. Arnott and C. Osborne (London: UCL University Press), 151–72.

30. Jean-Luc Marais, *Histoire du Don en France de 1800 à 1939: Dons et legs charitables, pieux et philanthropiques* (Rennes: Presses universitaires de Rennes, 2015).

31. Peter Gurney, "'The Sublime of the Bazaar': A Moment in the Making of a Consumer Culture in Mid-Nineteenth Century England," *Journal of Social History* 40, no. 2 (2007): 385–405.

32. Kennett Barrington allegedly died of saving a woman in a balloon crash after a long humanitarian career. Sir Vincent Kennett-Barrington, *The Times*, July, 14, 1903, 11; Peter Morris, *First Aid to the Battle Front: Life and Letters of Sir Vincent Kennett-Barrington (1844–1903)* (Stroud, U.K.: Alan Sutton, 1992).

33. Ian Stevenson, "The Nurse and Her Patient in Long-Term Cases," *American Journal of Nursing* 54, no. 12 (1954): 1462–64.

34. Frank P. Lamendola, "Keeping Your Compassion Alive," *American Journal of Nursing* 96, no. 11 (November 1996): 16R+16T; Charles R Figley, ed., *Compassion Fatigue: Coping with Secondary Traumatic Stress Disorder in Those Who Treat the Traumatized* (New York: Routledge, 1995), 23; Emanuel Miller, "Psychiatric Casualties: Among Officers and Men from Normandy Distribution of Aetiological Factors," *The Lancet* 245, no. 6343 (1945): 364–66.

35. On stress, see the work of Mark Jackson, *The Age of Stress: Science and the Search for Stability* (Oxford: Oxford University Press, 2013).

36. Charles R. Figley, *Trauma and Its Wake* (London: Routledge, 2013), vol. 1; Charles R. Figley, "Compassion Fatigue: Psychotherapists' Chronic Lack of Self Care," *Journal of Clinical Psychology* 58, no. 11 (2002): 1433–41; Charles R. Figley, ed., *Treating Compassion Fatigue* (London: Routledge, 2002).

37. Didier Fassin and Richard Rechtman, *L'Empire du traumatisme: Enquête sur la condition de victime* (Paris: Flammarion, 2010).

38. S. Proust, "Prévenir l'épuisement professionnel par la mobilisation des ressources psychosociales: L'organisation du travail dans son rôle potentiellement bienveillant," *Psycho-Oncologie* 9, no. 2 (2015): 69–75.

39. Philippe Zawieja, "Fatigue compassionnelle," *Dictionnaire des risques Psychosociaux* (Paris: Le Seuil, 2014), 316–19 ; Carlton D. Craig, and Ginny Sprang, "Compassion Satisfaction, Compassion Fatigue, and Burnout in a National Sample of Trauma Treatment Therapists," *Anxiety, Stress, and Coping* 23, no. 3 (2010): 319–39.

40. Herbert J. Freudenberger, "Staff Burn Out," *Journal of Social Issues* 30, 1 (1974): 159–65.

41. Alfried Längle, "Burnout: Existential Meaning and Possibilities of Prevention," *European Psychotherapy* 4, no. 1 (2003): 107–21, 108; María Luisa Vecina Jiménez and

Fernando Chacón Fuentes, "Motivation and Burnout in Volunteerism," *Psychology in Spain* 4 (2000): 75–81.

42. Natasha Tassell and Ross Flett, "Obsessive Passion as an Explanation for Burnout: An Alternative Theoretical Perspective Applied to Humanitarian Work," *Australian Journal of Rehabilitation Counselling* 13, no. 2 (2007): 106.

43. Matthew J. Hoffarth, "The Making of Burnout: From Social Change to Self-Awareness in the Postwar United States," *History of the Human Sciences* 5 (2017): 30–45. Hoffarth argues that the diagnostic of burnout put the emphasis solely on the employee and turned away from the broader politics of social change. This is not completely accurate in relation to voluntary organisation and their rising doubts on the "resilience" of their processes.

44. Joan L. Arches, "Burnout and Social Action," *Journal of Progressive Human Services* 8, no. 2 (1997): 51–62.

45. John H. Ehrenreich and Teri L. Elliott, "Managing Stress in Humanitarian Aid Workers: A Survey of Humanitarian Aid Agencies' Psychosocial Training and Support of Staff," *Peace and Conflict: Journal of Peace Psychology* 10, no. 1 (2004): 53; Mark A. Stebnicki, "Stress and Grief Reactions among Rehabilitation Professionals: Dealing Effectively with Empathy Fatigue," *Journal of Rehabilitation* 66, no. 1 (2000): 23.

46. Cynthia B. Eriksson, Jeff P. Bjorck, Linnea C. Larson, Sherry M. Walling, Gary A. Trice, John Fawcett, Alexis D. Abernethy, and David W. Foy, "Social Support, Organisational Support, and Religious Support in Relation to Burnout in Expatriate Humanitarian Aid Workers," *Mental Health, Religion and Culture* 12, no. 7 (2009): 671–86; Barbara Lopes Cardozo, Carol Gotway Crawford, Cynthia Eriksson, Julia Zhu, Miriam Sabin, Alastair Ager, David Foy et al., "Psychological Distress, Depression, Anxiety, and Burnout among International Humanitarian Aid Workers: A Longitudinal Study," *PloS one* 7, no. 9 (2012): e44948.

47. Della W. Stewart, "Casualties of War: Compassion Fatigue and Health Care Providers," *Medsurg Nursing* 18, no. 2, (2009): 91.

48. Herbert J. Freudenberger, "Burn-Out: The Organizational Menace," *Training and Development Journal* 31, no. 7 (1977): 26–27.

49. Bertrand Taithe, "The Cradle of the New Humanitarian System? International Work and European Volunteers at the Cambodian Border Camps," *Contemporary European History* 25, no. 2 (2016): 335–58.

50. Della W. Stewart, "Casualties of War: Compassion Fatigue and Health Care Providers," *Medsurg Nursing* 18, no. 2 (2009): 94.

51. Eg. Laura Landro, "When Nurses Catch Compassion Fatigue, Patients Suffer," *Wall Street Journal*, January, 3, 2012. http://www.wsj.com/articles/SB10001424052970204720204577128882104188856. Many other examples could be cited.

52. Chantal Brazeau, Robin Schroeder, Sue Rovi, and Linda Boyd, "Relationships between Medical Student Burnout, Empathy, and Professionalism Climate," *Academic Medicine* 85, no. 10 (2010): S33–S36; Sara T. Fry, Rose M. Harvey, Ann C. Hurley, and Barbara Jo Foley "Development of a Model of Moral Distress in Military Nursing," *Nursing Ethics* 9, no. 4 (2002): 373–87.

53. Susan D. Moeller, *Compassion Fatigue: How the Media Sells Disease, Famine, War and Death* (London: Routledge, 1999); Ornri Elisha, "Moral Ambitions of Grace: The Paradox of Compassion and Accountability in Evangelical Faith-Based Activism," *Cultural Anthropology* 23, no. 1 (2008): 54–189.

54. Charles Lavigerie, *Oeuvres choisies de son eminence le Cardinal Lavigerie, archêveque d'Alger* (Paris: Pouissielgue Frères), 154, also in Vincent Burozet, *Histoire des Désordres de l'Algérie 1866–1867–1869, sautarelles, tremblement de terre, choléra, famine* (Algiers: Garaudel, 1968); this originated from a report by the curé of Tenes, AGMA, Papiers Lavigerie, B7–240 1.

55. William Ian Miller has reflected on some of the political implications of disgust which apply here: *The Anatomy of Disgust* (Cambridge, Mass.: Harvard University Press, 1997), 207–10.

56. Halttunen, "Humanitarianism," 303–34.

57. Luc Boltanski, *La Souffrance à Distance: Morale Humanitaire, Médias et Politique* (Paris: Métailié, 1993); Moeller, *Compassion Fatigue*; Didier Fassin, *Humanitarian Reason: A Moral History of the Present* (Berkeley: University of California Press, 2012).

58. Susan Sontag, *On Photography* (New York: Farrar Strauss and Giroux, 1977), 19; and *Regarding the Pain of Others* (London: Penguin, 2003).

59. S. Nissinen, "Dilemmas of Ethical Practice in the Production of Contemporary Humanitarian Photography," in Fehrenbach and Rodogno, *Humanitarian Photography*, 297–322. Caroline Caron, "Humaniser le Regard: Du Photojournalisme Humanitaire à l'Usage Humanitaire de la Photographie," *Composite* 1 (2007): 1–19; Julien Stallabrass, ed., *Memory of Fire: Images of War and the War of Images* (Brighton: Photoworks, 2013).

60. Marie-Luce Desgrandchamps, "L'humanitaire en guerre civile: Une histoire des opérations de secours au Nigeria-Biafra (1967–1970)," (PhD diss., Université de Genève, 2014).

61. Kevin O'Sullivan, "Humanitarian Encounters: Biafra, NGOs and Imaginings of the Third World in Britain and Ireland, 1967—70," *Journal of Genocide Research* 16, nos. 2–3 (2014): 299–315.

62. Lasse Heerten and A. Dirk Moses, "The Nigeria—Biafra War: Postcolonial Conflict and the Question of Genocide," *Journal of Genocide Research* 16, nos. 2–3 (2014): 169–203.

63. Johannes Paulmann, "Conjunctures in the History of International Humanitarian Aid during the Twentieth Century," *Humanity: An International Journal of Human Rights, Humanitarianism, and Development*, 4, no. 2 (2013): 215–38.

64. Darell M. West, "Angelina, Mia, and Bono: Celebrities and International Development," *Global Development* 2 (2008): 74–84.

65. Suzanne Franks, "Getting into Bed with Charity," *British Journalism Review* 19, no. 3 (2008): 27–32

66. Tanja Müller, "The Ethiopian Famine Revisited: Band Aid and the Antipolitics of Celebrity Humanitarian Action," *Disasters* 37, no. 1 (2013): 61–79.

67. Michael Buerk interviewed in "The Reunion," BBC Radio 4 (September, 4, 2009).

68. Suzanne Franks, *Reporting Disasters: Famine, Aid, Politics and the Media: Famine, Aid, Politics and the Media* (London: Hurst, 2014).

69. Francine Saillant, Marie-Ève Drouin, and Nathalie Gordon, "Formes, Contenus et Usages Témoignage dans les ONG d'Aide Internationale: La Vérité à l'Épreuve du Marketing," *Alterstice* 1, no. 2 (2012): 35–46.

70. Eoin Devereux, "Good Causes, God's Poor and Telethon Television," *Media, Culture and Society* 18, no. 1 (1996): 47–68.

71. Elizabeth McAlister, "Soundscapes of Disaster and Humanitarianism: Survival Singing, Relief Telethons, and the Haiti Earthquake," *Small Axe* 16, no. 339, (2012): 22–38.

72. David King, "The New Internationalists: World Vision and the Revival of American Evangelical Humanitarianism, 1950–2010," *Religions* 3, no. 4 (2012): 922–49.

73. Lilie Chouliaraki, "The Theatricality of Humanitarianism: A Critique of Celebrity Advocacy," *Communication and Critical/Cultural Studies* 9, no. 1 (2012): 1–21.

74. Yung Soo Kim and James D. Kelly, "Photojournalist on the Edge: Reactions to Kevin Carter's Sudan Famine Photo," *Visual Communication Quarterly* 20, no. 4 (2013): 205–19.

75. Jock Stirrat, Jock, "Competitive Humanitarianism: Relief and the Tsunami in Sri Lanka," *Anthropology Today* 22, no. 5 (2006): 11–16; Toby Lanzer, "Has the Tsunami Affected Funding for Other Crises," *Forced Migration Review* 17 (2005), http://www.fmreview.org/sites/fmr/files/FMRdownloads/en/FMRpdfs/Tsunami/full.pdf.

76. Gilles Carbonnier, "Reason, Emotion, Compassion: Can Altruism Survive Professionalisation in the Humanitarian Sector?," *Disasters* 39, no 2 (2015): 189–207.

77. Margie Buchanan-Smith, *How the Sphere Project Came into Being: A Case Study of Policy-Making in the Humanitarian Aid Sector and the Relative Influence of Research* (London: Overseas Development Institute, 2003).

78. Philippe Calain, "Ethics and Images of Suffering Bodies in Humanitarian Medicine," *Social Science and Medicine* 98 (2013): 278–85.

79. Gilles Carbonnier, *Humanitarian Economics: War, Disaster and the Global Aid Market* (London: Hurst, 2015).

Afterword

After the death of his mother, Roland Barthes turned to the photographs they had kept in the house. He was trying to find her in the images, but looking at photographs became a frustrating enterprise. Some images were not her at all; most of them were *almost* her.[1] Suddenly, Barthes found his mother in a Photograph taken when she was five years old. He had not met his mother as she looked like in the image, but the Photograph of the *Jardin d'Hiver* was her to him.[2] What made the recognition possible was not the resemblance of the subject of the image. The connection he felt with the Photograph was not representational but material: the chemicals on the plate had captured the light that literally emanated from her mother, when she had posed in front of the camera. He had "the certainty that the photographed body touches me with its own rays" because the Photograph certified that she had been there.[3] Barthes called this phenomenon *ça-a-été* (this-has-been) and identified it as the essence of Photography.[4] Far from a banal statement that simply described the indexical nature of photography, Barthes's ça-a-été referred to a material and temporal relationship between the photographed subject, the viewer, and the photograph.[5]

The encounter between Barthes and the Photograph described in *Camera Lucida* presents a great occasion to rethink the creation of what we have called in this book *emotional bodies*, just as the performative "I love you" of *A Lover's Discourse* did. What made Barthes find his mother in the Photograph of the *Jardin d'Hiver* was his grief; a raw feeling of grief that had not yet been processed into mourning rituals. "The Photograph—my Photograph—is without culture: when it is painful, nothing in it can transform grief into mourning."[6]

Barthes's relationship to the Photograph was not based on intellectual or aesthetic reasons (what he called the *studium*) but on the *punctum*: the element that "shoots out of it like an arrow and pierces me," a "wound."[7] The Photograph was painful because it "pricked" him. Grief, materialized in the doing of an action (sorting out and looking at photographs), and pain, which was the result of the encounter between a body in grief and a photograph of someone who had been there, were at the origin of Barthes's emotional body. As Maggie Nelson notes, this body is still a gendered one: "the mother remains the (photographed) object; the son, the (writing) subject. 'The writer is someone who plays with his mother's body,' Barthes wrote."[8]

The fact that this volume on the history of emotions starts and finishes with Barthes might be surprising.[9] This is not a Barthesian book, and his presence has faded in the chapters. Our theoretical framework goes beyond semiotics and phenomenology, but Barthes's writings on love and photography touch on core concepts of this book, as they have enabled us to feel words as well as images in their making.[10] Both "I-love-you" and the *punctum* thus appear as perfect examples of the performativity of emotions and how emotions do and undo us in a performative way. In the introduction we argue that the utterance "*Je t'aime*/I love you" not only shapes lovers' bodies, it also makes us vulnerable to others' emotional reactions in a radical way. Something similar happens in the Photograph. The *punctum* makes us vulnerable, experiencing emotions such as grief, which transform us into a suffering body, which is, of course, an emotional one.

Chapters in this book have examined very different aspects of this process in diverse periods and geographical locations. Some chapters have focused on the *type* of emotional body. Boddice, León-Sanz, and Vidor have disentangled the bodily effects of emotions in individuals, while Nagy and Martín-Moruno have turned to collectivities and the role of emotions in building social bodies. As these chapters show, emotional bodies are not only flesh-and-bone bodies in pain or affected by body-image issues, but they are also groups of people who come together in a particular social context. This book has also paid attention to the *means* through which emotional bodies come to being. Fernández-Fontecha, Pichel, and Rosón have explored the ways in which discourses, photographic practices, and memories can create emotional bodies, focusing on the role of objects and images in this process. Finally, Arrizabalaga, Hutchinson, and Taithe have demonstrated that humanitarian bodies are the result of the performative work of emotions such as compassion, which are able to connect to distant people around the world.

In spite of the differences in topics, methodologies, periods, and geographies, there is a common thread that unites all the chapters of this book. In all the case studies, emotions do and undo the subject. The subject and its identity are the result of the performative work of emotions, not the other way around. This subject is necessarily ephemeral: it is a particular configuration of matter in which the doing of emotions is the driving force. The wide variety of approaches in this book has always been central to its aims. We can find emotional bodies in the Middle Ages as well as in contemporary humanitarian organizations, but they will necessarily be articulated in different ways according to their particular circumstances. A universal definition of *emotional body* is impossible, as emotions, bodies, and, ultimately, matter are constructions, which are necessarily contingent from a historical point of view. When we propose the concept "emotional body," we do so with an awareness of the giants on whose shoulders we are standing. The fact that there are traces of emotional bodies in Barthes's writing, in Butler and Barad, and, of course, in Nagy, Reddy, Scheer, or Labanyi indicates that the idea of emotions doing bodies has been around for a long time. The aim of this book is, therefore, to provide a more coherent framework to the historical performativity of emotions, exploring its potential from myriad points of view. Now is the time for other scholars to use this concept and explore its possibilities in the most Barthesian direction: by providing it "inflections, which will be forever new."[11]

Notes

1. Roland Barthes, *Camera Lucida: Reflections on Photography*, trans. by Richard Howard (London: Vintage, 1993), 66.

2. Ibid., 67. Barthes distinguishes between Photograph with capital P, which refers to this particular photograph, from photograph in lower case, which refers to the rest of photographs. The same goes for Photography, which refers to the universal concept, and photography, which refers to the individual practices.

3. Ibid., 81.

4. Ibid., 76–77.

5. "The important thing is that the photograph possesses an evidential force, and that its testimony bears not on the object but on time," Ibid., 88.

6. Ibid., 90.

7. Ibid., 26, 73.

8. Maggie Nelson, *The Argonauts* (Minneapolis, Minn.: Graywolf, 2015), 49.

9. On Barthes and the affective power of photography see also Elspeth H. Brown and Thy Pu, eds. *Feeling Photography* (Durham, N.C.: Duke University Press, 2014), 1–25.

10. On the pivotal role of emotions in Barthes see Patrizia Lombardo, *The Three Paradoxes of Roland Barthes* (Athens: University of Georgia Press, 1989).

11. Nelson, *Argonauts*, 5.

Selected Bibliography

Abruzzo, Margaret. *Polemical Pain: Slavery, Cruelty, and the Rise of Humanitarianism.* Baltimore, Md.: John Hopkins University Press, 2011.

Ahmed, Sarah. *The Cultural Politics of Emotion.* New York: Routledge, 2004.

Alberti, Fay Bound. *Matters of the Heart: History, Medicine and Emotion.* Oxford: Oxford University Press, 2010.

———, ed. *Medicine, Emotion and Disease 1700–1950.* Basingstoke: Palgrave Macmillan, 2005.

———. *This Mortal Coil: The Human Body in History and Culture.* Oxford: Oxford University Press, 2016.

Ambroise-Rendu, Anne-Claude, and Christian Delporte. *L'indignation: Histoire d'une émotion, XIXe-XXe siècle.* Paris: Nouveau Monde, 2008.

Barclay, Katie. "New Materialism and the New History of Emotions." *Emotions: History, Culture, Society* 1, no. 1 (2017):161–83.

Barthes, Roland. *Camera Lucida: Reflections on Photography.* Translated by Richard Howard. London: Vintage, 1993.

———. *A Lover's Discourse. Fragments.* Translated by Richard Howard. New York: Hill and Wang, 1978.

Biro, David. *The Language of Pain: Finding Words, Compassion, and Relief.* New York: Norton, 2010.

Bleiker, Roland, David Campbell, and Emma Hutchison. "Imaging Catastrophe: The Politics of Representing Humanitarian Crises." In *Negotiating Relief: The Dialectics of Humanitarian Space,* edited by Michele Acuto, 47–58. Oxford: Oxford University Press, 2013.

Boddice, Rob. *The History of Emotions.* Manchester: Manchester University Press, 2018.

———. "The History of Emotions: Past, Present and Future." *Revista de Estudios Sociales,* no. 62 (October–December, 2017): 10–15.

———. *A History of Feelings*. London: Reaktion, 2019.

———, ed. *Pain and Emotion in Modern History*. Houndmills: Palgrave Macmillan, 2014.

Boltanski, Luc. *Distant Suffering: Morality, Media and Politics*. Translated by Graham Burhell. Cambridge: Cambridge University Press, 1999.

Boquet, Damien, and Piroska Nagy, eds. *Politiques des émotions au Moyen Âge*. Florence: SISMEL, Edizioni del Galluzo, 2011.

———. *Sensible Moyen Âge: Une histoire des émotions dans l'Occident médiéval*. Paris: Seuil, 2015.

Bourke, Joanna. *Fear. A Cultural History*. London: Virago, 2005.

———. "Phantom Suffering: Amputees, Stump Pain and Phantom Sensations in Modern Britain." In Boddice, *Pain and Emotion in Modern History*, 66–89.

———. *The Story of Pain: From Prayer to Painkillers*. Oxford: Oxford University Press, 2014.

Braddick, Michael. "Introduction: The Politics of Gestures." Special issue, "The Politics of Gestures," *Past and Present*, 203, no. 4 (2009): 9–35.

Braunmühl, Caroline. "Theorizing Emotions with Judith Butler: Within and beyond the Courtroom." *Rethinking History* 16, no. 2 (2012): 221–40.

Brown, Elspeth H., and Thy Pu, eds. *Feeling Photography*. Durham, N.C.: Duke University Press, 2014.

Brudholm, Thomas, ed. *Emotions and War Atrocities: Philosophical and Theoretical Explorations*. Cambridge: Cambridge University Press, 2018.

Butler, Judith. *Gender Trouble: Feminism and the Subversion of Identity*. London: Routledge, 1990.

Carrera, Elena, ed. *Emotions and Health: 1200–1700*. Leiden: Brill, 2013.

Coakley, Sarah, and Kay Kaufman Shelemay, eds. *Pain and Its Transformations: The Interface of Biology and Culture*. Cambridge, Mass.: Harvard University Press.

Cohen, Esther. *The Modulated Scream: Pain in Late Medieval Culture*. Chicago: University of Chicago Press, 2010.

Darwin, Charles. *The Expression of Emotions in Man and Animals*. London: Murray, 1872.

Daston, Lorraine, and Peter Galison. *Objectivity*. New York: Zone, 2007.

Delgado, Luisa Elena, Pura Fernández, and Jo Labanyi, eds. *Engaging the Emotions in Spanish Culture and History*. Nashville, Tenn.: Vanderbilt University Press, 2016.

Didi-Huberman, Georges. *The Invention of Hysteria: Charcot and the Photographic Iconography of the Salpêtrière*. Translated by Alisa Hartz. Cambridge, Mass.: MIT Press, 2003.

Dixon, Thomas. *From Passions to Emotions: The Creation of a Secular Psychological Category*. Cambridge: Cambridge University Press, 2003.

Dolan, Alice, and Sally Holloway. "Emotional Textiles: An Introduction." *Textile* 14, no. 2 (2016): 152–59.

Downes, Stephanie, Sally Holloway, and Sara Randles. *Feeling Things: Objects and Emotions through History*. Oxford: Oxford University Press, 2018.

Dror, Otniel. "The Affect of Experiment: The Turn to Emotions in Anglo-American Physiology, 1900–1940." *Isis* 90, no. 2 (1999): 205–37.

———. "The Scientific Image of Emotion: Experience and Technologies of Inscription." *Configurations* 7, no. 3 (1999): 355–401.

———. "Seeing the Blush: Feeling Emotions." In *Histories of Scientific Observation*. Edited by Lorraine Daston and Elizabeth Lunbeck, 326–48. Chicago: The University of Chicago Press, 2011.

Dror, Otniel, Bettina Hitzer, Anja Laukotter, and Pilar Leon Sanz. "An Introduction to *History of Sciences and the Emotions*." In *History of Science and the Emotions*, edited by Otniel Dror, Bettina Hitzer, Anja Laukötter, and Pilar León-Sanz, 1–18. *Osiris* 31, no. 1 (2016).

Duchenne de Boulogne. *Mécanisme de la physionomie humaine, ou analyse électro-physiologique de l'expression des passions*. Paris: Renouard, 1862.

Eitler, Pascal, and Monique Scheer. "Emotionengeschichte als Körpergeschichte: Eine heuristische Perspektive auf religiöse Konversionen im 19. und 20. Jahrhundert." *Geschichte und Gesellschaft* 35, no. 2 (2009): 282–313.

Fassin, Didier. *Humanitarian Reason: A Moral History of the Present*. Translated by Rachel Gomme. Berkley: California University Press, 2012.

Febvre, Lucien. "Sensibility and History: How to Reconstitute the Emotional Life of the Past?" In *A New Kind of History: From the Writings of Febvre*, edited by Peter Burke, 12–26. Translated by K. Folca. London: Routledge and Keagan Paul, 1973.

Feldman Barrett, Lisa. *How Emotions Are Made: The Secret Life of the Brain*. New York: Houghton Mifflin Harcourt, 2017.

Fernández-Fontecha, Leticia. "Signos, legibilidad y diagnóstico: El problema del dolor en la infancia, 1870–1920." *Cuadernos de Historia Contemporánea* 36 (2014): 89–112.

Fiering, Norman S. "Irresistible Compassion: An Aspect of Eighteenth-Century Sympathy and Humanitarianism." *Journal of the History of Ideas* 37, no. 2 (1976): 195–218.

Frevert, Ute. *Emotions in History: Lost and Found*. Budapest: Central European University Press, 2011.

Gill, Rebecca. "Networks of Concern, Boundaries of Compassion: British Relief in the South African War." *Journal of Imperial and Commonwealth History* 40, no. 5 (2010): 827–44.

Gilman, Sander L. "The Image of the Hysteric." In *Hysteria beyond Freud*, edited by Sander L. Gilman, Helen King, Roy Porter, G. S. Rousseau, and Elaine Showalter, 345–452. Berkeley: University of California Press, 1993.

Goldberg, Daniel. "Pain, Objectivity and History: Understanding Pain Stigma." *Medical Humanities* 43 (2017): 238–43.

———. "Pain without Lesion: Debate among American Neurologists, 1850–1900." *19: Interdisciplinary Studies in the Long Nineteenth Century* 15 (2012).

Gouk, Penelope, and Helen Hills, eds. *Representing Emotions: New Connections in the Histories of Art, Music and Medicine*. London: Routledge, 2005.

Grahek, Nikola. *Feeling Pain and Being in Pain*. 2nd ed. Cambridge, Mass.: MIT Press, 2007.

Halttunnen, Karen. "Humanitarianism and the Pornography of Pain in Anglo-American Culture." *American Historical Review* 100, no. 2 (1995): 303–34.

Harrington, Anne. "Mother Love and Mental Illness: An Emotional History." In *History of Science and the Emotions*, edited by Otniel Dror, Bettina Hitzer, Anja Laukötter, and Pilar León-Sanz, 94–115. *Osiris* 31, no. 1 (2016).

Haskell, Thomas L. "Capitalism and the Origins of the Humanitarian Sensibility." *American Historical Review* 90, nos. 2 and 3, pts. 1 and 2 (1985): 339–61, 547–66.

Hide, Louise, Joanna Bourke, and Carmen Mangion, "Perspectives on Pain: Introduction." *19: Interdisciplinary Studies in the Long Nineteenth Century* 15 (2012).

Hirsch, Marianne. "Surviving Images: Holocaust Photographs and the Work of Postmemory." *Yale Journal of Criticism* 14, no. 1 (2001): 5–37.

Hitzer, Bettina. "Healing Emotions." In *Emotional Lexicons: Continuity and Change in the Vocabulary of Feeling, 1700–2000*, edited by Ute Frevert, 118–50. Oxford: Oxford University Press, 2014.

———. "Oncomotions: Experience and Debates in West Germany and United States after 1945." In *Science and Emotions after 1945: A Transatlantic Perspective*, edited by Frank Biess and Donald M. Gross, 157–78. Chicago: University of Chicago Press, 2014.

Hitzer, Bettina, and Pilar León-Sanz. "The Feeling Body and Its Diseases: How Cancer Went Psychosomatic in Twentieth-Century Germany." In *History of Science and the Emotions*, edited by Otniel Dror, Bettina Hitzer, Anja Laukötter, and Pilar León-Sanz, 67–93. *Osiris* 31, no. 1 (2016).

Hochschild, Arlie Russell. *The Managed Heart: Commercialization of Human Feeling*. Berkeley: University of California Press, 2012.

Hutchison, Emma. *Affective Communities in World Politics: Collective Emotions after Trauma*. Cambridge: Cambridge University Press, 2016.

———. "A Global Politics of Pity? Disaster Imagery and the Emotional Construction of Solidarity after the 2004 Asian Tsunami." *International Political Sociology* 8, no. 1 (2014): 1–19.

Illouz, Eva. *Consuming the Romantic Utopia: Love and the Cultural Contradictions of Capitalism*. Berkeley: University of California Press, 1977.

———. *Why Love Hurts: A Sociological Explanation*. Cambridge: Polity, 2011.

Jonasdottir, Anna G., and Ferguson, Ann, eds. *Love: A Question for Feminism in the Twenty-First Century*. London: Routledge, 2014.

Jones, Colin. "The Emotional Turn in the History of Medicine and the View from the Queen Mary University of London." Virtual issue, "Emotions, Health, and Wellbeing," *Social History of Medicine* 1 (2014): 1–2

———. *The Smile Revolution in Eighteenth Century Paris*. Oxford: Oxford University Press, 2014.

Käpylä, Juha, and Denis Kennedy. "Cruel to Care? Investigating the Governance of Compassion in the Humanitarian Imaginary." *International Theory* 6, no. 2 (2014): 255–92.

Knepper Paul, and P. J. Ystehede, eds. *The Cesare Lombroso Handbook*. London: Routledge 2013.

Konstan, David. *Pity Transformed*. London: Duckworth, 2001.

Labanyi, Jo. "Doing Things: Emotions, Affect and Materiality." *Journal of Spanish Cultural Studies* 11, nos. 3–4 (2010): 223–33.

Langford, Martha. *Suspended Conversations: The Afterlife of Memory in Photographic Album*. Montreal: McGill-Queen's University Press, 2008.

Laqueur, Thomas W. "Bodies, Details, and Humanitarian Narratives." In *The New Cultural History*, edited by Lynn Hunt, 176–204. Berkeley: University of California Press, 1989.

León Sanz, Pilar. "El carácter terapéutico de la relación médico-paciente." In *Emociones y estilos de vida: Radiografía de nuestro tiempo*, edited by Lourdes Flamarique and Madalena D'Oliveira, 101–30. Madrid: Biblioteca Nueva, 2013.

Leys, Ruth. *From Guilt to Shame: Auschwitz and After*. Princeton, N.J.: Princeton University Press, 2007.

———. "The Turn to Affect: A Critique." *Critical Inquiry* 37, no. 3 (2011): 434–72.

Leys, Ruth, and Marlene Goldman. "Navigating the Genealogies of Trauma, Guilt, and Affect: An Interview with Ruth Leys." *University of Toronto Quarterly* 79, no. 2 (2010): 656–79.

Lutz, Catherine. "Feminist Theories and the Science of Emotion." In *Science and Emotions after 1945: A Transatlantic Perspective*, edited by Frank Biess and Daniel M. Gross, 342–64. Chicago: Chicago University Press, 2014.

———. *Unnatural Emotions: Everyday Sentiments on a Micronesian Atoll and Their Challenge to Western Theory*. Chicago: University of Chicago Press, 1988.

Martín-Moruno, Dolores. "Love in the Time of Darwinism: Paolo Mantegazza and the Emergence of Sexuality." *Medicina and Storia* 10, nos. 19–20 (2010): 147–64.

———. "On Resentment." In *On Resentment: Past and Present*, edited by Bernardino Fantini, Dolores Martín-Moruno and Javier Moscoso, 1–16. Newcastle-upon-Tyne: Cambridge Scholars, 2013.

———. "Pain as Practice in Paolo Mantegazza Science of Emotions." In Otniel Dror, Bettina Hitzer, Anja Laukötter, and Pilar León-Sanz, *History of Science and the Emotions*, 137–62.

Micale, Mark. *Approaching Hysteria: Disease and Its Interpretations*. Princeton, N.J.: Princeton University Press, 1995.

———. *Hysterical Men: The Hidden History of Male Nervous Illness*. Cambridge, Mass.: Harvard University Press, 2008.

Miller, William Ian. *The Anatomy of Disgust*. Cambridge, Mass.: Harvard University Press, 1997.

Möller, Susan D. *Compassion Fatigue: How the Media Sell Disease, Famine, War and Death*. Routledge: New York, 1999.

Moran, Anna, and Sorcha O'Brien, eds. *Love Objects: Emotion, Design and Material Culture*. London: Bloomsbury, 2014.

Morris, David B. *The Culture of Pain*. Berkeley: University of California Press, 1991.
Moyn, Samuel. "Empathy in History: Empathizing with Humanity." *History and Theory* 45, no. 3 (2006): 397–415.
Musumeci, Emilia. *Emozioni, crimine, giustizia: Un'indagine storico-giuridica tra Otto e Novecento*. Milano: Franco Angeli, 2015.
Nelson, Maggie. *The Argonauts*. Minneapolis: Graywolf, 2015.
Newton, Hannah. *The Sick Child in Early Modern England, 1580–1720*. Oxford University Press: Oxford, 2012.
Norton, Matthew. "Narrative Structure and Emotions Mobilization in Humanitarian Representations: The Case of the Congo Reform Movement, 1903–1912." *Journal of Human Rights* 10, no. 3 (2011): 311–38.
Pedwell, Carolyn. *Affective Relations: The Transnational Politics of Empathy*. Milton Park, U.K.: Palgrave Macmillan, 2014.
Pichel, Beatriz. "From Facial Expressions to Bodily Gestures: Passions, Photography and Movement in French Nineteenth-Century Sciences." *History of the Human Sciences* 29, no. 1 (2016): 27–48.
Plamper, Jan. "The History of Emotions: An Interview with William Reddy, Barbara Rosenwein, and Peter Stearns." *History and Theory* 49 (2010): 237–65.
———. *The History of Emotions: An Introduction*. Translated by Keith Tribe. Oxford: Oxford University Press, 2015.
Reddy, William. *The Navigation of Feeling. A Framework for the History of Emotions*. Cambridge: Cambridge University Press, 2001.
Rees, Danny. "Down in the Mouth: Faces of Pain." In *Pain and Emotion in Modern History*, edited by Rob Boddice, 164–86. Houndmills: Palgrave, 2014.
Rey, Roselyne. *The History of Pain*. Cambridge: Harvard University Press, 1995.
Rosaldo, Michelle Z. "Toward an Anthropology of Self and Feeling." In *Culture Theory: Essay on Mind, Self and Emotion*, edited by Richard A. Shweder and Robert A. LeVine, 137–57. Cambridge: Cambridge University Press, 1995.
Rosenwein, Barbara H. *Emotional Communities in the Middle Ages*. Ithaca, N.Y.: Cornell University Press, 2007.
———. "Theories of Change in the History of Emotions." In *A History of Emotions, 1200–1800*, edited by Jonas Liliequist, 7–20. London: Pickering and Chatto, 2012.
———. "Worrying about Emotions in History." *American Historical Review* 107 (2002): 821–45.
Rosón, María, and Rosa Medina-Domenech. "Emotional Resistances: Spaces and Presences of Intimacy in the Historic Archive." *Arenal* 24, no. 2 (2017): 407–39.
Rozenblatt, Daphne. "Madness and Method: Enrico Morselli and the Social Politics of Psychiatry, 1852–1929." PhD diss., University of California, 2014.
———. "Scientific Expertise and the Politics of Emotions in the 1902 Trial of Giuseppe Musolino." *History of the Human Sciences* 30, no. 3 (2017): 25–49.
Scarry, Elaine. *The Body in Pain: The Making and Unmaking of the World*. New York: Oxford University Press, 1985.
Scheer, Monique. "Are Emotions a Kind of Practice (And Is That What Makes Them

Have a History?): A Bourdieuian Approach to Understanding Emotion." *History and Theory* 51, no. 2 (2012): 193–220.

Sedgwick, Eve Kosofsky. *Touching Feeling: Affect Pedagogy, Performativity*. Durham, N.C.: Duke University Press, 2003.

Showalter, Elaine. *The Female Malady: Women, Madness and English Culture, 1830–1980*. London: Virago, 1985.

Sontag, Susan. *On Photography*. New York: Anchor Doubleday, 1989.

Stearns, Peter, and Carol Stearns. "Emotionology: Clarifying the History of Emotions and Emotional Standards." *American Historical Review* 90, no. 4 (1985): 813–36.

Taithe, Bertrand. "'Cold Calculation in the Faces of Horrors?' Pity, Compassion and the Making of Humanitarian Protocols." In Alberti, *Medicine, Emotion and Disease*, 79–99. London: Palgrave Macmillan, 2006.

———. "Empathies, soins et compassions: Les émotions humanitaires." In *Histoire des émotions: De la fin du XIXe siècle à nos jours*, edited by Alain Corbin, Jean-Jacques Courtine, and Georges Vigarello, 364–81. Paris: Sous-sol, 2017.

Velten, Hans Rudolf. "Performativity and Performance." In *Travelling Concepts for the Study of Culture*, edited by Birgit Neumann and Ansgar Nünning, 249–66. Berlin: De Gruyter, 2012.

Vicinus, Martha, ed. *Suffer and Be Still: Women in the Victorian Age*. Indiana University Press, 1972.

Vidor, Gian Marco. "The Press, the Audience, and Emotions in Italian Courtrooms (1860s-1910s)." *Journal of Social History* 51, no. 2 (2017): 1–24

Wall, Patrick. *Pain: The Science of Suffering*. New York, Columbia University Press, 2002.

White, Paul "Introduction." *Isis* (Focus: The Emotional Economy of Science) 100, no. 4 (2009): 792–97.

Whyman, Rose. "The Actor's Second Nature: Stanislavski and Willian James." *New Theatre Quarterly* 23, no. 2 (2007): 115–23.

Wilson, Richard Ashby, and Richard D. Brown, eds. *Humanitarianism and Suffering: The Mobilization of Empathy*. Cambridge: Cambridge University Press, 2009.

Contributors

JON ARRIZABALAGA is a research professor in history of science at the Spanish National Research Council (CSIC), Institución Milà I Fontanals (IMF), Barcelona, Spain. His research is mostly focused on humanitarian action and war medicine in modern Spain, and on medicine, health, and disease in premodern Europe. His most recent publications include "War, Empire, Science, Progress, Humanitarianism: Debate and Practice within the International Red Cross Movement from 1863 to the Interwar Period" (*Asclepio* 66, no. 1 [2014]) and the volumes *Nicasio Landa, 'Muertos y heridos,' y otros textos* (edited with Guillermo Sánchez, Pamplona, Pamiela, 2016) and *"It All Depends on the Dose": Poisons and Medicines in European History* (edited with Ole P. Grell and Andrew Cunningham [London, Routledge, 2018]).

ROB BODDICE is a Marie-Skłodowska-Curie Global Fellow, based at Freie Universität Berlin and McGill University. Boddice has published extensively in the fields of history of medicine, history of science, and the history of emotions. His recent books include *The Science of Sympathy: Morality, Evolution, and Victorian Civilization* (University of Illinois Press, 2016), *Pain: A Very Short Introduction* (Oxford University Press, 2017), *The History of Emotions* (Manchester University Press, 2018), and *A History of Feelings* (Reaktion, 2019).

LETICIA FERNÁNDEZ-FONTECHA is a visiting scholar at the European Institute, Columbia University, New York. She specializes in the history of pain, the history of medicine and medical humanities, the history of childhood, and the history of emotions. Her current project, "Humanitarianism, The Spanish Civil War and the Cultural Work of Displaced Children," explores children's experiences of the war and the impact of wartime humanitarian ideas on the future of education in Spain. She is author of *They Still Draw Pictures* (La Uña Rota, 2018) and the poetry collection *La Piel o el Cuerpo* (Pre-textos, 2018), which won the National Spanish Poetry Prize Unicaja.

EMMA HUTCHISON is a University of Queensland research fellow and Australian Research Council DECRA fellow in the School of Political Science and International Studies at the University of Queensland. Her work focuses on emotions and trauma in world politics, particularly in relation to security, humanitarianism, and international aid. She has published in numerous academic journals and scholarly books. Her book *Affective Communities in World Politics: Collective Emotions After Trauma* (Cambridge University Press, 2016) was awarded the British International Studies Association Susan Strange Book Prize as well as the International Studies Association Theory Section Best Book Award.

PILAR LEÓN-SANZ is a professor of the history of medicine and medical ethics at the University of Navarra, member of the project "Emotional Culture and Identity" at the Institute of Culture and Society (UN). Her research interests include the medicine in eighteenth-century Spain, especially music therapy, and the practices and healthcare professionals during nineteenth and twentieth centuries; she is studying the concept of emotion and its place in medical knowledge. Her publications include History of Science and the Emotions, co-edited with Bettina Hitzer, Anja Laukötter, and Otniel Dror (*Osiris* 31, Chicago: University of Chicago Press, 2016); *La Tarantola Spagnola: Empirismo e tradizione nel XVIII secolo* (Besa Ed., 2008); "The Feeling Body and Its Diseases: How Cancer Went Psychosomatic in Twentieth-Century Germany," with B. Hitzer (*Osiris* 31 (Chicago: University of Chicago Press, 2016), 67–93, and "From Claims to Rights: Patient Complaints and the Evolution of a Mutual Aid Society (*La Conciliación*, 1902–1936), in *Complaints, Controversies and Grievances in Medicine: Historical and Social Science Perspectives* (Routledge, 2015), among others.

DOLORES MARTÍN-MORUNO is an assistant professor at the Institute for Ethics, History, and the Humanities, based in the Geneva Medical School (University of Geneva). She has published "Love in the Times of Darwinism: Paolo Mantegazza and the Emergence of Sexuality" (2011, Firenze University Press); *On Resentment: Past and Present* (Cambridge Scholars, 2013); and "Pain as Practice in Paolo Mantegazza's Science of Emotions" (*Osiris*, 2016). Her current research project, "Those Women Who Performed Humanitarian Action: A Gendered History of Compassion from the Franco-Prussian

War to WWII," was awarded a Swiss National Science Foundation Professorship in 2017.

PIROSKA NAGY is a professor of medieval history at the Université du Québec à Montréal. Her research, especially around the history and historiography of emotions, has been conducted for years with Damien Boquet in the project EMMA, Emotions in the Middle Ages (http://emma.hypotheses.org). Presently, she explores collective emotions, events, and change in the central Middle Ages, and also medieval affective anthropology, especially embodied religious emotions, experience, and charismas. She is author of *Le don des larmes au Moyen Age: Un instrument spirituel en quête d'institution, Ve—XIIIe siècle* (Albin Michel, 2000) and co-author, with Damien Boquet, of *Sensible Moyen Age: Une histoire des émotions dans l'Occident médiéval* (Seuil, 2015), translated in English with the title *Medieval Sensibilities: A History of Emotions in the Middle Ages* (Polity, 2018). Among her recent publications, with Naama Cohen-Hanegbi (eds.), is *Pleasure in the Middle Ages* (Turnhout, Brepols, 2018).

BEATRIZ PICHEL is a VC2020 lecturer in photographic history at the Photographic History Research Centre, De Montfort University, Leicester, U.K. She specializes in photographic history, the history of medicine and medical humanities, the history of emotion, and the cultural history of the war. Her current project, "Photography and the Making of Modern Medicine in France 1860–1914," funded by the British Academy, explores the role of photographic practices in the emergence and consolidation of medical specialties in the late nineteenth century. She is writing a monograph on photographic practices during World War I in France, and her work has been published in *History of the Human Sciences, Media History,* and the *Journal of War and Culture Studies,* among others.

MARÍA ROSÓN received her doctorate from Universidad Autónoma de Madrid (History of Art Department) in 2014 and currently works as a postdoctoral researcher in Valencia University's Department of Language Theory and Communication Science. She has been a visiting researcher at Southampton University, New York University, University of Oxford, and Leeds University and was awarded a research fellowship at the Museo Reina Sofía, Collection Department. María has also curated the exhibitions *José Ortiz Echagüe: Depicting Women, Types and Stereotypes* (Madrid Community, 2010) and *Women under Suspicion: Memory and Sexuality* (UNED, 2013). Her research is especially concerned with twentieth-century Spanish visual culture in intersection with gender studies. She has published *Género, memoria y cultura visual en el primer franquismo (materiales cotidianos, más allá del arte)* (Madrid: Cátedra, 2016).

BERTRAND TAITHE is a professor of cultural history at the University of Manchester and a specialist in the history of medical humanitarianism. He edits the *European Review of History* and is the chair of the editorial committee at Manchester University Press. His publications include *The Charity Market and Humanitarianism in Britain, 1870–1912* (Bloomsbury, 2018, with Sarah Roddy and Julie-Marie Strange), "Empathie, soins et compassions: Les émotions humanitaires," in Corbin, Courtine, and Vigarello, *Histoire des émotions, vol. III* (Seuil, 2017), *The Impact of History? Histories at the Beginning of the Twenty-First Century* (Routledge, 2015, edited with Pedro Ramos Pinto), *The Killer Trail: A Colonial Scandal in the Heart of Africa* (Oxford University Press, 2009), *Citizenship and Wars: France in Turmoil, 1870–1871* (Routledge, 2001), and *Defeated Flesh: Welfare, Warfare and the Making of Modern France* (Manchester University Press, 1999).

GIAN MARCO VIDOR is a research associate at the Institute for Ethics, History and Humanities at the University of Geneva. He was a researcher at the Center for the History of Emotions at the Max Planck Institute for Human Development in Berlin and a MaxNetAging fellow at the Max Planck Institute for Demographic Research in Rostock. His recent publications include a special section "Law and Emotions" (with Laura Kounine) in the *Journal of Social History* 51, no. 2 (2017), and the article "Rhetorical Engineering of Emotions in the Courtroom: The Case of Lawyers in Modern France," *Rechtsgeschichte—Legal History* 25 (2017).

Index

abolitionism, 224–27, 225, 226
"Abolition of the Slave Trade, The," 224–25, 225
action of emotions shared, 153
actors, photography of, 107–11, *109–10*, *112–13*
Adler, Alfred, 54–55
agential realism, 6
Ahmed, Sarah, 1, 5, 175
Alberti, Fay Bound, 5, 16
Alexander, Franz, 53, 55
Alfonso XII, 201
American Civil War, 211
American Pediatric Society, 86
American Psychosomatic Medicine/Association, 53, 54, 57, 62, 63
"Am I Not a Man and a Brother?" 226
Arch of Hysteria, The, 29
"Are Emotions a Kind of Practice?" 5
Arenal, Concepción: building humanitarian narrative at war, 201–3; on moving the population toward compassion, 208–10; on who deserves humanitarian relief, 205–7
Arendt, Hannah, 196, 229
Arrizabalaga, Jon, 196, 264
atavism, 38
Aubert, Charles, 98
Austin, John L., 2, 153
authentic embodiments and emotional pain, 29–32
Aznar, José María, 185–86

Balagny, M., 107–9
Band Aid, 253
Barad, Karen, 1, 6, 99, 114
Barclay, Katie, 6–7
Bardi dossal, 152–53, *155*, *157*, 162
Barnett, Michael, 228
Barrington, Vincent Kennett, 248
Barthes, Roland, 1–2, 9, 73, 120, 263–64
Bell, Charles, 23–24, *24*, 98
Bending, Lucy, 91
Bernard of Clairvaux, 156, 159
Bernhardt, Sarah, 97, 107
Bickford, Susan, 7, 19–20, 30–31
Biess, Frank, 60
"biographical pathology," 54
Biographical Sketch of an Infant, A, 79–80
Blair, Tony, 185
Blanqui, Louis Auguste, 178
Boddice, Rob, 7, 15, 74, 264
Body Experience in Fantasy and Behavior, 57
body image, 53–56; attitudes and, 65; body spatial axis and, 60; building a concept of, 57–59; in emotional bodies' performativity and disease, 62–65; and emotions in cancer patients, 59–60; Freud on, 55; key theorists on, 56–57; measures of emotions and, 60–62; relation between life stories or socialization process and, 63–64
Body Image and Personality, 56
body-image-oriented theory, 54–55
body reactivity, 57–58, 62–63; body spatial axis and, 60

body spatial axis, 60
Bohr, Niels, 6
Boltanski, Luc, 199, 253
Bonanno, Giuseppe, 40–41, 44
Borch-Jacobsen, Mikkel, 25
Bourdieu, Pierre, 5
Bourgeois, Louise, 29–30
Bourke, Joanna, 15, 77, 85
Braunmühl, Caroline, 7–8
British Anti-Slavery Society, 227
British Journal of Photography, 90
British Journal of Surgery, 28
Brocher, Victorine, 180
Brown, Elspeth, 74
Buerk, Michael, 253
burnout, 249–50
Bush, George W., 185
Butler, Judith, 1, 6, 175; on love, 2–3

Calnestrini, Silvio, 83
Camera Lucida, 73, 120, 263
cancer patients, measuring the influence of emotions and body image in, 59–60, 85
caregiver fatigue, 248–52
Carlist Wars, Spain, 196, 214–15; building humanitarian narratives during, 201–3; determining who deserved humanitarian relief during, 203–7; moving the population toward compassion during, 207–10
Carrara, Francesco, 42
Carrara, Mario, 39
Carrera, Elena, 16
Carter, Kevin, 254
Castañeda, Claudia, 84
Cervino, José Manuel, 138
Charcot, Jean-Martin, 24–26, 28, 29, 47, 100, 103, 105
Charity Organization Society, 247
children's pain, 74, 77–79, 91–93; Darwin on, 77, 79–85, 88, 91–92; infant-pain denial and, 80–81; performance of, 88–91; photographs of, 78–79, 88–91, 92–93; questions about communication of, 78–79; sick body and, 85–88
Christmas in Greccio and Saint Francis of Assisi, 148, 151–54; emotional community created by, 165–69; emotions expressed in, 161–62; grandeur-nature crib constructed for, 157–58; Greccio as setting for, 154–58, 155, 157; historiography of emotion and, 153–54; inner conversion and, 161; meaning and chronology of, 163–65;

mellifluous voice of, 160; as sharing a sensory and emotional event, 158–63
chronophotography, 111–14
Clark, Elizabeth, 221–22
classic school, 36, 38
Cleveland, Sidney E., 17, 55–56, 62–63; on body-image boundary, 65; on body reactivity, 57–58, 62–63; on body spatial axis, 60; building a body-image concept, 57–59; on emotions and body image in cancer patients, 59–60; on fantasies, 64; tests used for measures of emotions and body image and, 60–62
Cold War, the, 243–44
compassion fatigue, 242–44; in caregivers, 248–52; exhaustion of giving in, 252–55; humanitarian excess and, 244–48
Coulson, Sarah, 89
criminal anthropology, 36–37, 182
Criminal for Passion, 40
Criminal Man, 182
criminals of passion, 16–17, 47–48; Ferri's five main categories of criminals and, 42; fictional characters and the scientific construction of, 44–47; Lombroso on, 36–37; origins of views on, 36–38; performativity of emotions in defining, 41–44; premeditation in, 43; rarity of actual, 43–44; rise of criminal anthropology and, 36–37; role of the body in defining, 38–41
Criminal Woman, the Prostitute and the Normal Woman, 183
Cruikshank, Isaac, 224–25, 225
Cuadros de la Guerra, 203
Cultural Politics of Emotions, The, 5

Darwin, Charles, 245; on children's pain, 77, 79–85, 88, 91–92; on expression of emotions, 77, 79, 98
Darwin, William, 79, 80
Datson, Lorraine, 15
decolonization, 221
de la Tourette, Gilles, 100
Delgado, Luisa Elena, 5
demoniacs, 23–26
Development and Structure of the Body Image, 53, 57
Didi-Huberman, Georges, 99
disease and emotional bodies' performativity, 62–65
divorce, 44
Dixon, Thomas, 104

doing emotions, 4–8
"Doing Emotions: Affect, Culture and Materiality," 5
Dror, Otniel, 15, 63
du Bois-Reymond, Emil, 40
Du Camp, Maxime, 184
Duchenne de Boulogne, 103, 105
Dunant, Henri, 195, 246–47

Earl Dalhousie (ship), accounts of hysteria in passengers of, 19–21, 30–32
Edinburgh Ladies Emancipation Society, 226
Edwards, Elizabeth, 74
ego, 54, 56
El Cuartel Real, 211
embodied thoughts, 4–5
emotional bodies, 1, 264, 265; disease and, 62–65; doing emotions, 4–8; love and, 1–3; material entanglements in exploring, 8–10; pain in (*see* pain); performed in photography, 114–15; photographs of, 99–100; stabilized in emotional communities, 154
emotional communities, 4, 148; created by Saint Francis of Assisi, 165–69; emotional bodies stabilized in, 154
emotional pain and authentic embodiments, 29–32
emotional practices, 5
emotional refuge, 25–26, 29; medical gaze outside, 26–29
emotional regimes, 4, 26
emotionology, 4, 147
emotions: body image and physiological responses to, 57–59; and body image in cancer patients, 59–60; chronophotography and physiology of, 111–14; doing, 4–8; doing us, 4–8; historiography of, 153–54; humanitarian (*see* humanitarian emotions); love, 1–3, 264; materiality of, 6–7; performativity of (*see* performativity); pity, 196, 229, 233, 245; sympathy, 223, 233
Emotions, Bodies and Disease, 5
emotives, 153, 154
empathy, 251
Engaging Emotions in Spanish Culture and Society, 5
ETA (Basque separatists), 185–86
Eternal Sunshine of the Spotless Mind, The, 3
Euvrie, Julia Béatrix, 180
Evans, Elida, 60
Evanson, Richard Tonson, 87
exhaustion of giving, 252–55
Expression of the Emotions in Man and Animals, The, 77, 79, 81, 82, 98, 245

fantasies, 64
Fassin, Didier, 251
Faulkner, Robert, 90
Favre, Jules, 178
Fear, 182
Febvre, Lucien, 4, 147
Feeling Photography, 74
Fernández, Pura, 5
Fernández-Fontecha, Leticia, 74, 264
Ferri, Enrico, 36, 38–41; on born criminals, 44; on divorce, 44; on fictional characters as criminals of passion, 45, 46–47; five main categories of criminals, 42; on premeditation, 43; on Shakespeare's characters, 47
Figley, Charles, 249
Fisher, Seymour, 17, 53, 55–57; on body-image boundary, 65; on body reactivity, 57–58, 62–63; on body spatial axis, 60; building a body-image concept, 57–59; on emotions and body image in cancer patients, 59–60; on fantasies, 64; tests used for measures of emotions and body image and, 60–62
Flechsig, Paul Emil, 74, 83
Flourens, Gustave, 178
France. *See* Paris Commune
Francis of Assisi. *See* Christmas in Greccio and Saint Francis of Assisi
Franco-Prussian War, 178, 200, 202, 210–14
Franks, Susan, 253
Fredenberger, Herbert, 249–50
French Annales' School, 4
Freud, S., 28, 54, 56
Frevert, Ute, 148
Frugoni, Chiara, 156
Fulci, Ludovico, 45–46
fundraising, 252–55

Galison, Peter, 15
Garofalo, Raffaele, 36
Gazette des Tribunaux, 179, 181–82
gendering: of cancer pathogenesis, 64; of disaster, 230, 230–31; of hysteria, 26–29. *See also* women
Geneva Convention, 200–201, 203–4, 210, 211

Genzmer, Alfred, 74, 82–83, 85, 92
gestures: hallucination and, 105–6; photography for understanding meaning and materiality of, 98–99
Gilman, Sander, 24
"Ginx's Baby," 77, 79
Giraudet, Alfred, 98
Glasby, Anna M., 20–21
González Duro, 134
Gordon, Rae Beth, 99
Gougaud, Louis, 156
Great Ormond Street Hospital, 78–79, 86, 88, 92
Greccio, hermitage of, 154–58, *155, 157*. See also Christmas in Greccio and Saint Francis of Assisi
Gregory the Great, 159
Gross, Daniel M., 60
Guarnieri, Patrizia, 47–48
Guerola, Antonio, 202–3
Guide for the Diagnosis of Madness, 40
Guild of Help, 247
Guinon, Georges, 100–106

habitus, 5
hallucination, 105–6
Halttunen, Karen, 252–53
Haraway, Donna, 6
Harrington, Anne, 16
Haskell, Thomas, 199
Head, Henry, 56
Heyer, Heather, 175
Hiller, Jonathan, 47
Hirsch, Marianne, 73–74
historiography, 153–54
Hochschild, Arlie Russell, 223
Holocaust photography, 73–74, 147
Holt, Luther, 87–88
Honorius III, 163
Hudson, J., 19–21, 31–32
humanitarian emotions, 219–21; compassion fatigue and, 242–56; and images in contemporary humanitarianism, 228–33, *230, 232*; performativity and, 234–35; shifting conceptions of suffering over time and, 221–23; visualizing suffering and the historical emergence of, 223–28, *225, 226*
humanitarianism, 195–97; dangers in, 247; determining who deserves relief through, 203–7; emotions and images in contemporary, 228–33, *230, 232*; emotions in (*see* humanitarian emotions); excess, 244–48; fundraising in, 252–55; moving populations toward compassion and, 207–10; origins of, 199–200, 221–23; principles of, 219; rise of NGOs and, 244; Spanish Red Cross and (*see* Spanish Red Cross); volunteer vs. professional, 246–47; in wartime, 201–15
Hutchison, Emma, 196, 264
hypnosis at La Salpêtrière, 100–104, *101*
Hypnotisme expérimental: Les émotions dans l'etat d'hypnotisme, 103
hysteria: aboard the *Earl Dalhousie*, 19–21, 30–32; embodied sign of, 29–30; gendering of, 26–29; hypnosis at La Salpêtrière for, 100–104, *101*; pain viewed as, 22–23; as performance, 30; photographs capturing symptoms of, 106–7; presentation and representation of demons, tetanus, and, 21–26; tetanus and, 26–29
hysterical tetanus, 21–22, 30; medical gaze outside emotional refuge, 26–29

Iconographie photographique de la Salpêtrière, 100
"I Love You," 2–3, 9, 264; as performative practice, 5, 7
imagery in contemporary humanitarianism, 228–33, *230, 232*
Impallomeni, Giovanni Battista, 38
infant-pain denial, 80–81
Innocent III, 156
Institut de Droit International, 202
Institute of Child Health, 78
Investigations on the Psychic Function of the Newborn, 82–83
Irigaray, Pedro, 205
Isis, 15
Italian School, 36

Jaclard, Anna, 180
James, William, 113
Jardin des Plantes, 185, 187
Jasen, Patricia, 64
"Je-t'aime." *See* "I Love You"
Jewell, J. S., 27
Jones, Sydney, 88–90, *89*
Jung, Carl, 60

Kennedy, David, 234
Kennedy, Denis, 228
Kindermann, Herr, *81*
Konstan, David, 245
Kroner, Traugott, 83

282   Index

Kubie, Lawrence S., 55, 62
Kussmaul, Adolf, 80–81, 82

Labanyi, Jo, 1, 5
Laboulaye, Édouard, 211
La Caridad en la Guerra, 202, 204, 208, 211
La Nature, 107, 108
Lancet, The, 19, 21, 27, 31, 85–86
Landa, Nicasio: building humanitarian narrative at war, 201–2; moving populations toward compassion, 208; on SRC's services during the Franco-Prussian War, 210–14; on who deserves humanitarian relief, 204–5
Lange, Carl Georg, 41
language of emotion, 4
La photographie à la lumière artificielle, 108, 112
La photographie médicale, 98–99, 106, 111
Laquer, Thomas, 195
La Salpêtrière hospital, 75, 98–99; experimenting with hypnosis at, 100–104, *101*
La Sociale, 181
La Voz de la Caridad, 202, 203
Le Bon, Gustave, 184
Lecomte, Claude, 178
Légion des Fédérées, 180
Léo, André, 180, 181
León-Sanz, Pilar, 17, 264
Les convulsions de Paris, 184
Le Théâtre, 97–98; photography of actors in, 107–11, *109–10*
life stories and body image, 63–64
Lombroso, Cesare, 36–37, 39, 42–44; literary references in work of, 46; on the Paris Commune, 182–84
Londe, Albert, 106–7, 109; photographic cameras developed by, 111–12; photographs at La Salpêtrière hospital, 75, 98–100; photographs of actors, 109–11
love, 1–3
Lover's Discourse, A, 2
Lucas, Prosper, 37
Lumière brothers, 109
L'Union des femmes pour la défense de Paris et les soins aux blessés (The Women's Union for the Defense of Paris and Aid to the Wounded), 180
Luys, Jules Bernard, 103, 105

MacMahon, Patrice, 179
Madrid Red Cross, 211–12

Mantegazza, Paolo, 40
Manzano, José Luis, 136–37
Manzo, Kate, 229–30
Mareschal, G., 107–8
Marey, Étienne-Jules, 112
Martín-Moruno, Dolores, 7, 56, 148, 264
Masling, Joseph, 61, 62
materiality of emotions, 6–7
Mayhew, Henry, 37
Méchanisme de la physiognomie humanie, 105
Médecins Sans Frontières (MSF), 255
medical holism, 53
medicine, 15–17; cancer patients and, 59–60; on demoniacs, 23–26; gendering of, 26–29, 64; hypnosis in, 100–104, *101*; on hysteria (*see* hysteria); and medical gaze outside the emotional refuge, 26–29; performativity of medical photographs and experiments and, 104–7; psychosomatic (*see* psychosomatic medicine); view of hysteria in, 19–26
Memory of Solferino, A, 195
Mental Evolution in Man, 84
Micale, Mark, 26
Michel, Louise, 148, 177, 178–81, 185; memoirs of, 186–87; trial of, 181–82, 185, 187
Middlesex Hospital, 86
Millet, Kate, 2
Mind, 79
MMPI test, 60
Moeller, Susan, 253, 254
Morel, Bénédict Augustine, 37
Morselli, Enrico, 40
Mosso, Angelo, 40, 41, 182
Muertos y heridos (Dead and Wounded), 202
Munn, W. P., 27–28
Muybridge, Eadweard, 112

Nagy, Piroska, 148, 176
Navas, Ignacio, 75, 120–22. See also *Yolanda*
Nazi Germany. See Holocaust photography
Nightingale, Florence, 246, 256
nongovernmental organizations (NGOs), rise of, 243–44, 251
Nouvelle iconographie de la Salpêtrière, 98
nymphomania, 20, 30–31

On the Origins of Species, 84
"organic neuroses," 54
Osiris, 15
Othello, 45–46, 47

Index   283

Pagliacci, 47
pain, 15–16; authentic embodiments and emotional, 29–32; in children, 74, 77–93; Darwin on, 77, 79–82, 88, 91–92; humanitarianism and understanding of, 221–23; origins of humanitarianism based on suffering and, 221–22; as output of the brain, 22–23. *See also* suffering
Paris Commune, 7, 148–49, 176, 186–87; Lombroso's theory of criminals and, 182–84; Louise Michel and, 148, 177, 178–81; making of the women incendiaries of, 181–85; politics of emotion and, 176–77; prostitutes and, 180–81
performativity: of children's pain, 88–91; disease and emotional bodies', 62–65; of emotions in defining a criminal of passion, 41–44; of expressions in the theater, 97–115; humanitarianism and, 234–35; of hysteria, 30; of medical photographs and experiments, 104–7; in metaphysics, 6
Perrin, George M., 62
Perry, Loring Isaac, *230*
pétroleuses. *See* Paris Commune
photography, 73, 263–64; of actors, 107–11, *109–10*, *112–13*; cameras, chronophotography, and physiology of emotions and, 111–14; capturing symptoms of hysteria, 106–7; of children in pain, 78–79, 88–91, 92–93; Holocaust, 73–74, 147; humanitarianism and, 196; at La Salpêtrière, 75, 98–99, 98–104, *101*; performativity of actors and, 112–13; performativity of medical experiments and, 104–7; performing the emotional body in, 114–15; for understanding meaning and materiality of gestures, 98–99; in *Yolanda* (*see Yolanda*)
Photo-Journal, 112
physiological responses to emotion, 57–59
Pichel, Beatriz, 7, 56, 75, 264
Pierce, Irene R., 62
Pitres, Albert, 103, 105
pity, 196, 229, 233, 245
Poland, Alfred, 27
politics of emotion, 176
politics of pity, 196, 229, 233
Pope, Benjamin, 62
pornography, 252–53
Porter, Roy, 6, 64
Positivist School, 36, 38, 39, 41, 42–43, 46–48, 182
premeditation of crime, 43

Preyer, William Thierry, 83, 85, 92
Proudhon, Pierre-Joseph, 181
Psychological Study of Cancer, A, 60
psychosomatic medicine, 53–56; key theorists in, 56–57
psychotherapy, 28
Pu, Thy, 74

Rechtman, Richard, 251
Red Cross (RC), 195, 200, 211, 243, 246; founding of, 200; in Spain (*see* Spanish Red Cross)
Reddy, William, 4, 23, 25–26, 148, 153, 154
Regarding the Pain of Others, 196
Reign of Terror, 176
Rejlander, Oscar, 77, *81*, *82*
Representation of Bodily Pain in Late Nineteenth-Century English Culture, The, 91
Revue photographique des hospitaux de Paris, 100
Ribot, Théodule, 104–5, 113
Richer, Paul, 24, 99, 100, 103, 105, 112
Romanes, George, 84–85, 91
Rorschach test, 60
Rosaldo, Michelle, 4–5
Rosenberg, Charles E., 53
Rosenwein, Barbara, 4, 8, 148, 153–54
Rosón, María, 75, 264
Rostand, Edmond, 97
Rotch, Thomas, 86
Royal Hospital for Sick Children. *See* Great Ormond Street Hospital

Saint Francis of Assisi. *See* Christmas in Greccio and Saint Francis of Assisi
Sánchez Léon, Pablo, 132–33, 139
Santo Nilo libera un ossesso, 23
Sarcey, Francisque, 97–98, 108
Scheer, Monique, 1, 5, 16
Schilder, Paul, 55, 56, 62
sexuality, women's: link between cancer and, 64; Lombroso on criminality and, 182–84; prostitution and, 180–81; viewed as depravity (hysteria), 20
Shakespeare, William, 45–47
Shinn, Millicent Washburn, 84
Showalter, Elaine, 15
sick body in childhood illness, 85–88
Social Darwinism, 182
social egoism, 42
socialization processes and body image, 63–64

somatopsyche, 56
Sontag, Susan, 73, 196, 253
Soul of the Child, The, 83
South Australian Chronicle, 19
Spain: ETA (Basque separatists) in, 185–86; Red Cross in (*see* Spanish Red Cross)
Spanish Red Cross (SRC), 196, 200–201, 214–15; caring for the sick and wounded during the Franco-Prussian War, 210–14; determination of who deserves humanitarian relief by, 204–7; medical intervention services by, 202; moving the population toward compassion, 207–10; people building humanitarian narratives at war and, 201–3
Spencer, Herbert, 182
Sphere Project, 256
Stanislavski, Constantin, 113–14
Starr, Louis, 87–88
state terrorism, 185–87
Stearns, Carol, 4, 147
Stearns, Peter, 4, 147
Stevenson, Maria, 20
Story of Pain, The, 77
subjectivity, 7–8
suffering: historical emergence of humanitarian emotions and visualizing of, 223–28, *225*, *226*; mental, in humanitarian narrative, 242–43; shifting conceptions of, 221–23. *See also* pain
sympathy, 223, 233
System of Surgery, 27

Taine, Hippolyte, 184
Taithe, Bertrand, 195, 196–97, 199, 264
Tarde, Gabriel, 184–85
Taylor, John, 254
terrorism: fear of, 175–77; state, 185–87. *See also* Paris Commune
tetanus, hysterical, 21–22, 26–29, 30
theater: performing expressions in, 97–100; photography of actors in, 107–11, *109–10*
Thiers, Adolphe, 178, 184, 185, 186, 187
Third Republic, terrorism and. *See* Paris Commune

Thomas, Edith, 176
Thomas, Jacques-Léonard Clément, 178
Thomas of Celano, 151, 159, 160–62
Times, The (London), 19
Titanic disaster, 247
Transfiguration, 23
Turner, Victor, 162

United Nations, 244
Untersuchungen über das Seelenleben des Neugeborenen Menschen (Investigations of the Mental Life of the Newborn Child), 81

Vellita, Giovanni, 151–52
Vidor, Gian Marco, 16, 264
Vincent, Ralph, 88
visualization of suffering, 223–28, *225*, *226*
Vita prima, 152
volunteering, 246–47, 249
von Bismarck, Otto, 178

Wahler, H. J., 61
Wedgwood, Josiah, 225–27, *226*
Weiss, Thomas, 228
West, Charles, 86
Whyman, Rose, 113
Wickham, Harriet, 21, 31–32
Wolff, Harold, 54, 55
Woltke, Sophie, 100–103, 105–6
women: hysteria in (*see* hysteria); of the Paris Commune (*see* Paris Commune); portrayed as passive and in distress, *230*, 230–31; as prostitutes, 180–81; sexuality of (*see* sexuality, women's); suffering and pain in, disregarded by society, 227. *See also* gendering
World Vision, 254

Yolanda, 75, 120–22, 141–42; forms and memories, 122–31, *123*, *125*, *127*, *130*; youth, heroin, and disenchantment explored in, 132–41, *137*, *140*

History of Emotions

Doing Emotions History   Edited by Susan J. Matt and Peter N. Stearns
Driven by Fear: Epidemics and Isolation in San Francisco's House of Pestilence
   Guenter B. Risse
The Science of Sympathy: Morality, Evolution, and Victorian Civilization
   Rob Boddice
Shame: A Brief History   Peter N. Stearns
Emotional Bodies: The Historical Performativity of Emotions   Edited by Dolores
   Martín-Moruno and Beatriz Pichel

The University of Illinois Press
is a founding member of the
Association of University Presses.
———————————————

Composed in 10.5/13 Adobe Minion Pro
with Helvetica Neue Extended display
by Jim Proefrock
at the University of Illinois Press
Cover designed by Becca Alexander
Cover image: Photo by Shelby Miller on Unsplash

University of Illinois Press
1325 South Oak Street
Champaign, IL 61820-6903
www.press.uillinois.edu

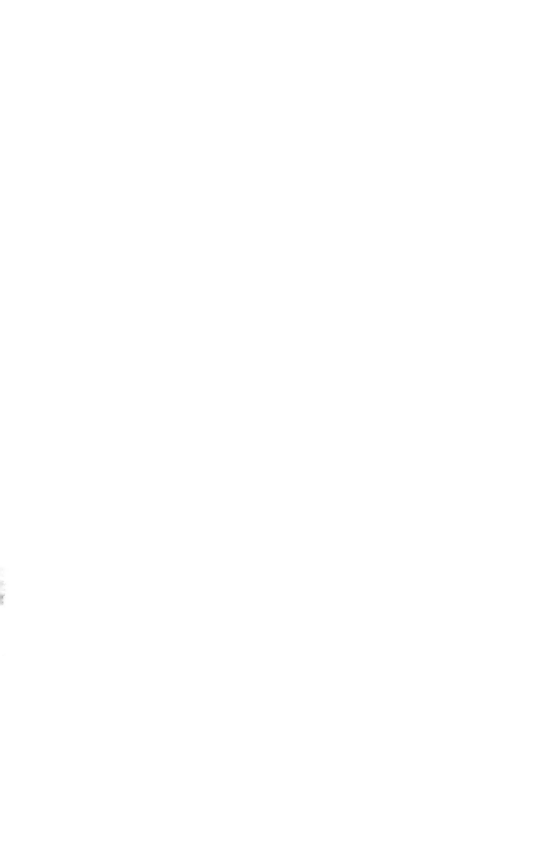